"In the tradition of Hippocrates, Dr. Susan Blum reestablishes food as the most fundamental and powerful mediator of health and wellness. *The Immune System Recovery Plan* provides a wealth of information, based on leading-edge science, that will surely have a profoundly positive impact on the vitality and longevity of its readers."

—David Perlmutter, M.D., F.A.C.N., author of *Grain Brain: The Surprising Truth About Wheat, Carbs, and Sugar—Your Brain's Silent Killers*

"A must-read for everyone with autoimmune disease. Dr. Blum masterfully presents the latest scientific information and gives patients practical, natural, and safe ways to help the immune system heal."

—Joel M. Evans, M.D., founder and director of the Center for Women's Health, Stamford, CT, and author of *The Whole Pregnancy Handbook*

"A godsend for the millions suffering from autoimmune disorders. This book's information is life-changing!"

—Christiane Northrup, M.D., author of *Women's Bodies, Women's Wisdom* and *The Wisdom of Menopause*

"Remarkable. Those who take the journey delineated between the covers of *The Immune System Recovery Plan* end up with a map that can actually lead to recovery, not just palliation of symptoms. Dr. Blum [brings] hope and skill to the treatment of pain and guidance toward the fundamental elements of healing."

—David S. Jones, M.D., president of the Institute for Functional Medicine

"Insightful. Medicine pioneer Blum asserts that reversing chronic illnesses . . . is not only possible but that improvement can happen as soon as they begin her program. [She] provides detailed explanations for how the immune system works, tests needed for self-diagnosis, questionnaires, and personalized treatment plans, as well as recipes."

—*Publishers Weekly*

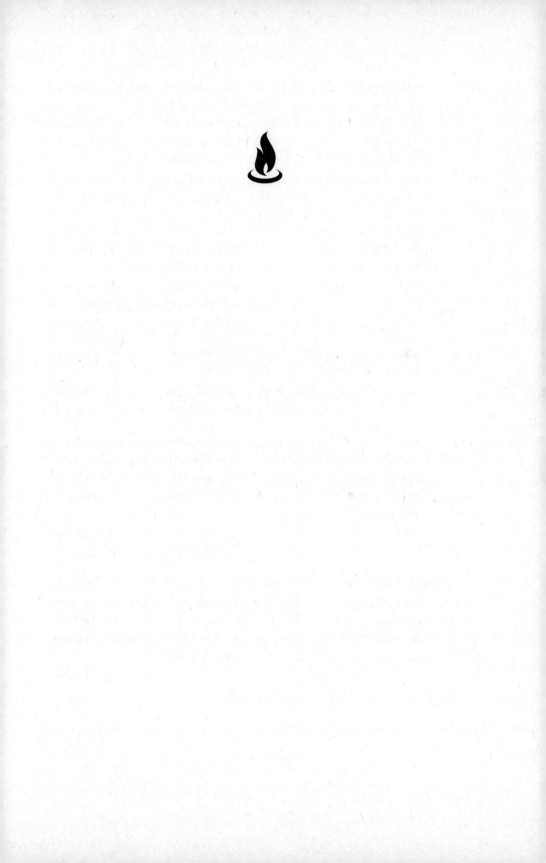

THE IMMUNE SYSTEM RECOVERY PLAN

A Doctor's 4-Step Plan to:

- Achieve Optimal Health and Feel Your Best
- Strengthen Your Immune System
- Treat Autoimmune Disease
- See Immediate Results

Susan S. Blum, M.D., M.P.H.

with Michele Bender

SCRIBNER

New York   London   Toronto   Sydney   New Delhi

This book contains the opinions and ideas of the author. It is intended to provide helpful general information on the subjects that it addresses. It is not in any way a substitute for the advice of the reader's own physician(s) or other medical professionals based on the reader's own individual conditions, symptoms, or concerns. If the reader needs personal medical, health, dietary, exercise, or other assistance or advice, the reader should consult a competent physician and/or other qualified health care professionals. The author and publisher specifically disclaim all responsibility for any injury, damage, or loss that the reader may incur as a direct or indirect consequence of following any directions or suggestions given in the book or participating in any programs described in the book.

SCRIBNER
A Division of Simon & Schuster, Inc.
1230 Avenue of the Americas
New York, NY 10020

Copyright © 2013 by Susan Blum, M.D.

First Scribner hardcover edition April 2013

SCRIBNER and design are registered trademarks of The Gale Group, Inc., used under license by Simon & Schuster, Inc., the publisher of this work.

For information about special discounts for bulk purchases, please contact Simon & Schuster Special Sales at 1-866-506-1949 or business@simonandschuster.com.

The Simon & Schuster Speakers Bureau can bring authors to your live event. For more information or to book an event contact the Simon & Schuster Speakers Bureau at 1-866-248-3049 or visit our website at www.simonspeakers.com.

Manufactured in the United States of America

15 17 19 20 18 16

Library of Congress Cataloging Control Number: 2012031929

ISBN 978-1-4516-9497-0
ISBN 978-1-4516-9500-7 (ebook)

*This book is dedicated
to the millions of people suffering
with autoimmune disease.
This is your message of hope.*

"If you do not change direction, you may end up where you are heading."

—Lao-tzu

Contents

Part IV:

SUPPORTING YOUR LIVER

Part V:

ADDITIONAL CONSIDERATIONS

Relief from a Hidden Epidemic of Pain and Suffering

What disease affects more women than heart disease and breast cancer combined?

What problem affects 24 million Americans but receives only 5.4 percent of the National Institutes of Health's (NIH) budget for this problem to study its potential causes?

The answer is autoimmune disease.

And it is mostly off the radar because it comes in so many flavors and types. Rheumatoid arthritis, lupus, multiple sclerosis, inflammatory bowel disease or colitis, diabetes, hypothyroidism, and psoriasis are all autoimmune diseases. We think of all these problems separately, when they are really just one disease with many different colors, depending on your age, sex, and genes. Autoimmune diseases affect our bodies at almost every level. Some affect our nervous system—like autism and maybe even depression—and others affect our joints and muscles, our skin, our endocrine glands, our hearts, and more. Autoimmune disease occurs when the body's immune system attacks its own tissues rather than a foreign molecule, such as a bacteria. There are more than one hundred different autoimmune diseases, and as anyone living with an autoimmune condition will tell you, it has a huge impact on quality of life.

The emerging science—and its practical application through functional medicine—points to just a few basic causes of autoimmune disease, most of which are ignored by conventional doctors, who try to shut off the immune system with powerful medications that have dangerous side effects.

But the truth is that the root causes of almost all autoimmune diseases are the same: microbes, environmental toxins, allergens, stress, and poor diet. By removing these root causes and supporting the body's optimal functioning through diet and lifestyle, you can actually recover from these conditions.

Dr. Susan Blum's groundbreaking book, *The Immune System Recovery Plan,* is a powerful guide to self-healing. Dr. Blum shows how you can address the root causes of disease and rebalance your immune system. She lays out a clear road map to recovery for the millions of people needlessly suffering from autoimmune disease and provides solutions for changes in diet, supplements, and environment that can help people deal with and even reverse autoimmune conditions. Dr. Blum's desire to find these answers was fueled by her own struggle with autoimmune disease, a condition she has successfully treated and recovered from by using the program described in this book.

Our conventional approach to autoimmune disease is to shut down the immune response with powerful medications including NSAIDs like Advil or Aleve, steroids like prednisone, anticancer drugs like methotrexate, and the new drugs like Enbrel, Humira, and Remicade that block the effects of a powerful inflammatory molecule called TNF alpha. But those new drugs slow down your immune system so powerfully that they increase your risk of cancer or life-threatening infections. And they have frequent and serious side effects and often give only partial relief.

These drugs may be lifesaving for some in the short term, but in the long term they do *nothing* to address the causes of disease.

Dr. Blum and I use the principles of functional medicine, which takes us to the root of the problem. We have treated hundreds of patients with autoimmune diseases successfully by addressing the underlying causes, including toxins, infections, allergens, poor diet, and stress.

I have even benefited from these methods myself. Chronic fatigue syndrome has autoimmune features and my blood tests clearly showed my body was attacking itself. Getting rid of my mercury poisoning reversed my chronic fatigue and autoimmune problems.

And this has been true for so many patients. For each one, doctors like Dr. Blum and I find all the causes—toxins, allergens, infections, poor diet, and stress—and deal with all of them while adding back the things the body needs to function optimally—whole, clean food, nutrients, exercise, stress management, clean water and oxygen, community, connection, and meaning.

Here are some of the stories of recovery that are possible for you.

- One ten-year-old girl came to see me with mixed connective tissue disease—her skin, joints, liver, and blood cells were all ravaged by inflammation. Doctors attempted but failed to control her symptoms with horse doses of intravenous steroids and immune-suppressing chemo drugs. No one asked "why." Why was she inflamed? What caused the overactivity of her immune system? They simply wanted to shut it down. After two months on a gluten- and dairy-free diet, clearing out all the yeast in her gut and restoring her nutrition with whole food and supplements, she was dramatically better. After a year, she had no symptoms and was off all her medications and her autoantibodies returned to normal. This type of disease reversal is not seen in conventional practice, but it is possible and available to everyone now through Dr. Blum's book, *The Immune System Recovery Plan.*

- One woman had crippling psoriasis and related arthritis. She was forty-two and couldn't walk up and down stairs or get into a bathtub by herself, nor could she properly care for her children. Nine months after we started treatment, including eliminating gluten and other food allergens, removing her heavy metals, and balancing her immune system, she walked back into my office not only thirty pounds lighter (being inflamed makes you fat) but completely free of pain and psoriasis.

- Another man suffered for years with the bloody diarrhea and pain of ulcerative colitis. Dietary changes and various digestive support helped but he never got better until we cleared out the bad bacteria from his gut and got him off gluten.

- And a recent patient with debilitating fatigue and multiple sclerosis and little white inflammatory scars on her brain experienced nearly complete relief of her symptoms after she had the mercury dental fillings removed and went on a comprehensive detoxification program. And when she repeated her MRI, all of the white scars from the MS were gone!

Functional medicine practices around the country are helping countless patients to recover from autoimmune disease. Dr. Susan Blum is the visionary behind one such practice, and at Blum Center for Health, she has improved the lives of thousands of people. The approach of finding and removing triggers of disease, such as hidden microbes, toxins, or allergens, and supporting the body's function with nutrients, herbs, and "pro" drugs such as probiotics is a movement that is now being practiced by practitioners at the cutting edge of medicine. It is an approach called functional medicine and has helped tens of thousands of patients worldwide. The valuable wisdom of functional medicine is described clearly and thoroughly in *The Immune System Recovery Plan.* By following the straightforward, revolutionary program described in this book, you, too, can treat the causes of autoimmune disease, reverse your condition, and give yourself the gift of health and well-being.

Functional medicine gives us the knowledge and the methods. Now you just need to apply them.

Mark Hyman, M.D.
West Stockbridge, MA
September 2012

Getting Started: A New Partnership

There's a growing epidemic in our country. It doesn't grab newspaper headlines or make the evening news, but it's there and it is debilitating and potentially deadly. It is the epidemic of autoimmune disease. **Autoimmune diseases are among the most prevalent forms of chronic illness in this country, now affecting an estimated 23.5 million Americans.** More people suffer from this group of chronic illnesses than from cancer or heart disease, yet most people don't even know what these conditions are. This lack of awareness is killing us—literally. It's causing severe pain, disability, and even death. Worse yet, many people with autoimmune conditions suffer with their symptoms because conventional doctors either can't figure out what's wrong or can't get to the root of the problem.

The answer is functional medicine, a medical specialty that has come of age in the past ten years and focuses on reversing these chronic conditions. Hope is here. You're holding it in your hands.

WHY A BOOK ON AUTOIMMUNE DISEASE?

There are more than one hundred different autoimmune conditions, and they are all serious chronic diseases caused by an underlying problem in the immune system. This book is a call to alarm: **these diseases are reversible and curable if caught early, before they progress and cause severe pain, disability, and even death.** The first symptoms might be vague feelings of fatigue, muscle or joint pain, or a nagging feeling that something isn't right. With simple blood tests, you can be diagnosed at this early stage, and then, by following the steps in this book, your immune system can be brought back into balance before irreversible damage is done to your brain, joints, thyroid, blood vessels, and other vital organs. If you have been suffering from an autoimmune condition for some time and you have already experienced some tissue damage, this book will help you feel better in general, show how you can actually reverse the effects of the disease, and help prevent your specific tissue damage from getting worse. As a doctor, I have long been aware of autoimmune conditions such as Graves' disease, rheumatoid arthritis (RA), Crohn's disease, ulcerative colitis, lupus, multiple sclerosis (MS), Hashimoto's thyroiditis, psoriasis, alopecia areata, vitiligo, Sjögren's syndrome, and scleroderma, among others. But when I was diagnosed with one of these illnesses, it changed both my personal and professional lives forever.

MY STORY

Before I go any further, let me introduce myself the way I would if you were one of the patients in my office. I'm Dr. Susan Blum, a board-certified physician in preventive medicine and an assistant clinical professor in the Department of Preventive Medicine at the Mount Sinai School of Medicine in New York City. I am also the founder of Blum Center for Health in Rye Brook, New York.

In medical school, I started down the road of traditional medicine. Then during my internal medicine residency, I quickly realized that I didn't want to focus just on illness or disease; I wanted to focus on *preventing* those conditions in the first place. But back then preventive medicine consisted mostly of screening tests and public health programs. It wasn't part of a doctor's everyday practice. Physicians just weren't given the tools in medical school to help their patients change their behavior, such as how to get people to eat healthfully or reduce stress. I knew I had to take a different route as a doctor, so I sought training from institutions that were considered "outside the box" at the time. In particular, I was interested in the relationship between stress, nutrition, and illness.

I moved off the beaten path of traditional medicine toward a more holistic approach and into an emerging field called functional medicine. First I completed a program at the Center for Mind-Body Medicine in Washington, D.C., where I learned tools for stress management and methods to reverse the effects of stress on the body. Then, at the Institute for Functional Medicine, I learned how food affects these processes, either promoting health or causing diseases. When I started applying what I had learned about stress management and nutrition in my own practice, I saw firsthand how these methods helped people to prevent and actually *reverse* chronic diseases. These two ideas—prevention and reversal of chronic disease—became my passions and are at the core of my medical practice today. But there is one area where these techniques are truly life-changing: autoimmune diseases.

I know this not only because I have seen the benefits for my patients who suffer from autoimmune diseases but also because I saw the impact on myself when I was diagnosed with an autoimmune disease.

I discovered it more than a decade ago when a friend asked me why my hands were so yellow. I actually hadn't noticed this before, but she was right, so I immediately had blood work done to find out why.

"You have hypothyroidism," my doctor told me after the lab results came back. *Me?* A thyroid problem? I couldn't believe it. Hypothyroidism is a condition in which the thyroid gland doesn't produce enough thyroid hormone. This hormone is necessary to help the body convert beta-carotene, a nutrient found in yellow and orange fruits and vegetables, into vitamin A. Because this conversion wasn't happening, all the beta-carotene from my healthful diet wasn't being properly processed. Instead, these nutrients were building up in my body, and one symptom of this was my yellow hands. In retrospect, I realized that this wasn't the only one. Another was the fact that I had to work really hard to keep from gaining weight, and a third was that I was often very tired. But at the time I didn't realize these were signs of a problem. They had been part of my life for so long that I considered them "normal."

Further testing revealed even more bad news. I had an autoimmune disease called Hashimoto's thyroiditis. In other words, my immune system, which is normally the body's defense in the daily battle against infection and invaders, was no longer protecting or defending me. In fact, my immune cells had turned against my thyroid, attacking it and damaging it to the point where it was struggling unsuccessfully to make enough thyroid hormone. I was shocked. I had become a vegetarian years earlier, I exercised regularly, I practiced yoga and meditation, and I had cultivated a strong, spiritual faith. I had faced my demons in psychotherapy and was finally content with my life. Because I was doing what I thought were all the right things already, being diagnosed with an autoimmune disease was shocking and frightening. I was also a medical doctor, so I just couldn't believe that something was going on inside my body that I didn't know about.

But my primary care physician just shrugged off this upsetting news. "It's no big deal," he said. "You'll just take thyroid hormone replacement medication and be fine." No big deal? Maybe not to him, but my intuition told me something wasn't right. My body was out of balance, and I wanted answers. Why did *I* have this disease? And why *now*? To understand my illness, I decided to use it as an opportunity to explore all that traditional and nontraditional medicine had to offer me. **I didn't want to take a pill that would only mask the problem and just *manage* my symptoms. I wanted to know *why* those symptoms were there in the first place.**

HOW FUNCTIONAL MEDICINE HELPED ME

The journey that I began after my diagnosis of Hashimoto's disease led me deeper into the unique and, at the time, relatively new field of functional medicine, an approach that considers the whole person, not just his or her symptoms. After receiving my diagnosis, I began using the principles I learned at the Institute for Functional Medicine to treat myself. As a result, I discovered that because of a genetic predisposition, I'm at high risk for autoimmune diseases. I also learned that my body has trouble removing mercury from my system. (Mercury is a toxin that's damaging to tissue in our bodies and a potential cause of autoimmune diseases.) I went on a gluten-free diet and reduced my mercury exposure by no longer eating fish high in this heavy metal (such as tuna, swordfish, eel, and striped bass), and over the course of two years I had my many dental amalgam fillings removed. I began to drink protein shakes that reduce inflammation and enhance the function of the liver. (Since the liver is the body's main detoxifying organ, this helps it clear mercury and other toxins from the body.) Two years after I learned I had Hashimoto's and started the journey to treat my autoimmune disease using functional medicine, my antibody levels were normal and my disease was cured. I was taking a small amount of thyroid hormone (called levothyroxine), and I had great energy and my weight was easy to maintain. I was thrilled and excited to share what I had learned with my patients.

That was the first step. Because my thyroid was already damaged when I was first diagnosed, my next goal was healing my thyroid, which can take a variable amount of time for each person, depending on how long it has been under attack by the autoimmune disease. Since my thyroid gland was quite damaged from the Hashimoto's, I still needed, and continue to need, thyroid hormone replacement. That said, I now take half the dose that I was taking ten years ago. Today I feel healthier and more energetic than I ever have. My health journey has taught me what my body needs, how to ask, and how to listen. **Reversing a chronic disease takes time and effort, but it *can* be done.** My story is proof of that. I did it for myself and made the professional decision to help other people living with autoimmune diseases do it, too.

Years ago I gave a lecture to an audience full of health care professionals at the Center for Mind-Body Medicine's professional training program. During that lecture, I talked about the importance of using food as medicine and how simple things such as breathing and relaxation can work to help heal disease. I was stunned to find that these important, life-changing concepts were new to most of the two hundred people in the audience. And they were health care professionals! I couldn't believe it. How could these doctors teach these things to their patients if they didn't understand them and weren't practicing them themselves? It was then that I realized it was time to get the word out more broadly than simply to my patients and the people who attended that lecture and other talks I continue to give.

HOW FUNCTIONAL MEDICINE CAN HELP YOU

In 2010, after several years of planning (and many more spent dreaming about such an opportunity), I opened Blum Center for Health in Rye Brook, New York, where the focus is on a comprehensive integration of functional medicine, mind-body medicine, and preventive medicine. It includes a cooking school to teach patients and clients how to eat for their health and a mind-body-spirit center that teaches an array of relaxation techniques not only to prevent chronic health conditions but also to reverse them. This, combined with the functional medicine treatment I offer as a medical doctor, has created extraordinary, life-changing results for my patients.

I'm not the only person who has been told to simply pop a few pills and move on. And I'm certainly not the only one who thought that there should be a better way. Today, in my functional medicine practice at Blum Center for Health, patients often share with me what their traditional medical doctors have said after diagnosing them with an autoimmune disease: "Get used to the painkillers. You'll need them for the rest of your life," "We don't know why people get these diseases," and "Your immune system can't be treated." These are just a few examples, but the recurring theme is generally one of hopelessness. The idea is that you should just accept your diagnosis and the inevitable lifelong battle with painkillers, drugs that suppress your immune system, and the side effects of both (some of which can be devastating and long-term). I simply refused to accept that there was nothing I could do for myself or the other 23.5 million Americans currently living with autoimmune diseases. But with the prevalence of autoimmune diseases on the rise, I know that there are many, many people living with these conditions who will never make it to my office. I wrote this book so I could offer this plan—an effective and healthy approach—to a broader audience.

Many traditional doctors have an attitude of "just give in to your illness," which only leads you to feel utterly powerless. **It also makes your disease worse because it undermines the body's natural healing process. The mind-body connection is real and powerful.** There are many studies that show that the more control a person feels he or she has over a situation, the higher the rate of healing. People do better, feel better, and live better with various health conditions if they have a sense that there is something they can do for themselves. And there is! That is one of the core principles of functional medicine, and as an expert in the field, I'm here to show you how much control *you* can have over your own health and well-being.

So what exactly is a functional medicine expert? First, let me tell you what it is not. Most traditional doctors take note of your symptoms and figure out what diagnosis they can bundle those symptoms into. This usually dictates your treatment. Therefore, if you and a friend have the same symptoms, you often get the same diagnosis and then the same treatment. This works for trauma and for health issues such as appendicitis or a broken leg, where certain things such as surgery can remedy an immediate problem or symptom. Unfortunately, this approach doesn't work when you're trying to treat and prevent complex, chronic illnesses such as autoimmune diseases.

A functional medicine expert is like a medical detective gathering all the clues of your past (where you grew up, your family situation, traumatic events, health history, etc.) and your present (potential toxins in your environment, social life, stress level, relationships, diet, workout regimen, sleep habits, symptoms, etc.). Armed with this information, a functional medicine expert tries to uncover how and why your body is not functioning well. This type of detective work is what I offer all of my patients at Blum Center for Health and what I used to cure myself of the serious autoimmune condition that I had. It is exactly what I will offer you with the interactive elements that run throughout this book.

Sidney Baker, M.D., a well-known preventive medicine specialist who is often called the father of functional medicine, once said, "If you are sitting on a tack, the answer is not to treat the pain. The solution is to find the tack and remove it." *The Immune System Recovery Plan* will help you find the "tacks" that are causing your immune system to malfunction and remove them one by one. It will take you through the four critical steps that will remove things from the body that are bad for the immune system and then make sure the body has exactly what it needs to function properly.

THE IMMUNE SYSTEM RECOVERY PLAN

I wrote *The Immune System Recovery Plan* to share an important message of hope and healing. **Shockingly, there is no other book on the market that tells the average person how the immune system works and shows how to fix it.** And that's exactly what I'll detail in these pages. I will explain how I have helped *hundreds* of people with autoimmune diseases such as lupus, rheumatoid arthritis, Sjögren's syndrome, Hashimoto's disease, and Graves' disease, among others, reverse their symptoms and reduce their antibodies.

Antibodies are molecules normally made by your immune cells to attack and destroy foreign invaders, but in autoimmune diseases, these antibodies are misdirected and attack and damage your own tissue. Many of these conditions are chronic, debilitating, and potentially life-threatening. In fact, autoimmune diseases are one of the top ten leading causes of death in girls and in women up to sixty-four years of age.

The Immune System Recovery Plan will help you figure out *what* you're feeling, *why* you're experiencing certain symptoms, and *how* you can treat the underlying causes of those symptoms so you can reverse your autoimmune disease. How can one book address whatever autoimmune condition you have? Because most of these conditions have similar underlying imbalances. Through the interactive aspects in *The Immune System Recovery Plan*, which include checklists, questionnaires, and self-assessments, you will be able to do with this book what my patients do with me in my office. Naturally, you won't be doing your own blood work or stool tests (since those require a health care professional), but by using the four steps in this book, you will learn how to treat whatever autoimmune condition you have. The four steps to healing and preventing autoimmune disease are:

- Step 1: Using food as medicine
- Step 2: Understanding the stress connection
- Step 3: Healing your gut
- Step 4: Supporting your liver

I suggest you do the four steps in order, which will help you reap the most benefit from this book. However, each one can also stand alone, so you can target one area at a time if you prefer. *The Immune System Recovery Plan* is divided into four parts, corresponding to the four steps. Each part is divided into three chapters:

- The first chapter in each part offers **a clear explanation about how the immune system is affected** by the topic at hand—for example, how the immune system responds to stress or how digestive health influences the immune system.
- The second chapter is **a workbook with self-assessments.** Using the results of these assessments, I will help you personalize your own treatment plan. This chapter will provide all the information you need to implement the plan, including specific instructions on how to integrate these tools into daily life and how to make permanent lifestyle changes.
- The third chapter provides **recipes** that show you how to use food as part of your personalized treatment plan. Each recipe includes foods specifically targeted to each of the four steps.

As we move through the four steps, I will explain why each is important and show you how quickly you can begin to feel better. By following each of the four steps, either alone or together, you will begin to improve your immune system immediately. These steps are the foundation that I use in the treatment plan I create for every one of my patients and are the simplest and most effective "medicine."

The Immune System Recovery Plan will answer the following questions and many more:

- How the five A's (antacids, antibiotics, Advil, alcohol, and animal foods) make you sick
- Why the most common foods in the standard American diet are commonly mistaken by your body as invaders, causing your immune system to attack your own body
- How exposure to mercury and other toxins changes the composition of your tissues, causing your immune system to attack your own body
- How common viruses—such as the Epstein-Barr virus, which causes mono—can provoke an ongoing immune reaction that causes you to feel chronically swollen, stiff, puffy, and tired
- How conventional treatments, which shut off the body's immune response, have serious side effects including insomnia, weight gain, muscle pain, increased blood pressure, and depression
- How the functional medicine approach can be used in conjunction with traditional treatments to offer big benefits and very little risk

- How every virus you've ever had—including cold sores, chicken pox, shingles, hepatitis, Epstein-Barr, and more—leaves residual particles in your body that can develop into autoimmune disease, and how to make sure that those conditions aren't created in your body
- How 70 percent of your immune system lives in your gut, and why balancing the good and bad bacteria in your digestive tract can lead to optimal immune function
- How having the right amount of bacteria in your gut reduces the incidence of allergies and autoimmune disease

HELP FOR US ALL

One thing I'd like to note is that although this book highlights autoimmune conditions/diseases, *The Immune System Recovery Plan* **will help anyone wishing to have a healthier, more balanced immune system.** The steps outlined here have helped my patients who suffer from asthma and allergies, as well as people who feel they catch every flu or cold bug that they encounter.

More people today than ever before have autoimmune diseases, and this epidemic is partially the result of an environment that bombards us with toxic food, stress, chemicals, and heavy metals. And while we cannot live in a bubble, we *can* protect our health by becoming more aware and changing what comes into our homes, into our families, and into our bodies. Every single one of us has both a choice *and* a responsibility to care for ourselves.

What's most important to know is that we *do* have control over what happens to us. Yes, **being diagnosed with an autoimmune disease is something to take seriously. But it is *not* a life sentence and should not be treated as one.** You don't have to live in pain or take debilitating medication for the rest of your life. You can heal your own immune system. I know this not only because I've experienced this with many of my patients but also because I have lived it.

The Immune System Recovery Plan gives you tools for treating and even reversing your autoimmune conditions as well as the tools for preventing them in the first place. My goal for you while reading this book is to see that autoimmune disorders *are* treatable and that permanent solutions *do* exist beyond a lifetime of taking pills. There *is* hope and so much that you—yes, *you*—can do to be the facilitator of your own healing. And you are not alone. I am here to guide you on this journey, so let's get started!

According to the National Institutes of Health (NIH), "Research discoveries of the last decade have made autoimmune research one of the most promising new areas of discovery."

BEFORE YOU BEGIN

I realize that this book contains technical information that can sometimes feel overwhelming and treatment plans that are asking you to make many changes in your diet and your life. But as you read through it all, take a deep breath and look past the trees. I want you to see the forest. I want you to know that there are options that don't involve medication—options that can actually help you heal your immune system. While you *do* need to focus on the trees, which are the details of each of the four steps in this book, keep your eye on the big picture of what we are trying to accomplish: healing your body on the deepest level.

My goals for this book are threefold. First, I want you to realize that an enormous body of scientific literature supports this approach to healing and balancing the immune system. You may come up against physicians who are unfamiliar with functional medicine and unfamiliar with some of the studies I share with you in this book. But just because your doctor doesn't know about this information doesn't mean it is wrong. My goal in this book is to empower you to take charge of your own health. I also want you to have the confidence to share this information with others.

My second goal is to offer you treatment like what you might get at my office. There are millions of you and only one of me. This is why I created a workbook. It is broken up into sections so that you can put it down and pick it up later, working through at your own pace. It is a lot to do at once, and you don't have to do it all in one week or even one month. Don't get overwhelmed. You can do it. And remember, help is always close by: you can get help from our website, or you can find a functional medicine doctor to help you figure some of this out if it is too much for you. (See the appendix for resources.)

My third goal for this book is to offer a message of hope. My heart sings at the opportunity to let you know that you don't need to give up and give in to a life of chronic suffering and medication. I sincerely wish each of you a healing journey as you make these changes that I know will help you feel better.

CHAPTER 1

Autoimmune Disease Basics

A HEALTHY IMMUNE SYSTEM

Your immune system includes a group of cells in your body that protect you against infections and illness. This is why the immune system is often referred to as an "army" of cells. Every day when you're exposed to things that could cause infection and illness—such as viruses, bacteria, mold, parasites, and foreign proteins in food—your immune system takes action. To do so, it calls upon many different kinds of soldiers, but to understand autoimmune disease, we will focus on one battalion in particular, called lymphocytes. Lymphocytes are a type of white blood cell that is responsible for protecting you from harmful foreigners like infections. However, if they aren't working right, lymphocytes are the cells that cause autoimmune diseases. There are two kinds of "soldiers" that make up the lymphocyte battalion. The first is killer T cells, which directly attack anything they don't recognize and which they perceive as an invader. I think of this direct attack as cell-to-cell combat. The other kind of soldier is called a B cell. These cells produce antibodies, which are molecules that grab on to anything that your immune system thinks is foreign and dangerous. After these molecules get hold of the foreigner, your immune system initiates a bigger response that causes an inflammatory reaction. When this happens, new compounds are released that attack the foreigner in order to kill it and clear it out of your body. You can think of antibodies as bullets released from the B cells to kill the invader. Both kinds of soldiers of the immune system, antibody-producing B cells and killer T cells, start a process that results in inflammation throughout the body. Though the process may begin somewhat differently, the end result you feel is the same for the most part. The first definition of a competent and healthy immune system is one in which the killer T cells and the antibody-producing B cells are in balance so that the immune response is balanced, too.

Depending on the invader, sometimes you actually feel something is happening when your immune system takes action and sometimes you don't. Examples of these foreign invaders include bacteria and viruses. If you get a sinus or ear infection, which is caused by bacteria, you may experience your immune system taking action by having a stuffed nose and pain in your ear or sinus area. If you get the flu, which is from a virus, you might have a high fever. These symptoms are the result of your immune system trying to fight the bacteria or virus. You might have a strong reaction and the inflammation might be felt in your muscles or in your joints, like arthritis. All of these are signs that the immune system is working to fend off the infection. If your immune system is strong, this war within you should stop after a week or two at the most. Once its job is done, the immune system will relax and go back to its normal state of watching and waiting for the next offender, and the inflammation goes away. In someone with a healthy immune system, this is a good, normal process, and we need these killer T cells and antibodies to keep us healthy.

There is more than one type of T cell. The killer T and B cells are told what to do by the T helpers and the T regulators, which either turn on or turn off the immune response. The different types of T cells need to be in balance for the immune system to turn off properly after it is activated and the job is done. This balance is the second definition of a healthy immune system.

While your immune system needs to be vigilant in order to guard against infections and toxins, it also has to be very careful not to hurt your own tissues by mistaking your own cells for the invader. During their earliest development, your immune cells have to learn the difference between something that is a natural part of your body, or "self," and

---

Three things that define a healthy immune system:

1. Balance between killer T cells and antibody-producing B cells
2. Balance between T helpers and T regulators to turn on and off the immune system
3. The immune system's ability to differentiate foreign invaders (such as viruses or bacteria) from natural parts of your body (such as cells and tissues)

a foreign substance, or "not self." Being able to make this distinction is called tolerance. The third definition of a healthy immune system is one that attacks only invaders and not itself.

AN IMMUNE SYSTEM GONE AWRY

An autoimmune problem develops when the immune system fails at all three of these definitions of health. The body begins to make too many killer T cells or too many antibodies (this varies depending on the auto-immune disease and will be discussed in depth later) and then fails to turn off, so the immune reaction doesn't stop. (These first two problems can also be seen in people with asthma and allergies, because they have an overactive immune response to substances called allergens. Symptoms such as wheezing and sniffling, and even life-threatening tongue swelling and throat tightness, are caused by the immune response, not the allergen itself.) But most important for those of you with autoimmune diseases, the immune cells are attacking your body's own tissues when they should *only* be attacking outside invaders. Put all three problems together and the result is inflammation and damage to your cells and organs.

WHAT ARE AUTOIMMUNE DISEASES?

"Autoimmune" represents a *category* of at least one hundred diseases, not one specific illness. This can be confusing and is probably why many people aren't familiar with autoimmune diseases or are unsure which illnesses fall into this category. Furthermore, the names of these con-ditions, which include Hashimoto's thyroiditis, rheumatoid arthritis, systemic lupus erythematosus, Sjögren's syndrome, celiac disease, and multiple sclerosis, among others, don't have the word "autoimmune" in them. This is unlike diseases such as the various forms of cancer, where their names contain the word "cancer" and the area where the malignant tumor(s) are found. For example, breast cancer is a tumor in the breast, colon cancer a tumor in the colon, and skin cancer a tumor on the skin. Without the word "autoimmune" as part of their names, autoimmune conditions sound like they are distinctly different diseases. However, that couldn't be further from the truth.

What can also be confusing is that the names of autoimmune condi-tions don't tell you *where* the disease is located in the body. Some autoim-mune conditions are *systemic*, meaning that the attack spreads throughout the body to all tissues, as in lupus. Others are organ specific, where the attack occurs in a specific area or organ, like Hashimoto's, which occurs in the thyroid. In either case, the name isn't a helpful indicator of where the problem actually exists. For example, Hashimoto's and Graves' disease are in the thyroid, multiple sclerosis is in the brain and spinal cord, vitiligo is in the skin, and pernicious anemia is in the blood cells. Although the affected areas are different, we now know that the underlying problems in all of these diseases are very similar. In fact, the focus of recent research has switched from looking at the specific organ affected by the disease to determining the underlying mechanisms for how these diseases begin. This idea—that all of these conditions have similar origins—is critical to our approach for treating and reversing them.

More than one hundred different autoimmune conditions have similar characteristics. They are all serious chronic diseases with an underlying problem in the immune system. Another thing they have in common is inflammation, which is irritation and swelling *inside* your body, in any part including your brain. Inflammation can cause a wide range of symptoms, including fatigue, puffiness, muscle or joint pain, abdominal discomfort including diarrhea, and difficulty concentrating or "brain fog." Or you may just have a vague, nagging feeling that something isn't right, even if your doctor can't find anything wrong with you.

By using a functional medicine approach and focusing on the primary cause of the immune dysfunction, research has uncovered many potential triggers for these diseases. (A trigger is anything that starts an unhealthy immune response.) **It turns out that many autoimmune diseases are set off by similar things, such as gluten, heavy metals, toxins, infections, and stress.** The main difference between each disease is that the immune cells target and attack tissue in different parts of the body. Essentially, most autoimmune conditions are more alike than they are different. And it turns out that fixing the foundational systems—which are your diet, stress hormones, gut health, and body's toxic load—will heal the immune system and help them all. This is the revolutionary approach I detail in *The Immune System Recovery Plan* and why the treatment program it contains can benefit and target *all* autoimmune diseases.

WHAT CAUSES AUTOIMMUNE DISEASE?

The National Institutes of Health estimates that up to 23.5 million Americans suffer from autoimmune disease and that the prevalence is rising. With the numbers increasing every year, many experts have questioned what causes autoimmune disease and have been studying this to find out.

As a result, there are many thoughts and ideas about how you "get" an autoimmune disease. Here are the explanations with the most evidence behind them.

Potential Trigger: Our Modern-Day Diets

Gluten

Modern-day agricultural practices include something called genetic modification. This means that the genes in the seeds for crops like corn, soy, and wheat are altered in a laboratory so that these plants can grow larger or resist disease more effectively. The result of altering our crops this way is that they now contain proteins that are not natural to the plant. Animal studies have found that these proteins are extremely difficult for us to digest, which causes symptoms such as:

- Heartburn
- Reflux
- Gas
- Bloating after eating

We have also seen evidence that these proteins cause immune reactions in the gut that can promote the development of autoimmunity. Autoimmunity means that the cells of your immune system are damaged and then make a mistake and attack your own tissues. Gluten is a protein found in wheat, barley, kamut, and spelt, and genetic modification has made it stronger and more concentrated in the grains we eat. This higher concentration of gluten in our food has been linked to the increase in food allergies over the last few decades. Why? Because gluten is a relatively new component of our diets.

Originally, our ancestors were hunter-gatherers, so they ate animals, nuts, seeds, and berries, rather than grains. Then they settled down to farming (only ten generations ago) and ate seasonally, rotating their food to eat what was available during that time of year. The benefit of this is that you are constantly varying your diet, whereas eating the same thing all the time increases your risk of developing an allergic reaction. Processed foods, which are those that have been altered by manufacturers so they no longer look like you just grew them, often have all the fiber and many of the nutrients removed. This process was created to give these foods a longer shelf life and make more food available to more people, but we now know that this is not a nutritious way to eat. Today, people who eat the standard American diet eat white flour at most meals, often to the exclusion of healthier, whole foods. Instead, you should choose whole foods, which look like they did when you picked them.

The problem with gluten is that it's hard to digest, and when a lot of large pieces get into the bloodstream, the immune system goes on high alert, seeing the gluten as a foreigner and producing antibodies to attack it. Unfortunately, when these antibodies attack the gluten, they mistakenly attack our tissues as well. **This is called molecular mimicry and is one way gluten is believed to cause autoimmune disease.** Molecular mimicry is not specific to gluten. It can occur when your immune system mistakes your own tissue for any foreigner.

The other way food can trigger inflammation and autoimmune reactions is called immune-complex disease. Using gluten as our example, the antibodies bind to the gluten and form a complex that travels around the body. These are called immune complexes and are a common, important way that your immune system deals with foreigners. You need immune complexes for the normal functioning of your immune system. Normally the immune system clears these complexes out of the blood, but if there are too many of them, they settle in different organs, causing local inflammation, tissue damage, and autoimmune reactions. This can cause swollen, painful joints and is thought to be one of the processes for developing rheumatoid arthritis.

Am I saying that gluten is the main reason you have an autoimmune disease? For some people, it is; for others, it is a big piece of the puzzle. I like to use the puzzle analogy for this because there are often several causes of your autoimmune disease or immune dysfunction, and my approach is to address one piece at a time. I have chosen the four sections of this book to deal with the biggest, most common pieces. One part is food, but you must also address your stress system, make sure your gut is healthy (don't forget that is part two of the gluten story, because the gluten might not have caused a problem if your intestinal barrier was doing its job), and make sure you aren't overloaded with toxins. Once you address all these pieces, your puzzle will be complete, and when you look at it you will see a picture of health.

Fiber, Fat, and Immune-System-Supporting Nutrients

Other edibles besides gluten also impact your immune system. A diet high in animal-based foods such as dairy, eggs, and beef can promote inflammation and throw off the balance of good bacteria that live in your digestive tract. Fiber and vegetables are also critical for this bacterial balance and to nourish the liver so that it's able to effectively remove toxins from your body. (As you'll read later in Chapter 11, "Supporting Your Liver," toxins put your immune system at risk, too.) Unfortunately, many people don't eat enough fiber and vegetables to reap these benefits.

There are many nutrients that you must include in your diet in order to have a healthy immune system—some examples include vitamin D, vitamin A, selenium, zinc, and healthy fats—but these are often missing in the standard American diet. For example, processed foods fill us up with bad fats that cause many problems besides damage to the immune cells. We'll talk about this in detail in the next chapter, "Using Food as Medicine."

Potential Trigger: Chronic Stress and Hormone Imbalance

Some people don't feel stressed emotionally, but they are skipping meals, not sleeping enough, or overexercising. These behaviors tax your body, causing it to secrete the stress hormone cortisol from your adrenal glands. Other people may be taking good care of their bodies, but they are anxious, worried, upset, or depressed, or they have severe, ongoing emotional trauma. These behaviors cause the same cortisol response from your adrenal glands. The adrenal glands are small nodules that sit on top of your kidneys and make all of your stress hormones. I want to be clear that not all stress is bad. For example, in an emergency situation, your adrenal glands release cortisol and adrenaline, which provide you with the energy to move quickly to get help. Or before an important talk, it gives you the energy to focus and think.

But *chronic* stress means your levels of cortisol are constantly elevated, something that can damage your immune system and prevent it from healing. Chronic stress can also lead to what is called adrenal fatigue, which is when your adrenal glands get exhausted and don't produce the hormones required to keep your body running properly, including adrenaline, DHEA, and testosterone. Adrenal fatigue results in:

- Unexplained exhaustion
- Feeling like you can't get up in the morning even after a good night's sleep
- A burst of energy between 4:00 and 6:00 p.m.
- Feeling overwhelmed
- Cravings for sweet or salty food

- Low blood pressure
- Low blood sugar
- Irritability

Adrenal fatigue (also known as adrenal exhaustion and adrenal burn-out) is associated with inflammation and autoimmune disease, which is why it's so important to understand and better manage the stress in your life.

Stress can also have a negative effect on the levels of good bacteria in your digestive tract, which itself can cause autoimmune disease. Stress hormones may also be the problem if you are fatigued all the time, get sick often, have developed arthritis, experience irregular periods, are going through a difficult menopause, or have trouble losing weight. This will be discussed in detail in Chapter 5, "Understanding the Stress Connection."

Potential Trigger: An Imbalance of Good Bacteria in Your Gut

Your immune cells, specifically the killer T cells and B cells, are the most central to the autoimmune problem. It is when these cells don't work right that the body starts attacking itself and doesn't stop. In order to help these cells function better, it's important to understand how they develop. When you are an adult, immune cells are made in your bone marrow and then migrate to the thymus (a small organ under your breastbone), your lymph nodes, and an area called the gut-associated lymphoid tissue (GALT, just under the surface of the intestinal lining). The thymus was very active when you were in your mother's womb, and when you were born, it was the main home of your immune cells. As you age, it still helps these cells mature and develop, but it becomes less and less active.

The lining of your intestines should contain good bacteria (also called flora) that are critical for helping the immune cells mature properly because they interact with the cells in your GALT. When these good bacteria aren't flourishing, the immune system is susceptible to dysfunction. Several things can impact your good bacteria. As I just mentioned, one is stress. Another is that we are a society living on what I call the five A's: antacids, antibiotics, alcohol, Advil, and animal foods. These things (along with infections and other medications) alter the beneficial bacteria in your intestines and damage the barrier of the intestinal wall so that food leaks into the GALT area below the intestinal lining, and then into your bloodstream. When this happens, the immune system recognizes the food particles in your blood as foreign invaders and develops antibodies to attack that food. As a result, you may have a reaction to a food that you've been eating all your life.

The other important role of the beneficial flora is that they help the killer T cells in the gut lining develop and learn the difference between a foreign substance (i.e., an infection or bacteria) and your body's own tissues. This is why healing your gut by making sure the beneficial bacteria and intestinal lining are the healthiest they can be is one of the fundamental ways to keep your immune system healthy. We'll talk more about this in Chapter 8, "Healing Your Gut," but it's important to know that **a healthy gut is critical for a balanced and well-functioning immune system.** It can help prevent autoimmune disease *and* has the potential to treat your symptoms and heal your immune system.

Potential Trigger: Toxins

A toxin is any environmental chemical, heavy metal, or other compound that is foreign to the body and causes a harmful reaction of any kind. This can also include mold because it commonly gives off dangerous toxins. Environmental exposure to toxins, which can damage both the immune system and other cells in your body and lead to autoimmune disease, is something we're experiencing today at unprecedented levels. In fact, the Center for Disease Control's (CDC) Fourth National Report on Human Exposure to Environmental Chemicals tested 212 chemicals and found that *all* of them were in the blood and urine of most Americans.[1] This is not surprising, since we're routinely exposed to toxins through food, pesticides, groundwater, industrial waste, and industrial chemicals. With respect to autoimmune disease, we are particularly concerned with any toxin that changes the chemical structure of our DNA, its sister genetic material called RNA, and the proteins in your cells because this can stimulate an immune response in your body. In other words, the toxin changes your tissue structure, leading your body to see your own tissue as a foreign substance and then attack it.

The most well-studied toxin in relation to autoimmune disease is mercury. (Of the 212 toxins found in the CDC's report, this was in the top six.) Mercury exposure comes from silver-colored dental amalgam fillings used for cavities. It is also released into the atmosphere as a by-product of burning coal or wood for fuel and the incineration of mercury-containing material. Because this has been going on for many decades, the mercury from the air has settled into our soil, rivers, and oceans. As a result, it's in many of the fish we eat, such as swordfish, tuna, striped bass, and king mackerel. (Since mercury concentrates up the food chain, larger fish who eat the littler fish tend to contain the highest levels.) Studies have linked mercury to Hashimoto's thyroiditis, Graves' disease, lupus, and MS. It appears that mercury is one of the toxins that directly damages your tissues, making them look foreign to the immune system. By now you know that the immune system attacks anything that it doesn't recognize. **This is why a crucial part of *The Immune System Recovery Plan* is to assess your potential toxin exposure and then take steps to remove as many toxins as possible from your diet and environment.** This is what we will do in Part IV, "Supporting Your Liver."

Another crucial issue with toxin exposure is that when the body contains too many toxins, the liver, our main detoxifying organ, gets tired trying to clear them out. Think of it as liver fatigue. The liver has many detoxification pathways, enzyme systems that are responsible for removing toxins. Each one requires specific nutrients, and if there are too many toxins and not enough nutrients, the liver gets depleted and toxins accumulate. The liver is also responsible for helping process the hormones your body creates naturally. When the liver gets exhausted due to high levels of toxins in the body, it also struggles with its daily job of processing our own hormones and the chemicals naturally created by the body. Estrogen in particular is metabolized through the liver, which contains specific enzyme systems that need to be working well in order for this hormone to be processed and properly removed from the body. However, if the liver is stressed, the estrogen builds up and the body actually produces *more* toxic estrogen, which can cause DNA damage and promote an immune reaction. In fact, toxic estrogens are thought to play an important role in both lupus and rheumatoid arthritis. As you will learn in Part IV, "Supporting Your Liver," specific food and supplements can help hormones, chemicals, and toxins flow through the liver more efficiently and effectively.

Potential Trigger: Infections

There is a lot of literature linking viruses to autoimmune disease, and I will discuss the potential linkages later. But the solution is not to blame the virus. All of us have viruses in our bodies; it's our immune system's job to keep them in remission. By this I mean that the viruses are supposed to be disabled so that they don't make us sick. However, if a virus is active, the immune system remains on a heightened state of alert and this means ongoing inflammation in the body. This is a problem. Symptoms of this tend to be very general, such as feeling puffy, swollen, stiff, and tired and/or having difficulty thinking and remembering things. For example, this is very common with the virus that causes mononucleosis (mono), which has been implicated in autoimmune disease. Called the Epstein-Barr virus, it stays in your body forever, sometimes undetected, at other times causing problems. I have many patients tell me that they never felt quite the same after having mono and when I test their blood for the Epstein-Barr virus, I often find that it is still active.

The solution to this is to understand *why* your immune system has failed to suppress the viruses. This is exactly what we will do in *The Immune System Recovery Plan* as we work to strengthen and balance the fundamental foundations of a healthy immune system (diet, stress, gut health, and reducing your toxic load). As a result, your immune system can disable the viruses and prevent them from persistently stimulating it.

HOW TO USE THIS BOOK:
YOUR GOOD HEALTH DREAM TEAM

As I mentioned earlier, autoimmune diseases have become the most prevalent form of chronic illness in our country. Yet there still hasn't been enough attention paid to them. I think this is why people view these conditions as different illnesses. The endocrinologist sees the patients with Hashimoto's thyroiditis and Graves' disease; the rheumatologist sees the patients with rheumatoid arthritis and lupus; the gastroenterologist sees those diagnosed with celiac disease; and the neurologist sees the multiple sclerosis patients. As a result, there is not one unified approach, which I believe has slowed the advancement of a better understanding of autoimmune diseases and more appropriate treatments of their root causes.

Another issue is that most conventional treatment for these conditions focuses on controlling symptoms with medications that work by shutting off the body's immune response. This isn't always effective and is often accompanied by serious side effects. For example, steroids such as prednisone can cause insomnia, weight gain, increased blood pressure, muscle pain, and depression. Other drugs are used to disable the immune system and can have more severe effects on the digestive tract such as nausea and vomiting, but also fever, muscle pain, anemia, and recurring infections. They also can damage the liver, lungs, and kidneys. Because some of these drugs can stay in your body for up to two years *after* you've finished using them, they are very dangerous if you get pregnant within that time frame. This is a critical issue since autoimmune diseases affect women 75 percent of the time. This statistic has led many researchers to look at the role of sex hormones in the development of autoimmune diseases. I will share more about this topic when we talk about stress and stress hormones, detox, and estrogen metabolism through the liver, and when we talk about lupus in the last chapter.

But the most important problem with these drugs is that they are treating only the *symptoms* of your autoimmune condition, not the *cause* of it. They don't explain *why* your immune system is not working properly in the first place, and if you don't figure this out, you can only manage your symptoms rather than cure your condition completely.

If a traditional doctor suspects that you have an autoimmune disease, the first blood test he or she will do is what's called an anti-nuclear antibody (ANA) test. This doesn't look for any one specific autoimmune disease but is a general screening test for systemic autoimmune diseases such as lupus. Your doctor might also do some tests for different organ-specific diseases, such as Hashimoto's or Graves' disease. As I mentioned earlier, in a healthy immune system antibodies target and attack foreigners that can cause infections and illnesses. When an autoimmune condition develops, these antibodies target your *own* tissue, and often the first antibody to show up in laboratory tests is the anti-nuclear antibody. If the ANA test is positive, the doctor does specific tests for lupus, rheumatoid arthritis, Sjögren's syndrome, scleroderma, mixed connective tissue disease, polymyositis, or dermatomyositis. If all these tests are negative and you just have a positive ANA, you're not diagnosed with an autoimmune disease. At least not yet. The conventional medical approach is to watch and wait to see if your symptoms get worse and you test positive eventually. This is all with the expectation that someday you *will* develop one of the specific diseases.

This watch, wait, and do nothing approach is against all of the principles of preventive medicine and functional medicine because there is so much that we can do to *prevent* the development of full-blown autoimmune diseases. It turns out that you can have a positive ANA test for many years before you develop any of the actual diseases or before you have any symptoms. For example, you can have anti-thyroid antibodies for many years before you notice a problem with your thyroid function. You can have an immune reaction to gluten for many years before you show any signs of celiac disease such as damage to the small intestine. My goal, and that of preventive medicine and functional medicine, is to catch the antibodies early and then fix the immune system by discovering why it is dysfunctional. This way we can quiet down the killer T cells and the antibodies, preventing them from doing tissue damage and turning into a full-blown disease.

By now you understand that antibodies and killer T cells are good when they are made against bad things such as harmful bacteria, viruses, or cancer cells. But we don't want to have antibodies or killer T cells attacking our normal, healthy tissue because it will begin a cascade of damage, inflammation, and eventually impaired function. For example, in people with rheumatoid arthritis, the antibodies that deposit in the joints cause damage that deforms the joint itself, causing pain and impaired function. In lupus, antibodies can attack the cells lining the blood vessels, causing damage to the blood supply to the organ where this is happening. (People with lupus often get kidney damage this way.) This is why it is critical to find the antibodies early, *before* there is damage in joints, blood vessels, or anywhere else in the body. Research proves that this can be done, and I know it for certain because it is what I do daily with my patients in my office. It is how I cured myself, too. This book will show *you* how.

HOPE IS HERE

My goal in writing *The Immune System Recovery Plan* is to bring a message of hope. You don't have to sit and wait to get a disease that is preventable. And you don't have to sit and watch your disease get worse, thinking that there is nothing that can be done to reverse it. If you've already been diagnosed, it is not too late. You *do* have options besides taking prescription drugs for the rest of your life. And my goal is to help you see that. By following the steps in this book, you can feel healthy again (yes, healthy!) and reverse your disease.

But let me first make one thing very clear. I am not anti-medication. If you are having a flare of your disease, meaning your symptoms get worse and you're in terrible pain and feel very sick, conventional medication can be very helpful and necessary. But once this crisis has passed, your focus should shift to figuring out the root cause of the immune dysfunction and fixing *that*. Also, functional medicine is not an alternative approach. I am a medical doctor and I work with my patients and traditional physicians, even while my patients are taking medication. I work to fix the foundations of their immune systems so that all the symptoms and antibodies disappear. When they are ready, their doctor and I decide together how to go about tapering off the patients' medication.

In this book, I will present my four treatment programs for you to do on your own. If you're taking medication for your autoimmune disease, you can still do these programs. However, if you're concerned, talk to your doctor about these plans. Keep in mind that many of the suggestions and treatments are lifestyle changes and don't require you to do anything that would make you or your doctor uncomfortable. But also know that just because your doctor isn't familiar with some of the things I'm suggesting, that doesn't mean they're dangerous or bad for you. It may simply mean that your doctor hasn't read the studies and/or learned about this approach. Don't be discouraged by this. I've found that many of the doctors in my community who once were skeptical of functional medicine are now eager to send me patients and work with me to help them. Why? Because they see that this approach offers big benefits with very little risk. I am passionate about this because it is truly a logical approach to treating the cause of the autoimmune problem. This goes beyond simply treating symptoms. It means that there is real hope because there is something we can do to help you treat, reverse, and prevent disease.

THE MOST COMMON AUTOIMMUNE DISEASES

The most common autoimmune diseases that I see in my medical practice are Graves' disease, Hashimoto's disease (also known as Hashimoto's thyroiditis), lupus (more formally known as systemic lupus erythematosus), multiple sclerosis (MS), rheumatoid arthritis (RA), Sjögren's syndrome, and celiac disease. I also see other autoimmune diseases, including glomerulonephritis (a kidney condition), type 1 diabetes, pernicious anemia (destruction of red blood cells), and vitiligo (a skin condition). For our purposes, I am going to focus on the seven diseases I see most. Here is information on these common autoimmune diseases, their symptoms and important tests to get if you suspect you have one. But remember, it doesn't really matter if your condition is on my list or not. You still need to fix your foundational systems if you have an autoimmune disease.

CELIAC DISEASE

This is a disease caused by an allergy to gluten and is marked by destruction of the microscopic, finger-like protrusions called villi that line the small intestine. It may take many years of gluten exposure before the villi are damaged and a laboratory confirms that you have celiac disease, but in the meantime the gluten can cause other digestive and autoimmune issues before it is diagnosed. Celiac disease has become the most well-known autoimmune disease because so many people have developed sensitivities to gluten.

Symptoms of Celiac Disease

Gluten can cause autoimmune diseases in other organs in addition to the gut, so there are a wide range of symptoms, from numbness and tingling in the extremities to fatigue from low thyroid function. Some common symptoms include:

- Arthritis
- Generalized brain fog
- Generalized fatigue
- Digestive issues such as diarrhea, gas and bloating after eating, and heartburn
- Anemia

Tests to Request from Your Doctor or Health Care Professional

There is a lot of confusion about how to diagnose celiac disease. Gastroenterologists will give you this diagnosis only after a biopsy showing damage to the villi of the small intestine. This is very restrictive, since you might have what's called silent celiac disease for decades before this test is positive. Instead, ask your doctor for tests for anti-gliadin antibodies and anti-deamidated gliadin antibodies. These tests are more sensitive in picking up gluten allergies and can be positive for many years before there is any damage to your small intestine. If these are positive, it's a sign that an autoimmune attack is taking place somewhere in your body. In that case, you should assume you have very early celiac disease that hasn't affected your intestines yet but is doing plenty of damage in your body, perhaps showing up as Hashimoto's thyroiditis, Graves' disease, multiple sclerosis, or another autoimmune disease.

And just to add to the confusion, even if all the above tests are negative, you might *still* be sensitive to gluten. That's because these tests were designed to pick up celiac disease only and gluten can cause other autoimmune diseases as well. Therefore, if you have any autoimmune disease—not necessarily celiac disease—it is good to do the tests above, but if they are negative, you should still remove gluten from your diet, based on research showing a connection between gluten and many other autoimmune diseases.

GRAVES' DISEASE

Graves' disease happens when your body makes antibodies that stimulate your thyroid gland, causing it to secrete high levels of the hormone thyroxine (also known as T4). This condition is called hyperthyroidism.

Symptoms of Graves' Disease
- Weight loss
- Rapid pulse
- Protruding eyes
- Insomnia
- Feeling too warm
- Restlessness
- Diarrhea
- Irritability
- Heart palpitations

Tests to Request from Your Doctor or Health Care Professional
- Thyroid-stimulating hormone (TSH)
- Free T4
- Free T3
- Thyroid-stimulating immunoglobulins (TSI)
- TSH receptor antibody

Here is the pattern of test results you would expect if you have Graves':

- TSH is low, typically <0.5 mlu/L, often lower or undetectable.
- Free T4 is elevated, usually over 2.5 ng/dl.

- Free T3 might be normal but is usually over 4.0 pg/ml.
- Either the TSI or the TSH receptor antibody will be positive. If they are both normal, then you don't have Graves' disease.

The above pattern is what the numbers would look like in a typical, classic case of Graves' disease. However, sometimes only one of the numbers looks out of range, such as a high free T4 with a normal TSH. This is a sign that you might have caught the problem early, and it is the perfect time to go through the steps in this book and reverse the problem before the disease starts.

HASHIMOTO'S THYROIDITIS

Also called chronic autoimmune thyroiditis, this is the most common autoimmune disease. Here, the immune cells invade the thyroid. In early Hashimoto's thyroiditis, the thyroid still functions pretty well, so if your doctor is checking only your TSH and hasn't measured the antibodies, you might miss the early stages of this condition. This is unfortunate because early on is the perfect opportunity to reverse the antibodies and prevent thyroid damage. If the immune attack goes on for too long, the thyroid might become permanently damaged, requiring lifelong hormone replacement.

Symptoms of Hashimoto's Thyroiditis
- Enlarged thyroid (goiter)
- If your thyroid is actively inflamed, some people experience a sore throat.
- Fatigue
- Hair loss
- Weight gain

Tests to Request from Your Doctor or Health Care Professional
- TSH
- Free T4
- Free T3
- Anti-thyroglobulin and anti-thyroid peroxidase antibodies

Here is the pattern of test results you would expect if you have Hashimoto's:

- One of your antibody levels will be elevated, either thyroid peroxidase antibodies or anti-thyroglobulin antibodies. If these are normal, you don't have Hashimoto's.
- TSH, free T4, and free T3: If these levels are normal, you are not hypothyroid. In early Hashimoto's, you can have the autoimmune disease and the thyroid is still making adequate amounts of hormones. This is the perfect time to follow the steps in this book, because you have caught the problem early while it is reversible and can prevent damage to your thyroid gland. Here are my suggested normal values for the hormones for screening purposes:
  - TSH: <3.0 mlu/L
  - FT4: >1.0 ng/dl
  - FT3: >2.6 pg/ml
- If the TSH is over 3.0, or if the free T4 is under 1.0 and the free T3 is under 2.6, your thyroid might be starting to show signs of damage from the autoimmune disease. You can discuss with your doctor whether it is a good idea to take a prescription thyroid hormone replacement. I will talk more about treating Hashimoto's in Chapter 14, "Infections and Specific Autoimmune Conditions."

LUPUS

Lupus, which is more formally known as systemic lupus erythematosus, involves more tissues in the body than other autoimmune diseases because it is a condition in which the body creates antibodies against the DNA of the cells. As a result, you can end up with disease all over your body and can have fever, joint, and muscle pain. Keep in mind that the symptoms come and go, because the disease can cycle through being in remission and being active. Unfortunately, many lupus patients get very sick, often dying from the involvement of the small blood vessels, which gives them disease in all their organs, including the kidneys and heart. Lupus affects more women than men, especially those in their twenties and thirties, leading researchers to believe that estrogen plays a role in causing or triggering the disease. I will explain more about this in Chapter 11, "Supporting Your Liver."

Symptoms of Lupus

- Fatigue
- Muscle pain and weakness
- Fever when the disease is active
- Symptoms specific to the organ involved, such as joint pain, muscle pain, and difficulty breathing
- Butterfly rash over the cheeks and nose that appears after sun exposure
- Hair loss (but not baldness)
- Oral or nasal ulcers that are not painful
- Cold- or emotion-induced color changes of the fingers or feet

Tests to Request from Your Doctor or Health Care Professional

- Anti-nuclear antibodies
- Anti-phospholipid antibodies
- Antibodies to double-stranded DNA
- Anti-Smith (Sm) antibodies

The ANA test is the first screening test for lupus. As I have explained, a positive test doesn't mean you have lupus unless one of the other three tests is positive as well.

MULTIPLE SCLEROSIS (MS)

Myelin is the protective coating on the outside of all the nerves in your body. In those who have MS, the myelin in the brain and spinal cord is damaged. This damage is called sclerosis. MS primarily affects women who are of northern European descent and who are of childbearing age. The most common first symptom is an episode of central nervous system dysfunction, such as optic neuritis. This is eye pain that gets worse when you move your eye in any direction. Sometimes symptoms go away on their own. Each time they come back, it's called an episode or exacerbation of symptoms.

Symptoms of MS

- Eye pain
- Numbness, tingling, or pins-and-needles sensation anywhere in the body that doesn't go away after two weeks

- Swelling of the limbs or trunk
- Intense itching sensation, especially in the neck area

Tests to Request from Your Doctor or Health Care Professional

- There are no antibody tests for MS. Instead, it's diagnosed when lesions in the brain or spinal cord are seen on an MRI. It's important to note that the diagnosis is made only after having neurological symptoms twice or a second episode that shows a second lesion in the brain or spinal cord. One episode that resolves and never comes back is not considered MS.

RHEUMATOID ARTHRITIS (RA)

If you have arthritis, it's often difficult to tell the difference between symptoms of RA and common osteoarthritis pain and swelling that can occur with aging or after injury. Rheumatoid arthritis occurs when your immune cells attack your joints, causing tissue damage, inflammation, and pain. It is a very specific form of arthritis, and sometimes the only way to know which kind of arthritis you have is to do the blood tests listed below.

Symptoms of RA

- Muscle pain
- Fatigue
- Low-grade fever
- Weight loss
- Depression
- Morning stiffness that lasts at least one hour for at least six weeks
- Swelling of three or more joints for at least six weeks
- Swelling of wrist or fingers for at least six weeks
- Symmetric joint swelling
- Nodules or bumps under the skin and over an affected joint

Tests to Request from Your Doctor or Health Care Professional

- Hand X-ray
- Blood tests for ANA, rheumatoid factor (RF), and anti-citrullinated peptide/protein antibodies (anti-CCP)
- Blood tests for inflammation: ESR (erythrocyte sedimentation rate) and high-sensitivity C-reactive protein (sometimes called a Cardio CRP)

It is good to get all the above blood tests because they will deter-mine if you have rheumatoid arthritis. It is possible to have a posi-tive ANA with all the rest of the tests being negative. In that case, you don't have RA. The opposite can also be true: you can have RA because you have a positive RF or anti-CCP but have a normal ANA. The ESR and the Cardio CRP are indicators of how much inflamma-tion might be happening at the moment, helping to monitor flares in the disease.

SJÖGREN'S SYNDROME

Sjögren's syndrome, which can occur on its own or in conjunction with RA, is an attack on the mucus-secreting glands that causes a reduction in secretions. It is often felt first in the salivary glands, which are in the mouth, and lacrimal glands, those that secrete tears. Ninety percent of patients are female.

Symptoms for Sjögren's Syndrome
- Dry mouth and dry eyes
- Dryness in the vagina, skin, lungs, sinuses, and digestive tract
- Fatigue
- Joint pain
- Muscle pain
- Cognitive dysfunction

Tests to Request from Your Doctor or Health Care Professional
- ANA, anti-SSA, and anti-SSB antibodies

Elevated levels of anti-SSA or anti-SSB are diagnostic for Sjögren's.

SYMPTOMS TO TAKE SERIOUSLY

Below is a checklist of symptoms for common autoimmune diseases. If you have any of the boldfaced ones, you should go to your doctor and ask to be tested for the disease or diseases I have mentioned. The other (not boldfaced) symptoms in the following lists are nonspecific, meaning many other things besides autoimmune diseases can cause them. If you have four or more of the nonspecific symptoms and they are all consistent with one condition, then you should have the test suggested or an ANA screening. For example, if all your symptoms fit with lupus but you don't have any of the *specific* lupus symptoms, you should still get tested. This is very important because with many of these conditions, the symptoms don't make a diagnosis; the lab tests do. I have also included several additional autoimmune diseases in the checklist below because these are fairly easy to identify and get tested for.

General Symptoms

- Fatigue: all autoimmune diseases
- General discomfort, uneasiness, or feeling ill: all autoimmune diseases
- Insomnia: Graves'

Fever/Body Temperature

- **If you are having fevers but you don't have a virus or infection, or if you feel hot all the time: lupus, Graves', celiac disease, Sjögren's**
- If you feel hot when others are cold: Graves' thyroiditis with an overfunctioning thyroid gland
- If you feel cold when others are hot: Hashimoto's thyroiditis with a low-functioning thyroid gland

Hair

- **Hair loss, usually in patches or circles: alopecia areata (this is confirmed by examination; there is no blood test)**
- **Loss of all the hair on your body: alopecia universalis (this is confirmed by examination; there is no blood test)**
- Thinning of your hair or general hair loss: celiac, lupus, Hashimoto's with low-functioning thyroid gland

Skin

- Dry skin: Hashimoto's thyroiditis
- Bruising easily: celiac

- Itchy skin: celiac
- **Rash over your cheeks and bridge of the nose (butterfly rash), usually red with some bumpy texture (but no pimples), that gets worse in sunlight: very specific for lupus**
- Skin sensitivity to the sun: lupus
- General rash anywhere on the body: lupus
- **Fingers that change color when cold: Raynaud's phenomenon, lupus**
- **Nodules or bumps under the skin, usually on your hands or feet: rheumatoid arthritis**
- **Skin thickening: scleroderma**
- **Loss of skin pigmentation in blotchy patterns anywhere on the body: vitiligo (this is confirmed by examination; there is no blood test)**

Eyes
- Vision changes: lupus, MS
- **Dry, itching eyes or feeling like there is something in the eyes: Sjögren's, rheumatoid arthritis**
- **Double vision, eye discomfort, uncontrollable eye movements: MS**

Throat, Neck, Voice, and Mouth
- Swollen glands (lymph nodes): lupus, Sjögren's
- **Enlarged neck from an enlarged thyroid: Hashimoto's**
- Mouth sores or ulcers: lupus, celiac, Sjögren's
- Difficulty swallowing or speaking: Sjögren's, MS
- Loss of sense of taste: Sjögren's
- Hoarseness: Sjögren's
- **Dry mouth: Sjögren's, RA**
- **Excessive thirst: type 1 diabetes**

Muscles, Joints, and Tendons
- **Joint pain or joint swelling: RA, Sjögren's**
- Morning joint stiffness lasting more than one hour: RA
- Pain and tenderness throughout the body: Sjögren's, lupus
- Muscle weakness: Hashimoto's, Graves', MS
- Muscle cramps and joint pain: celiac
- Muscle spasms and twitching: MS

Weight Changes
- Unexplained weight loss: Graves', celiac, lupus, type 1 diabetes
- Unexplained weight gain: Hashimoto's, gluten sensitivity (not celiac), type 1 diabetes

Digestion/Gastrointestinal
- Constipation: Hashimoto's, celiac, MS
- Abdominal pain: celiac, lupus
- **Bloating, gas, or indigestion: celiac**
- **Diarrhea, either constant or on and off: celiac**
- Nausea and vomiting: celiac, lupus, Graves'
- Stools that float and are foul-smelling, bloody, or "fatty": malabsorption from celiac

Mood and Thinking
- Difficulty concentrating: Hashimoto's, MS, Graves'
- Depression: celiac, MS
- Irritability or anxiety: Graves', Hashimoto's

Balance and Neurological Symptoms
- **Numbness and/or tingling in the extremities: lupus, MS, celiac, type 1 diabetes**
- Headaches: lupus
- Seizures: lupus, celiac
- **Problems walking, loss of balance, coordination: MS**
- Tremor: MS, Graves'
- Dizziness, vertigo: MS

The public's interest in autoimmune diseases is extensive, and people are clamoring for more information. Proof of this is the fact that autoimmune diseases and disorders are the most popular health topics requested by callers to the Department of Health and Human Services' National Women's Health Information Center.

PART I

Using Food as Medicine

To map out a course of action and follow it to an end
requires some of the same courage that a soldier needs.
—Ralph Waldo Emerson

CHAPTER 2

Using Food as Medicine

Did you know that the molecules in the foods you eat actually tell your cells how to behave? Should the cells make inflammation? Should the immune cells defend your body against infection? This process of identification and instruction is called nutrigenomics, and it shows just how deeply connected our diets are to our health. Food is information that communicates with the body on a cellular level and tells it what to do as well or better than medicine can. Most people don't know that prescription drugs work for only 50–60 percent of people at best. Though we're just beginning to really understand why a drug works for one person and not another, it's clear that people have different biochemistry and genetics. This concept also applies to food and food sensitivities: because we are all biochemically unique and we have different genetics, we don't all respond to the same food the same way.

In this chapter, you will discover why food matters. You will learn how to evaluate and understand what makes *you* biochemically unique, and then I'll show you how to use this information to create your own personalized nutrition plan. We will explore your family history and genetics and create lists of foods that can be used to positively affect your biochemistry and genes. We will see which foods may trigger your autoimmune condition and figure out ways to remove them from your diet. Doing this has made a huge difference in my patients' autoimmune conditions and their health in general. For example, with one patient, Ilise, we cured her rheumatoid arthritis by changing what she ate. The first thing we did was remove gluten from her diet. As you'll see, this is something I do with most of my patients, and with good reason. Within days of doing so, Ilise's joint and muscle pain disappeared; within six months of eating in this new way, her laboratory tests were all normal (i.e., they didn't show antibodies for rheumatoid arthritis). Clearly gluten was the culprit (or at least a primary one), because any time she ate gluten-containing foods, she could barely walk the next morning.

Most people view food as either "good" or "bad." "I was so good today" or "I was so bad today" are phrases you've undoubtedly heard or said yourself in regard to something that you've eaten. Many of us also think that food's only impact on the body is to make it either gain weight or lose it. This couldn't be further from the truth. **Food is much more than calories.** What you choose to eat has a powerful impact on your health and how you feel each day. It can also have a big effect on the amount of inflammation in your body.

WHAT IS INFLAMMATION?

I mention inflammation in this book a lot because more and more we're finding out about its close link to many serious illnesses and conditions. So what is inflammation? Does inflammation have a purpose? Any benefits? Inflammation describes the release of chemicals and messengers in your body that create irritation and swelling inside you. Normally this is a good process and helps your body respond to a foreign microbe or to an injury. But if the process goes on too long or gets out of control with very high levels of these inflammatory chemicals, it can interfere with the normal function of your cells and cause tissue damage in your body. For example, inflammatory messengers can tell your fat cells to hold on to the fat and not let it go. Obviously this isn't good and will prevent you from shedding pounds or maintaining weight loss. Inflammatory messengers can also damage your blood vessel walls, increasing your risk of plaque, atherosclerosis, heart disease, and hypertension. And they can stimulate the immune system so that the immune cells keep releasing more and more chemicals.

This is one reason why it's so critical to figure out which foods are best for your unique biochemistry. We need to make sure you aren't eating foods that are causing inflammation. Once you do, you will feel better and your immune system will be stronger and happier. You will have less inflammation in your body, which can mean less joint pain, fewer headaches, and relief from bothersome stomach problems. And, though this is not a weight loss book, figuring out what foods are ideal for you will help your metabolism do its best work; as a result, you're likely to shed pounds along the way.

FOOD HAS A FUNCTION

This approach to eating is called *food as medicine*. Food actually has a function in the body way beyond calories. For example, some people think that one food with 100 calories has the same impact on the body as another food with the same number of calories. But 100 calories from an apple and 100 calories from a cookie do not behave the same way once they get into your system. The apple has nutrients in it that make your cells sparkle. The apple contains a lot of quercetin, a member of the flavonoid family that has been found to have anti-inflammatory and anti-allergy properties, among other functions. The cookie, on the other hand, is loaded with sugar and fat, two things that set off a chain of events that can create inflammation and, if you make sugar a mainstay in your diet, can cause serious diseases. So, let's see: an apple with anti-inflammatory quercetin versus a cookie with pro-inflammatory sugar. Which should you choose? While you probably knew the answer before, I hope you can see my point: that **you should choose food based on how it will affect your cells, not just based on calories.**

In this chapter, I am going to explain to you the ideas and concepts behind food as medicine and what we know about food and autoimmune diseases. In the two chapters that follow, "Using Food as Medicine Workbook" and "Using Food as Medicine Recipes," I am going to help you discover what makes your body unique and guide you in choosing the right foods for *your* immune system.

Earlier I mentioned my patient Ilise. After removing gluten from her diet, she was able to get out of bed pain free every morning for the first time in five years. But whenever she would eat gluten, she would experience extreme pain and immobility. Certainly, the gluten was doing something in her body that goes way beyond the calories! And she is not alone. Gluten sensitivities and allergies are more prevalent today than ever before. This would be an obvious place to give you a statistic that demonstrates this prevalence, but there is currently no agreed way to measure gluten sensitivity. Still, the grocery store shelves are evidence of an increase, since more and more products tout the fact that they are gluten free. In fact, estimates are that global sales for gluten-free products topped out at over $2.5 billion in 2010.[1]

FOODS THAT CAUSE INFLAMMATION

There are many foods that can cause inflammation in the body. Later in this chapter I will describe the effects of sugar and fats, and I will explain food sensitivities. For now, keep in mind that every food has the potential to cause an immune reaction, not just gluten, although gluten is the most important for autoimmune diseases. But I want to be clear that it is not the calories in these foods that are the problem. It is the details, the *information* present in the foods, that your body sees, reads, and reacts to. When we talk about food sensitivities, it is the protein in the food that is providing the information to your immune system. Often removing products that contain these problem ingredients from your diet can quiet some or all of your symptoms, no matter what they are. I see this all the time in my practice and this is a perfect example of using food (or the removal of food) as your medicine. Of course, food offers the body beneficial information, too, telling it how to heal and repair itself and function optimally.

In the "Using Food as Medicine Workbook," which follows this chapter, I will show you how to figure out which foods are causing reactions in *your* body. This is the very first step to reversing autoimmune disease. What's exciting is that this is very easy to do on your own, yet it can have a big impact on your health and the way you feel.

"DIET" IS A FOUR-LETTER WORD

When it comes to weight loss, there is a seemingly endless array of programs and diets out there. Some are trendy, attention-grabbing plans that don't really work, while others are successful. What is important to realize about these programs is that while you might lose weight, you won't necessarily change your biochemistry and reduce inflammation on the *inside.* Now don't get me wrong—losing weight has an enormously positive effect on your risk for developing many chronic diseases such as cancer, diabetes, and heart disease. And there are some weight loss programs that *are* good for your insides, even though this isn't the goal that they set out to achieve. So if you have found a diet or nutrition program that works for you, that's great. You can combine the information that I'm going to give you with what you are already doing.

What makes any diet or nutrition program successful and what all of them have in common is that they help you become very mindful about the food (and exercise) choices you make during the day. This is great because it helps you begin to notice what you are eating. Most people munch mindlessly, slurping giant quantities of soda, nibbling on doughnuts during meetings, and having an entire meal from the drive-through in their car. Unfortunately, you might not realize you're doing this—it's like food amnesia—so you continue eating throughout your day. Not only does this cause weight gain, but it can also make you sick. Once you start paying attention, you become aware of all your bad habits—this is the first step to any lifestyle change. For example, once you start observing yourself throughout the day, it may become obvious that you are drinking too many sugary beverages, having too many late-night cookies, and digging too deep into the bread basket. By noticing these habits, you can then take steps to change them. The point here is that awareness and mindful eating come first. (I will share a helpful mindful eating exercise in the "Using Food as Medicine Workbook.")

During an initial visit with all my patients, I ask them to tell me what they ate the day before. Believe it or not, out of everything we discuss in our entire appointment, this is usually the hardest question for most people! But try it for yourself. Can *you* remember what you ate yesterday? How about two days ago? It turns out that the first step of any nutrition program, *paying attention and planning your food*, is the most important for a positive result, no matter what you are trying to achieve. While this is important for weight loss, this is especially critical for your autoimmune condition and health in general.

FOOD IS INFORMATION

What do I mean when I say that food is information? As I mentioned, the food you eat tells your cells how to behave by changing the way the enzymes work inside the cells. For example, sugar does a lot more than just provide calories—or, actually, empty calories that offer no nutrients. It causes the level of sugar in your blood (blood glucose, or just glucose) to spike, which gives you an energy high, followed by a hard energy crash. Additionally, the glucose in your blood that spikes after you eat sugar attaches to the cells in your body and initiates changes that begin deep inside those cells, at the nucleus, activating your genes to make enzymes that increase the amount of inflammation in the cell.

Deep within every cell in your body is a complete book of your life, your complete genetic code. Each cell has all your genes in it. To make this a little simpler to understand, think of your genes as a book with many, many chapters. At any given time, only some of the chapters are being read. So in your liver, the cells are reading the liver chapter; in your tongue, the cells are reading the tongue chapter; and in your heart they're reading the heart chapter. The genes that code for those cells are activated and direct all the activity of that cell so that it is doing its job properly. Some of these chapters are fixed on or off when you're a baby developing in your mother's uterus (like whether the cell will become a liver cell or heart cell). But throughout life there are many chapters that are not fixed, so they can be opened and read, or closed and ignored. A great example is how your cells respond to resveratrol. Studies have shown that when you eat food such as red grapes or drink red wine, the resveratrol from these foods travels into the cells in your body and straight to the nucleus of the cell, where it turns on what has been called the "longevity gene," because it makes enzymes that help the cell live longer. You can think of this gene as one of the chapters of the cell that would remain unread without the resveratrol.

This is why we say *food is information*—it can have a powerful effect on activating your immune system in a way that makes it work better or in a way that promotes autoimmune diseases. Going back to my example about eating sugar, when sugar binds to the surface of any cell in your body, it starts a chain reaction that changes the enzymes in the cell and causes the cell to make all sorts of inflammatory molecules that can make you sick if this goes on for too long, like when you eat doughnuts for breakfast and have two teaspoons of sugar in your coffee every day. While this process always happens when you eat sugar, if you indulge only on occasion, the inflammation goes away quickly and unnoticed.

This concept is called nutrigenomics, and it's so important that there are entire scientific journals dedicated to this field of study. If you break down the word, you can see that it is really a fancy term for the idea that the food you eat (*nutri-*) affects the genetic expression of your cells (*genomics*). How this works is that food affects which genes are activated. Genes direct your enzyme activity, and enzymes determine how a cell, tissue, or organ will function. I am so frustrated every time people tell me they are eating a "good" diet because they have those 100-calorie cookie packs for their snacks every day. They may be low in calories and help you control your portion sizes, but the ingredients they contain, including sugar and trans fats, are telling your cells to create inflammation and your body to gain weight. If instead you eat a handful of almonds, the beneficial fats these nuts contain will be telling your cells to *reduce* inflammation. (And we know inflammation is the driver for all chronic diseases, including autoimmune diseases.)

All this is evidence that the expression "You are what you eat" isn't far from the truth. Everything you eat is digested and absorbed and then ends up floating around in your blood, eventually arriving to feed all your cells. This is how every cell in your body is affected by your diet. When it comes to the immune system, these cells are supposed to be touching and bumping into everything you eat, which is why food has an important influence on anyone with immune dysfunction.

• • •

The rest of this chapter will be divided into two parts. In the first part, we will explore foods that need to be removed from your diet because they are potentially hurting your immune system. In the second part, we will look at foods that are really good for you, because science has shown that they help improve immune function and balance, specifically in people with autoimmune diseases.

FOODS THAT NEED TO BE REMOVED

What's in Our Food That Is Causing All These Problems?

Every food contains a combination of proteins, carbohydrates, and fats along with vitamins and minerals in varying amounts. Plants also contain a group of compounds called phytonutrients that are potent stimulators of cell function. Often there are bad things hitching a ride in your food, too, such as molds, bacteria, parasites, pesticide residues on fruits and vegetables, and antibiotic and hormone residues in animal foods; I will talk about these food toxins in Chapter 11, "Supporting Your Liver."

Let's talk about proteins first, because they have a powerful effect on your immune system. This nutrient is found in all the food you eat, with fruits and vegetables having less and animal food, like chicken and meat, having more. Your body tissues are all made of protein as well, which is why you need to make sure you are getting enough of it in your diet to provide raw material for the daily repair that your body is constantly going through. (A general formula for the recommended amount of protein you should eat daily is 1 gram for each kilogram of your body weight.)

Protein is made of building blocks, called amino acids, that are linked together. There are a total of twenty amino acids, of which nine are considered essential because you must get them from your diet as opposed to your body making them. A protein is identified not only by *which* amino acids are in its makeup but also by the three-dimensional structure they create when they are together. This is an important concept, especially for the immune system, because your immune cells attempt to recognize the different patterns of amino acids in everything they bump up against, in order to determine if it is friend or foe. In other words, your immune cells are consistently analyzing the protein that makes up the tissues in your body and the food you eat.

Every bacteria or virus has a known amino acid pattern on its outer surface, which I will call its "name tag." Your immune cells remember and are always vigilantly looking for known foreigners, which they identify by reading the bacteria's or virus's name tag. This surveillance system is what keeps you healthy. All of your own tissue has name tags, too, because they also are made of protein and amino acids. As you already know, your immune system should not attack your own tissues, but it should recognize and attack bad bacteria, yeast, viruses, and other infectious agents. It's when your immune system makes a mistake (when it misreads the name tag) that problems begin. The point is that the amino acid sequences are the foundation for how the immune system reads name tags in both foreign cells and in your own cells, and that's how they learn not to attack your own tissue. Because foods contain proteins, they have name tags, too, and have the potential to cause an alarm if your immune cells don't recognize them.

Do You Have a Food Sensitivity?

Normally, the food you eat is very well digested by the time it makes it down to your small intestine, where it will be absorbed. By this point, the food has been broken down into very small particles with the name tags pretty well digested, so they aren't recognizable. When this happens, there's no immune reaction. However, if the food is still in big pieces, then its name tags (amino acids) are recognizable by the immune cells. This is why good digestive power is so important and why taking antacids and proton pump inhibitors puts you at an increased risk of developing food sensitivities. (I will explain this in more detail in Chapter 8, "Healing Your Gut.") As long as your intestinal lining is strong and healthy, it forms a barrier keeping the immune cells on one side and the food on the other. Problems begin when the barrier is not intact, so big particles of food with foreign name tags seep through it. Then they encounter the immune cells on the other side. At this point, the immune cells read the name tags on the food particles and signal to your body how it should respond. When food leaks through a weak intestinal barrier, this is called leaky gut syndrome, and it explains how people can develop immune reactions, allergies, and sensitivities to food at any age. I will explore this concept and how to fix it in Chapter 8, "Healing Your Gut." My point in mentioning it here is just to explain how food proteins can become a problem for your immune system.

It is believed that foods can cause inflammation throughout your body by several different mechanisms. First, you can develop a food allergy, which is when your immune cells make antibodies against the food. There are four different kinds of antibodies, but for our discussion of food allergies, two are most important. When you go to the allergist, you'll be checked for IgE antibodies, which are the ones that cause hives, swelling of the tongue, or difficulty breathing. The other kind of food allergy, one your doctor might not test for, involves IgG antibodies, which play a role in causing immune-complex disease. This is when the food gets into your bloodstream and your immune system makes antibodies that attach to the food, making something called an antigen-antibody complex. Because this is a huge particle, it can settle out into your tissues and cause local inflammation and damage, which then results in an even bigger immune attack to this tissue. Your joints are very susceptible to deposits of immune complexes, and this is believed to be one of the main mechanisms behind the development of rheumatoid arthritis.

Because evidence suggests that all people with autoimmune diseases have leaky gut syndrome, it is likely you are having immune reactions to the food you eat, and I will help you identify and remove the foods that are causing problems. Having any kind of symptom from a food you eat is called a food sensitivity, and this is the way that food can cause inflammation. While food sensitivities are not true allergies because we can't confirm them with a blood test, they can't be taken lightly. In the absence of a blood test, I rely on whether the food is causing symptoms such as fatigue, feeling puffy and stiff all over, difficulty concentrating, joint or muscle pain, and any kind of digestive symptoms, such as reflux, gas and bloating after eating, diarrhea, or constipation. **The simplest way to figure out if you have a food sensitivity is to remove the particular food from your diet for three weeks and then reintroduce it, paying close attention to how your body reacts.** I will help you do this in our treatment section, "Using Food as Medicine Workbook." Now, let's move on to a very specific food protein, called gluten.

A CLOSE LOOK AT GLUTEN

While it is possible that there are several foods that are responsible for symptoms that you're having, such as joint and muscle pain, headaches, diarrhea, gas, bloating, fatigue, and difficulty concentrating, for autoimmune diseases the most important food to look at is gluten. Gluten is a protein found in the grains wheat, barley, rye, kamut, and spelt. Oats don't naturally contain gluten but are likely contaminated by it unless the label says they're gluten free, and rice, quinoa, buckwheat, and millet are naturally gluten free. While we talk about gluten, it is actually a composite of other proteins, the main ones being gliadin and glutenin. It might be simplest to think of glutenin and gliadin proteins as different "name tags" that your immune system sees when you eat these foods.

People often ask me why there is a bigger problem with gluten today than ever before and why so many people feel worse when they eat it. The answer is twofold. First, **you are exposed to more gluten today than ever before,** and second, if you are like most people, your digestive system is a mess, so partially digested gluten gets past your intestinal lining and absorbed in the bloodstream, where it runs amok throughout your body. (We'll get into this in detail in Chapter 8, "Healing Your Gut.") Why is there more gluten today? As I described in Chapter 1, there has been an increase in the use of genetic modification in the wheat grown in our country since the 1940s. The genetically modified wheat has been altered to have more gluten because it is thought to make the plant heartier. In addition, as we've seen, there are several different proteins that make up gluten, and it is the most toxic variety that has become more concentrated. But most important, with average Americans eating three to four servings of wheat products every day, we're eating highly concentrated gluten every day, too.

Is gluten new? In some ways the answer is yes. In Paleolithic times, which encompassed most of humans' history on earth, people were hunter-gatherers. This means that we ate what we could kill or forage for, including animals, nuts, leafy greens, seeds, and berries. This is what our bodies were used to. When farming became more common (which was only ten generations ago), people still ate with the seasons and rotated grains and crops. But then the field of agriculture expanded and humans learned to process and store grains. This made it easier to eat wheat all year round and in high quantities. At that time humans were still eating ancient forms of wheat (einkorn and emmer), which had different genes and different gluten than the wheat we eat today. I recently read a book called *Wheat Belly*, by William Davis, M.D., and he gives a fascinating and detailed chronicle of how wheat has changed over time. According to Dr. Davis, wheat really changed in 1943, when it was intentionally reengineered so that there would be more yield per acre, in a misguided effort to help end world hunger.[2] For our purposes, I want you to realize that this new wheat came along at the same time as when people started eating more processed food. Then we became a fast-food nation, and now a fast-food world. We were never meant to eat processed wheat with super-concentrated gluten several times a day, 365 days a year. And research clearly shows that overexposure to food proteins can cause immune reactions. I believe overexposure to this recently developed form of wheat is why we're now seeing increasing frequency and greater severity of physical reactions to gluten.

Celiac Disease

As a doctor, my job is to read the most current research to stay on top of all the newest evidence about a given condition or disease. In this literature, gluten is definitely making headlines, with many studies linking gluten to a number of diseases.

But first let's talk about celiac disease. Celiac disease, an autoimmune disease of the small intestine, is thought to be one of the most common disorders, affecting about 1 percent of the population in areas where most of the people are of European descent, such as Europe, North and South America, and Australia. It is also increasing in other regions, such as North Africa, the Middle East, and part of the Asian continent, because diets in those countries have become more westernized and the people living there are eating more wheat products than they did before. People with celiac disease have a strong genetic predisposition to the condition, and when their genetics combine with environmental triggers, they get the disease. Here the trigger is probably gluten, especially super-concentrated, genetically modified gluten.

What happens in this condition is that the immune cells attack and damage the villi, little finger-like projections that stick out from the wall of your digestive tract. A good way to visualize villi is to imagine a shag carpet lining the digestive tract. The villi are important because they increase the surface area of your intestinal wall, which allows you to finish digesting and absorbing all those nutrients that your body needs. If these attacks by the immune cells go untreated, the villi are destroyed and the intestinal wall ends up inflamed and looking flat, with all of the shaggy protrusions gone from the carpeting. What do you feel when this happens? Usually people with this kind of gluten reaction have digestive symptoms such as diarrhea, gas, and bloating. Also, they don't absorb nutrients such as protein, fat, vitamins, and minerals very well, so they can become anemic, tired, frequently sick, and lose hair, to name a few common symptoms. In children, celiac disease can cause stunted growth.

Traditional medicine holds that the only way to diagnose true celiac disease is with a blood test and a biopsy of the lining of the small intestine. The blood test is specific for damaged intestinal villi. **However, studies have now shown us that it is possible to have** *potential* **celiac disease, which means your body might be on its way to having the full-blown intestinal disease, even though the tests all come back normal.** This latent or quiet intestinal disease may not be evident now but might show up years from now if you keep eating gluten.

It is also possible that you have no gut symptoms right now but might be having a reaction in another part of your body from eating gluten. We can't see everything gluten is doing, and it actually can be decades before the damage shows up in your intestines as celiac disease. So the first disease you might get is a different autoimmune condition. This isn't surprising, since autoimmune thyroid disease, rheumatoid arthritis, and multiple sclerosis have all been associated with celiac disease. The thyroid, joints, and nervous system are damaged first, and this can be the initial sign that something is amiss, before any symptoms of celiac disease are evident. In fact, several studies have suggested that in some people, these conditions are part of the celiac disease spectrum.[3]

Gluten Sensitivity Versus Celiac Disease

Up until now, celiac disease was considered the only harmful physical reaction or disease caused by gluten. But in 2010, $2.5 billion was spent on gluten-free products around the world. This number shows us that it's not just those who suffer from celiac disease who are embracing a gluten-free diet. So what is going on? There's a relatively new condition called gluten sensitivity.[4] If you look at Figure 1, you can see the different kinds of reactions you can get from eating gluten. Celiac disease is one kind of reaction, and gluten sensitivity is the other.

Gluten sensitivity is determined when your lab tests are normal for celiac disease but your symptoms go away on a gluten-free diet. Research hasn't quite sorted out the mechanisms or figured out a laboratory test to determine if you have this sensitivity, but it is thought to be caused by an immune reaction that's different from the one associated with celiac disease. Symptoms of gluten sensitivity often include abdominal pain, bloating, diarrhea, constipation, foggy mind, tiredness, eczema or other skin rash, headache, joint and muscle pain, numbness of legs and arms, depression, and anemia, together with a normal or mildly abnormal lining of the small intestine. The best way to know if you have gluten sensitivity is to remove gluten from your diet and see if some of your

Figure 1

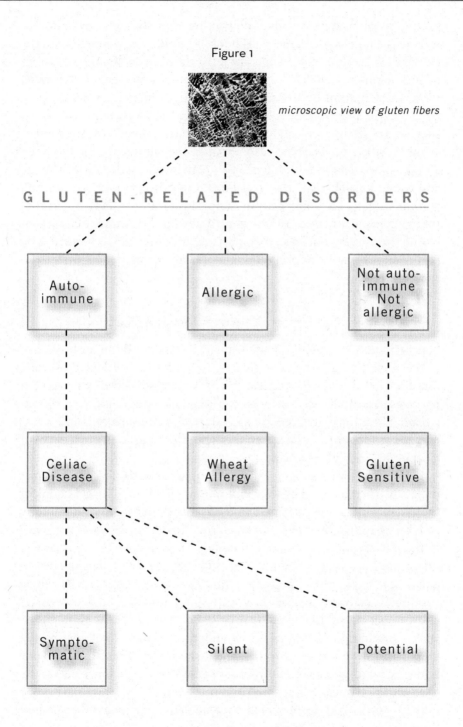

microscopic view of gluten fibers

GLUTEN-RELATED DISORDERS

symptoms go away. (I will give you specific directions on how to do this in "Using Food as Medicine Workbook.") I do this experiment with my patients all the time, and I am constantly astonished when I hear stories of how a gluten-free diet has helped. Not only do patients report relief from the symptoms on the list above, but they tell me they are sleeping better, are in a better mood, see improvement in menopause symptoms such as hot flashes and night sweats, and find relief from many other symptoms that I haven't yet read about in the latest scientific literature as being associated with gluten. I am convinced that food in general, and gluten in particular, is a critical factor in causing or exacerbating all chronic disease, including autoimmune disease. While there is no proof that gluten sensitivity causes or contributes to autoimmune disease, it has not been ruled out as a possibility. A gluten-free diet is a mandatory part of all my treatment programs, and it is my recommendation for you as well.

How Does Gluten Cause an Immune Reaction?

Let's say you eat a delicious gluten-filled croissant or bagel for breakfast. If your digestive power is not great or if you have a weakened or leaky intestinal lining, you are at a great risk of having partially digested gluten particles make their way past your intestinal lining and into your blood-stream. There the gluten bumps up against your immune cells and is recognized as foreign. (I will explain this, and how to fix it, in great detail in Chapter 8, "Healing Your Gut.")

Normally, gluten is digested and no longer recognizable as an intact molecule when it is seen by your immune system. But if a bigger chunk of the gluten particle sneaks in past your intestinal barrier and your immune cells bump into it, they send out an alarm. This alarm activates the genes in the nucleus of the immune cell and opens a "chapter" in the book of life in the cell. Now, a chain of events is unleashed that tells the cell to attack the gluten. If you keep eating this food, your immune cells will be continually activated, releasing all sorts of inflammatory molecules in an effort to get rid of the gluten. It is believed that one of the ways gluten causes autoimmune diseases is that gluten resembles—that is, it has an amino acid structure, or name tag, that is similar to—many tissues in our bodies. And so, while your body is busy attacking the gluten, it also starts to attack the tissues of your small intestine, your thyroid, myelin (in your nervous system), and your joints, thereby damaging these other tissues. (This process is called molecular mimicry.)

Testing Your Reaction to Gluten

Molecular mimicry is thought to be one of the mechanisms for how gluten can cause autoimmune disease. The fact that the name tag of gluten looks like the name tags of our own tissues causes the immune system to make this mistake. The immune attack resulting from this mixup is referred to as *molecular mimicry*. This reaction is driven by antibodies, and the tests that we currently use to measure these antibodies are called anti-gliadin antibody (AGA) and deamidated gliadin antibody (DGA) tests. This is the first test to become positive in celiac patients, even before any sign of damage to the intestines. I use this as a screening for all of my patients, and I find many of them are positive. In fact, these are the first tests you should ask for from your doctor.

I can't tell you how many times my patients have told me that their gastroenterologist said it was okay to eat gluten because their AGA test was positive, but the other celiac-specific tests were normal. Hearing this makes me really angry! Clearly these other doctors aren't reading the scientific literature that has shown that a positive AGA test could be the first, earliest sign of potential celiac disease. Before any intestinal damage occurs, these anti-gliadin antibodies can be attacking other tissues in your body. I really hit the roof if the person telling me this story *already* has a diagnosis of Hashimoto's disease, Graves' disease, multiple sclerosis or rheumatoid arthritis. These are the autoimmune diseases most often associated with celiac disease or preceding the onset of celiac disease. If you have a positive anti-gliadin or anti-deamidated gliadin antibody test, this should tell you to *stop* eating gluten.

Now, the majority of my autoimmune patients are not positive for this test, but that doesn't prevent me from recommending that everyone with an autoimmune disease stop eating gluten. **Just because modern medicine hasn't discovered the right laboratory test for you doesn't mean the gluten isn't wreaking havoc with your immune system.** There is enough evidence for it, and I have seen it time and again in my practice. What have you got to lose? At the very least, you need to read "Using Food as Medicine Workbook" and do the experiment so you can see for yourself if removing gluten improves your symptoms.

What Foods Are Bad for Your Immune System?

Food is filled with other compounds besides gluten that can cause a reaction from your immune system. Most of the time foods act subtly and gradually. This makes it hard to connect a particular food to how you feel because often these kinds of reactions are acting outside your gastrointestinal system. In other words, you don't have any symptoms such as gas, bloating, or a stomachache, but you may have other symptoms such as joint pain or a headache that you don't even realize are linked to what you ate. I have found that if you are feeling tired, are having difficulty concentrating, or have any joint or muscle pain or discomfort, food might be causing some of the problem.

Sugar

Gluten is not the only potential threat to your immune system; I also want to mention carbohydrates. One really dangerous type of carbohydrate is sugar. A diet containing processed sugar is associated with increased inflammation and impaired function of the immune cells called T cells and B cells. There are no specific studies looking at eating sugar and autoimmune diseases, but there is plenty of research on sugar and immune function.[5] A high-glycemic-index diet is one that contains foods that cause your blood sugar level to rise very quickly. Examples include foods filled with sugar and white flour. This kind of diet is very unhealthful and has been linked to heart disease, cancer, stroke, and diabetes. In fact, it's linked to all chronic disease. One goal of this book is to make sure that you are eating in a way that will help heal and balance your immune system. To do this, you must eliminate any food made with white flour or white sugar, such as bagels, bread, breakfast cereals, cakes, cookies, crackers, candy, and soft drinks. That said, you also have to watch out for other foods where sugar is hiding. For example, commercial fruit-flavored yogurt and fruit smoothies from fast-food places usually have added fruit syrup. I will go over this in our workbook, but for now it is important to keep in mind that as part of your Immune System Recovery Plan, white flour and white sugar will have to go.

Fats

Now let's talk fat, which I think is the most misunderstood nutrient of all. When it comes to fat, most of my patients are in one of two categories: either they are terrified of fat and avoid every type, or they are eating the standard American diet and, as a result, consuming tons of the bad fats (saturated animal fat and trans fats from processed foods). Both situations are a problem, because if you aren't eating any fat, you are missing the anti-inflammatory benefits of the good fats that are in foods such as fish, flax, avocado, coconut, nuts, seeds, and olive oil, and if you are eating too many bad fats, you are promoting inflammation and immune dysfunction. Here we'll talk about removing the bad fats, and then in the next section we will focus on adding foods that have been shown to help people with autoimmune disease.

One kind of bad saturated fat comes from cattle, in beef and dairy products. Our cattle are fed poor diets (mostly corn) that cause their bodies to make more saturated fats. When you eat beef and dairy products from corn-fed cattle, the fats they contain increase inflammation in *your* body. If you still want to eat beef and dairy foods, your best bet is to choose products from grass-fed, organically raised cattle if you can find them. Cattle that eat grass have healthier fat, and this transfers health benefits to you when you eat it.

Processed foods are filled with trans-fat-containing partially hydrogenated oils, which do not naturally occur in our environment. In fact, they are made in a laboratory. They were created to improve the shelf life of foods and to replace butter. Butter is a saturated fat, which was blamed for rising rates of heart disease back in the 1970s and 1980s. However, it turns out that trans fats have caused disease at a rate much higher than saturated fat in butter. Removing all the trans fats from your food is an important part of this program.

FOODS THAT IMPROVE IMMUNE FUNCTION AND BALANCE

The Anti-inflammatory Diet

I recommend that all of my patients adopt an anti-inflammatory approach to eating. This is not a meal plan but a way of life. Because inflammation is the driver for all chronic diseases, it just makes sense to eat more of the foods that decrease inflammation and to eliminate the foods that increase it, no matter whether you have an already diagnosed illness or simply you want to prevent one.

As you can see, the kinds of fat you are eating are really critical. When you eat bad fats, they create an increase in a molecule called arachidonic acid in your body, which in turn creates inflammatory molecules called eicosanoids. A study done in Germany showed that patients with rheumatoid arthritis who were treated with fish oil saw this condition improve more dramatically if they were also put on an anti-inflammatory diet, thus reducing the amount of arachidonic acid in their body at the same time.[6] The point is that it isn't good enough to take fish oil supplements and then continue to eat inflammation-producing foods; you won't get better. It's like trying to fill your car's gas tank with higher-octane gasoline when it is already full of lower-octane fuel that will clog up your engine. The bottom line? Fill your tank with anti-inflammatory foods and you will feel better.

The Good Stuff

Now that we've talked about what you shouldn't eat, let's talk about foods and nutrients that you should eat. Phytonutrients are compounds that give fruits and vegetables their color. Some that you've probably heard of include lutein, lycopene, and resveratrol, to name just a few. Research on resveratrol has shown clearly that it can activate what is called the longevity gene inside the cells, helping them to live longer. There have also been many studies looking at foods and nutrients that might help treat autoimmune diseases. So far, the best evidence has been found for essential fatty acids (the good fats), vitamin D, vitamin A, zinc, selenium, and green tea. I will also briefly mention mushroom extracts, because they are used so frequently in immune support formulas and I want you to understand how to use them. Keep in mind that the goal of *The Immune System Recovery Plan* is to fix the foundation of your immune system so that you can recover completely. Therefore, I will not detail all the different foods and supplements that support immune health in general, but will focus on those that have been demonstrated to reduce your immune imbalance and improve your symptoms. Here I will share with you what the current research tells us, and then in the next chapter I will give you the details about how much and what kinds of each food you should eat and which supplements you should take.

Essential Fatty Acids

Let's continue the discussion about good and bad fats. It is important that you not only remove all of the trans fats from your diet and cut down on the saturated animal fats but also increase the amounts of good fat you are eating. Some people think that the phrase "good fat" is an oxymoron, but it's simply not true. Good fats include essential fatty acids, which are fats that our bodies can't produce, so we need to eat foods that contain them (hence the word "essential"). Examples include omega-3 and omega-6 fats, which you probably hear about often. The important omega-3 fats EPA and DHA are the active ingredients in fish oil supplements. The omega-6 fat that is very important for your immune system is called GLA and can be found in evening primrose, black currant, and borage oil supplements. In the next chapter we will talk in detail about where to get these nutrients in food, but the most common sources are fish, such as wild salmon and sardines; nuts, such as almonds and walnuts; seeds, including sunflower and pumpkin seeds; and leafy greens, such as kale and Swiss chard—foods typically missing from the standard American diet. The other healthy fats are saturated fats such as those found in avocados, coconuts, and clarified butter (ghee). Unfortunately, these foods got a bad rap during the anti-fat revolution in the 1980s, and people continue to believe this myth. What I find interesting is that the prevalence of chronic disease has been rising ever since that period. I don't see that as a coincidence.

There are two primary ways that fats influence your immune system. Your cell membranes are made of fatty acids. If you eat a lot of omega-3 and -6 fats, the cell membranes will be loose and fluid, which is the way they work best. On the other hand, if you eat a lot of saturated fats and trans fats, they will go into your cell membranes and make them stiff, which has a negative effect on how the cell communicates with the messenger molecules it bumps into constantly. In fact, a study done at the University of Massachusetts Medical Center showed that rheumatoid arthritis patients who took borage oil, which contains gamma linoleic acid (GLA), showed improvements in their symptoms. Results revealed that the GLA was converted into a substance called DGLA in the body and then taken into the membranes of the overactive immune cells, where it reduced their activity.[7] What this means is that the GLA had a calming effect on the overstimulated immune cells. Since this overstimulation is a problem in all autoimmune diseases, it is important to think about the fats you are eating in your diet.

The second way fats can impact your immune system is that all the fats you eat are converted into important molecules called prostaglandins, the different types of which can either increase or decrease inflammation in your body. When you eat GLA-containing foods or take a GLA supplement, it increases the amount of a very good prostaglandin called PGE1. PGE1 has been found to do many wonderful things in patients with rheumatoid arthritis such as reduce inflammation, reduce circulating immune complexes, and decrease overactive T cells. **Studies using fish oil have also shown anti-inflammatory benefits for both rheuma-**

toid arthritis and lupus patients, most of whom have shown a reduction in symptoms and the severity of the disease.[8] Many patients have also found that they've been able to decrease the amount of medication they're taking to suppress their symptoms. It is very important to add these fats to your diet, and the workbook will offer both food and supplement recommendations.

Vitamin D

Vitamin D is the most-studied nutrient with respect to autoimmune diseases. Investigators researching multiple sclerosis first noticed that there was a much higher rate of this disease in the northern latitudes, where there is the lowest exposure to sunshine. Since this nutrient is made in the skin from exposure to sunlight, researchers very quickly found a relationship between low vitamin D levels in the blood and a risk of MS. In fact, low vitamin D levels have now been found to be associated not only with MS but also with other autoimmune diseases such as rheumatoid arthritis, lupus, insulin-dependent diabetes, and inflammatory bowel disease (IBD). While no one has proven that vitamin D deficiency *causes* any of these autoimmune diseases, having low levels puts you at risk, and treating people who are deficient in vitamin D reduces symptoms and slows the progression of their condition. A study done at Ohio State University regularly measured the vitamin D levels in a group of lupus patients and found that they were more likely to have a flare in their disease when these levels dropped in the winter.[9]

Despite its name, vitamin D is actually thought of as a hormone and not a vitamin. That's because, true to the definition of a hormone, it binds to many cell receptors all over the body, causing changes in cell function. Vitamins do not bind to cell receptors but instead act as helpers in enzyme reactions. The active form of vitamin D is called cholecalciferol, or D_3, but there is another kind of vitamin D, called ergocalciferol, or D_2, which is found in some plants. It is hard for your body to convert the plant kind, D_2, into the active kind, D_3, which is why we always recommend D_3 for supplementation. Whether you make D_3 in the skin from sunlight or take it as a supplement, it first goes to your liver and is made into 25-OH vitamin D, the vitamin D you should have measured in a blood test because it is the most reliable way to find out how much vitamin D is in your body. The 25-OH vitamin D is converted into 1,25-dihydroxyvitamin D. This is the most potent form of the hormone, because it goes into the cell, to the nucleus, and activates the genetic code, opening a chapter in the book of life that is all about your immune system.

Vitamin D and Your Immune System

1,25-dihydroxyvitamin D does the following:[10]

- Binds to dendritic cells in the body and astrocytes in the brain, which are the first-line immune cells that encounter anything foreign and send out an alarm. Vitamin D keeps them less reactive to self-antigens, meaning they stay tolerant and are less likely to attack the body's own tissues.
- Works on T cells so that they mature into T regulator cells, which are the healthiest kind, instead of Th1, Th2, or Th17, which can all drive autoimmune disease.
- Directly inhibits Th1 lymphocytes. This means that vitamin D will quiet down those hyped-up killer cells. Remember, in autoimmune diseases there can be a lopsided increase in these cells, and vitamin D helps them come back into balance.
- Decreases antibody production in activated B cells, which is another one of the imbalances we see in autoimmune diseases.

So if your 25-OH vitamin D levels are good (above 50 nm/l is the goal; some studies say 75 nm/l), it will help regulate your T cells so that they are more tolerant of your own tissues and won't get turned on and out of control. If you already have an autoimmune condition and you are low in vitamin D, taking a supplement will help destroy the killer cells that are already activated and prevent the production of more, thus reducing the inflammation and destruction caused by these cells.

How much vitamin D should you take? Studies have shown it is safe to take up to 4,000 IU/day, but your 25-OH vitamin D levels should be monitored every three months by a doctor or other health care professional.[11] Once you reach your desired levels (50–75 nm/l), you can cut back to 1,000–2,000 IU/day, with a doctor checking your blood levels to confirm the right maintenance dose for you.

Keep in mind, vitamin A is necessary for the absorption of vitamin D, and also helps regulate and support the healthy development of your immune cells. Vitamin A is an antioxidant, and the workbook will offer both food and supplement recommendations to help you increase your vitamin A and D intake.

Selenium and Zinc

Selenium and zinc are two important minerals that help your immune system function well. Several studies have suggested that being deficient in selenium may be a trigger for autoimmune thyroid disease. The reasoning goes something like this: selenium is a mineral that's necessary in order for your thyroid gland to function at its best. It is a required element for the enzymes that make thyroid hormone and for the glutathione peroxidase enzyme, which plays a critical antioxidant role and prevents damage to the thyroid follicles. If there is no selenium, your thyroid can't make hormones and the cells can be damaged by something called free radicals. (Free radicals are created in every cell by normal biochemical reactions and can be damaging if they're not deactivated or "quenched.") It is believed that one of the ways that autoimmunity develops is that the thyroid cells get damaged and look abnormal; then the immune system sees them and attacks, causing more damage and inflammation.

One study showed that giving 200 mcg of selenium per day decreased one of the primary antibodies in Hashimoto's thyroiditis.[12] There is also a strong link between selenium deficiency and celiac disease. People with celiac disease have malabsorption of many nutrients, selenium being one of them. Sometimes you can develop the autoimmune thyroid disease first and not even realize you have celiac disease until it's discovered later. In the next chapter, we'll talk more about my recommendations for getting selenium from your diet to make sure you don't become deficient and increase your risk of autoimmune thyroid disease.

While zinc is less well studied than selenium for its possible role in autoimmunity, studies on multiple sclerosis using mice have shown that zinc plays an important role in T cell and disease activity. Zinc is an essential trace element with a critical role in the normal development of the immune system and in keeping it in balance. Zinc deficiency impairs your immune system, but zinc supplementation can reverse this. A study done at the University of Connecticut showed that 30 mcg/day of zinc reduced the severity of multiple sclerosis in mice.[13] While this doesn't mean we can assume zinc will have the same impact on humans, I think it holds promise as one of the pieces to the puzzle. Why not make sure the immune system is working optimally? I think zinc is important and I always include it in my treatment programs because it is easy enough to get in foods such as sesame tahini, pumpkin seeds, and dark chocolate, as well as in a multivitamin/multimineral supplement.

Green Tea

The active component in green tea is something called epigallacatechin gallate (EGCG), and it has been getting a lot of attention lately. It has been shown to be beneficial in treating and preventing cancer, cardiovascular disease, weight loss, neurodegenerative diseases, and more. Now a recent study from Oregon State University has shown that EGCG has a powerful effect in increasing T regulator cells, which by now you know are critical for the maintenance of tolerance and prevention of autoimmunity.[14,15] While this study was done on mice, it suggests that green tea could be a helpful part of a nutritional approach to supporting the immune system in specific ways tailored for autoimmune patients.

In this chapter, you have learned that the food you eat provides information to your cells, and tells them how to behave. You now understand that food can be your medicine, because choosing foods that have an anti-inflammatory effect (such as the good fats) and removing foods that trigger inflammation (such as sugar and bad fats) can have a soothing effect on your immune system. Now it is time to move on to the workbook, so that you can identify your food sensitivities and discover what foods are good for *you*. And of course I will also help you find the nutrients that I talked about for your immune system, either in your food or in supplements if that is your preference.

CHAPTER 3

Using Food as Medicine Workbook

Like most of my new patients, Amy, a forty-eight-year-old Caucasian woman, walked into her first appointment at Blum Center for Health cradling a large file in her arms. The papers spilling out from it revealed an array of lab tests from conventional and functional medicine doctors she had seen over the previous two years. Her top complaints were painful, irregular periods with heavy bleeding, difficulty sleeping, hot flashes, and extreme anxiety—symptoms she had been experiencing for three years. Besides this, she had no history of health problems. In fact, until then, she had actually been very healthy, which was one reason why not feeling well now was so distressing to her. Adding to this was the frustrating fact that none of the doctors or experts she met with had been able to figure out exactly what was wrong with her and what she could do about it. First she had been given progesterone cream to regulate her period, and when this didn't work she was put on birth control pills.

When Amy came to see me, she was still on the pill, and while it was helping, she had gained ten pounds and her sex drive had plummeted. At our first meeting, she told me that she was hoping I could help her get off the pill. In fact, the first thing I did was tell her to stop the birth control pills so that they would no longer mask her symptoms and I could see what was really going on in her body. She was clearly in the beginning stages of menopause, called perimenopause, but no one had stopped to look at what else might be happening in addition to the changes in her levels of the hormones estrogen and progesterone.

When a woman is going through menopause, her hormones form what I call an endocrine orchestra. Each hormone interacts with the others and needs to be in balance for the entire body's systems to work well. Often I find that the thyroid hormones are a little too low or high or that the adrenal glands are fatigued (we will talk more about the adrenal glands in Chapter 5, "Understanding the Stress Connection") for women at this stage of life. I had a feeling that one of these hormone systems was out of balance, which would explain why Amy's transition into menopause was so difficult. My next steps were to check Amy's thyroid with a blood test and her adrenal glands with a saliva test. When the results came back, I was surprised to find her adrenal hormones were all in balance and working well. But I was not surprised that her levels of free T3 and free T4, which are the hormones made by the thyroid, were at the high end of the normal range and her thyroid-stimulating hormone (TSH), which is made by the brain, was a little low. As part of my initial screening tests, I always look for anti-thyroid antibodies, which are the hallmark of an autoimmune disease called Hashimoto's thyroiditis; I was pleased to see that Amy did not have them. However, the low TSH level and high free T3 and free T4 levels indicated to me that Amy had an overactive thyroid gland. Some doctors may call these results normal, but following a hunch, I sent her back to the lab to check for Graves' disease. Amy's results came back positive for this autoimmune condition, in which the body makes antibodies that stimulate the thyroid gland to produce too much hormone, which creates an unhealthy imbalance. Specifically, Amy was positive for something called thyroid-stimulating immunoglobulins (TSI). This was unexpected but exciting news, because at least now I knew what was wrong with Amy and how to help her. And I wasn't the only one who saw things this way. Amy felt relieved, too. Finally she had some answers.

Next I put Amy on a gluten-free diet, even though none of her tests came back positive for celiac disease (which I discussed in detail in the previous chapter). Why? Because I know that if you have an autoimmune thyroid disease, you're more likely to have celiac disease (and vice versa) even if laboratory tests are negative. For this reason, I told Amy to stop eating gluten.

In addition, Amy had a stool analysis and heavy metal testing to look for mercury and lead stored in her body. (Removing these toxins from the body are at the top of my checklist for reversing autoimmune disease, which is why they are the fourth step in this book.) Results revealed that Amy had parasites in her stool and moderately elevated levels of mercury in her body, but by the time we started treating those things, her Graves' disease antibodies disappeared as a result of the gluten-free diet alone. Better yet, once Amy went on a gluten-free diet, her hot flashes, insomnia, and anxiety all improved and her period became regular and easy. To be clear, I'm not sure if this happened because the extra thyroid hormones that we discovered in her body were interfering with her estrogen and once we corrected this her symptoms of perimenopause stopped, or if eating gluten was doing something directly to her brain and body's temperature control center, causing the hot flashes and other hormone symptoms. Either way, both Amy and I were thrilled that these symptoms and antibodies were disappearing. Her anxiety, though much improved, didn't completely resolve until I treated the parasites and gave her some extra vitamin B_{12}, folate, and SAMe supplements. I chose these specific vitamins because they are part of a group of nutrients called methyl donors, which are very important for supporting the brain chemical pathways involved in anxiety.

FOOD AND THE WAY YOU FEEL

Amy's story illustrates two very important points. First, gluten is a tricky food protein. You might have symptoms from eating gluten that seem completely unrelated to food—such as anxiety and hot flashes—but until you remove the gluten from your diet, you really don't know what its impact is on your body. The second is that removing gluten can improve your autoimmune antibodies. The only way to know this is by having a doctor or other health care professional repeat the lab tests that were done to look for antibodies, usually six months after the first lab test and after you begin a gluten-free diet. It is possible to see a change in your antibodies without a noticeable change in symptoms, which is why I am telling you to eat gluten free even if you don't think eating this way changes how you feel. Amy had both a change in her labs for the better and a resolution of bothersome symptoms. For her, making a gluten-free diet a permanent way of life was an easy decision.

Experts believe and studies suggest that anyone with an autoimmune disease has what is called leaky gut syndrome. Though I will discuss this in depth in Chapter 8, "Healing Your Gut," it's important to mention here that having a leaky gut causes you to develop food sensitivities. (This is why it is very likely that if you have an autoimmune disease, you are having symptoms and reactions to more than one food.) So what's the difference between a food allergy and food sensitivity? A food allergy is when a blood test and/or skin test confirms that you have an allergy to a specific food. But even if those allergy test results say that you are *not* allergic to a specific food, you may still have a reaction when you eat it. This is called a food sensitivity. **Food sensitivities still involve a reaction from your immune system, causing inflammation in your body, which is not good if you have autoimmune disease.** However, modern medicine just doesn't have the right tests yet to determine food sensitivities, so we have a different way to confirm if you are having a problem with a particular food. In this chapter, I am going to show you how to test yourself for sensitivities to gluten, dairy, corn, and soy, the foods that most commonly cause problems. Remember, a food sensitivity just means you feel worse when you eat the food and better when you don't. The food can cause any symptoms at all, from digestive symptoms such as reflux, gas and bloating after eating, constipation, or diarrhea to things such as fatigue, difficulty concentrating, headaches, joint pain, or muscle pain. Later in Chapter 12, "Supporting Your Liver Workbook," I will show you how to do a more complete elimination diet and we will test some additional foods as part of a detox program.

Now let's move on to finding out if you are sensitive to gluten, dairy, soy, or corn. Then I will show you how to incorporate what you learned and create a personalized anti-inflammatory diet to begin the treatment of your autoimmune disease or other immune imbalance.

Self-Assessment

Testing for Food Sensitivities

Because everyone is different, my goal here is to create a personalized program for you, based on your unique biochemistry. Your health right now is a result of your genetic predisposition interacting with your environment over the entire course of your life; the food you bring into your body is the largest environmental exposure you have. Also, perhaps there is someone else in your family with an autoimmune condition such as celiac disease or who you know is sensitive to gluten. This is important information for you because it means *you* are at an increased risk for these things, too.

In this section, I will show you how to start discovering the right foods for you, a concept called personalized nutrition. We are going to do this with my food elimination and challenge program, so called because first you will remove a food from your diet and then you will eat it again, which we call a food challenge. This will help you discover any food sensitivities to gluten, dairy, soy, or corn. As I noted, I have chosen these foods because people are the most sensitive to them. It will come as no surprise that the majority of the wheat, corn, and soy in our food supply is genetically modified and thus your body might see their genes and proteins as foreign. Also, wheat, corn, and soy have made their way insidiously into everything we eat, whether it's obvious foods such as pasta, corn chips, and soy sauce or less obvious forms such as soy lecithin and cornstarch. Another reason for these food sensitivities: you have been eating lots and lots of these foods, which increases your chances of having an immune reaction. Dairy is also removed because it causes symptoms such as sinus congestion, gas, bloating, and dark circles under your eyes. Other foods that might be a problem include eggs, shellfish, peanuts, and vegetables in the nightshade family (tomatoes, potatoes, eggplant, and peppers), plants that contain a substance that can irritate your joints, causing pain and inflammation. Don't worry about these foods right now because when we get to the fourth step of our program I will take you through a more comprehensive elimination and we will test the rest of these foods.

Getting Started

Get ready to change your diet. Remember, this is just for three weeks, not forever. We will review the list of foods to remove and show you how to make substitutions for the foods you usually eat. This is planning time, so take a look at the recipes in the next chapter (which are all free of gluten, dairy, soy, and corn) and review the pantry shopping list at the end of this chapter so that you can go food shopping and get what you need to start.

Set a date. Look at your calendar for a three-week stretch of time that you can dedicate to this elimination program. Timing is of the essence here because it will involve food shopping and preparing what you need. For example, you may need to bring your meals and snacks to work with you to avoid grabbing food filled with gluten and dairy (which is most fast food) when you're hungry or tempted by invitations to eat with colleagues.

Remember, the first two to three days are the hardest. It will get easier as you go along, and as you feel better, you will have more motivation and more energy to stick with it.

Part 1: Remove Gluten, Dairy, Corn, and Soy from Your Diet for Three Weeks

A lot of times my patients ask me why we are removing all four foods at once and whether it would be better or just as good to remove one at a time. The way the experiment works, first you remove the foods and feel better, then reintroduce each food one at a time to see if you feel worse. If you remove only one food, you might not feel better because you are still eating another problem food. Then you might not notice you feel worse when you reintroduce the food, because you never felt better in the first place. Therefore, it is best to remove all four foods at once, because this increases the likelihood that you will actually improve your symptoms from the diet change, and then you will be able to tell if you feel worse when you eat the food again.

But if removing four foods feels too overwhelming, I suggest you start with eliminating just two: gluten and dairy, which are the hardest because these are the foods that most people live on every day as part of the standard American diet.

Gluten

What Not to Eat

Gluten is a protein found in wheat, barley, kamut, rye, and spelt. Bread, cakes, cookies, pasta, and cereal are obvious places where you will find gluten, but it's also hiding in many, many other foods. As a result, you need to read food labels and look at the ingredient lists for wheat, barley, kamut, rye, or spelt. For example, did you know that soy sauce is made from wheat? Or that beer is made from barley? Probably not, and you're certainly not alone. Because it is not possible to list here all the foods that contain gluten, reading food labels is key. Oats are okay only if the label says they're gluten free.

What You Should Eat

Quinoa, millet, buckwheat, and rice contain no gluten. One good thing about the prevalence of gluten sensitivity these days is that you can actually find bread, pasta, crackers, and even cookies made from these ancient grains. Many foods say clearly on their packages that they are gluten free. (I've even noticed that some stores are starting to have gluten-free sections or aisles.) Some gluten-free foods, such as breads and muffins, are kept in the frozen section rather than the traditional bread or baked goods aisle. This is because without the usual chemical preservatives, they spoil much faster, so they are kept frozen. Also, while I want you to be enthusiastic about switching to gluten-free eating, I also want you to beware that just because a food says it's gluten free doesn't mean it's healthful. For example, gluten-free cookies still contain sugar so they may not be a healthy choice. The chart on page 69, "Menu Ideas During the Elimination Diet: No Deprivation!," will help you see that eating gluten free is actually pretty easy and that there are lots of gluten-free choices.

Dairy

What Not to Eat

This includes any milk product made from cow, goat, or sheep's milk, such as yogurt, cheese, milk, kefir, and butter. When we meet for the first time, many of my patients tell me that they are lactose intolerant because they get gassy and bloated when they eat dairy. But food sensitivities to dairy are caused by proteins called casein and whey, not lactose, the milk sugar that many people think is making them feel sick. Often after doing this elimination test, many patients realize that milk is causing other symptoms that go beyond their stomachs. These include chronic congestion and sinusitis, postnasal drip, ear infections, and more. The dairy industry would have you believe that your bones will wither away if you don't drink milk, but I assure you that is far from the truth. There is plenty of calcium in a whole-foods diet (for example, in sesame seeds, almonds, and dark green leafy vegetables such as kale and collard greens), so don't worry about giving up dairy because you think your bones are dependent on it.

What You Should Eat

Dairy alternatives include almond, rice, hemp, and coconut milk. These milk substitutes are also made into yogurt, kefir, and cheese. My favorite is coconut milk because it contains wonderful good fat for your gut and brain.

Corn

What Not to Eat

Just a few generations ago, corn in the United States was grown for our own personal consumption. Today, it's being grown as a commodity. By this I mean that it is used for other purposes, such as making an ingredient called high-fructose corn syrup that is used in many, many foods because it tastes sweeter and is cheaper than sugar. Corn is also used as feed for cows instead of the grass they are naturally meant to consume. The problem here? When cows eat grass, their meat is filled with healthy omega-3 fats, which we benefit from when we eat their meat. But when cows eat corn, their meat is filled with inflammatory saturated fats, which then cause inflammation in our bodies when we eat it. (I'll talk more about good and bad fats later in this chapter.)

Because corn has become a valuable commodity, farmers want to maximize how much they can grow, so they use genetically modified (GM) corn seeds. I'm not sure if it is this GM corn or the fact that we are overexposed to corn in our daily diets (meaning most people eating the standard American diet consume corn several times every day) that has caused so many people to be sensitive to it. Having a corn sensitivity means that you feel better when it is removed from your diet and worse when you eat it. We are going to help you find out if this describes you. Remember, you need to remove whole corn, whether on the cob, in a can, or frozen, and popcorn, too. You also need to be careful about reading labels. Look for cornstarch, corn syrup, corn syrup solids, corn flour, and high-fructose corn syrup—basically, anything with the word "corn" in it.

Soy

What Not to Eat

Soy is on the list here because it causes digestive upset and inflammation for many people, something I've seen in my practice over and over. I know that when I eat soy, it makes my hands feel swollen the next day. Unless it is organic and says "non-GMO" on the label, most soy is made from GM seeds, and this is always a concern. Soy is also used as an additive in many foods, especially packaged processed foods, so you must read labels and avoid anything that lists soy protein, soy lecithin, or soy oil in its ingredient list. When you start reading labels looking for these words, you will be shocked at how many foods contain them. This is the beginning of a very important food education for you.

I always have my patients remove soy from their diets and then reintroduce it, making sure that it doesn't make their symptoms worse. There is plenty of controversy around soy when it comes to its possible influence on thyroid function, and there is also concern about soy and breast cancer. While I won't go into that in detail because it goes beyond the scope of this book, based on what I've read in the latest scientific literature, my opinion is that unless you find you have a sensitivity to soy in the elimination challenge, it is perfectly fine in moderation for everyone. By "moderation" I mean eating soy foods one to three times a week. If you find that eating soy does not cause you any symptoms and you want to eat it as part of a balanced diet, then the most important thing to consider is what *kind* of soy you are eating. Focus on eating whole organic, non-GM soy foods such as tempeh, edamame, and tofu.

Eliminate and Replace

Here is a summary of the four food categories, what you should remove, and what you can eat as a substitute. (Obviously, if you already know you have an allergy or sensitivity to a particular food that's on the "Foods to Include" list, don't eat it.)

Type of Food	Food to Remove	Food to Include
Corn	Whole corn, corn syrup, cornstarch, and any ingredient containing the word "corn"	All other vegetables, steamed or sautéed in olive or coconut oil
Gluten	Wheat, barley, spelt, kamut, rye, and most oats	Rice, millet, buckwheat, and quinoa; oats are okay if they say "gluten free"
Soy	Tempeh, tofu, edamame, soy sauce, tamari, and any ingredient containing the word "soy"	Lentils, chickpeas, all other beans
Dairy	All cow, sheep, and goat's milk, yogurt, kefir, cheese, butter, and any ingredient containing the word "casein" or "whey"	Almond, rice, coconut, and hemp milk, yogurt, and kefir

Menu Ideas During the Elimination Diet: No Deprivation!		
	Menu Day 1	**Menu Day 2**	**Menu Day 3**
Breakfast	Gluten-free toast with almond or peanut butter	Eggs: boiled or poached Or Pesto Scrambled Eggs* or Weekend Frittata*	Hot cereal: gluten-free oatmeal or warm Quinoa Cereal with Fruit and Nuts* Or cold cereal: Gluten-Free Granola* with coconut, rice, or almond milk
Lunch	Salad with your favorite veggies, beans, grilled chicken, or fish, dressed with olive oil and lemon or vinegar	Quinoa Pasta with Peas, Arugula, and Sun-Dried Tomatoes* Or Soba Noodles Salad* with vegetables and chicken or shrimp Or Lentil Salad*	Sandwich made with gluten-free bread or wrap: turkey, avocado, chicken, peanut or almond butter, hummus and veggies
Snack	Nuts and fruit Or guacamole and rice chips	Tahini and veggies Or hummus and rice crackers	Almond Butter Granola bars* Or Almond Blueberry Muffins*
Dinner	Turkey Burgers* with Beet and Fennel Salad	Mediterranean Herb-Crusted Salmon* with Creamed Spinach* and Wild Mushroom Quinoa*	Chicken Stuffed with Peppers, Pine Nuts, and Spinach* with sweet potato and arugula salad
Dessert	Fruit or Blueberry Parfait*	Coconut yogurt or coconut milk ice cream	Chocolate Avocado Pudding*

* A recipe for this can be found in the recipe chapter of this book.

Part 2: Reintroduce Foods One at a Time

Once you have made it three weeks without eating gluten, dairy, corn, and soy, you have completed the first part of the Elimination Diet. Now, you begin the second and final step, which is the reintroduction of these foods one at a time. This is when you will gather all the information about whether the food is good for you or not and you'll uncover some food sensitivities. Below is a form you can fill out to help you keep track. You can also easily download this form from my website, www.immuneprogram.com. Think about your health and the symptoms you might be experiencing, even if they seem unrelated to food. Write them down in the left column. (I listed some common symptoms below just to give you an example of how to fill out the chart.)

For each food that you reintroduce, think about the symptoms on your list and use the words "none," "mild," "moderate," or "severe" to describe your reaction to it in the boxes provided. This will help you remember later when you look back.

Symptom	Gluten	Dairy	Soy	Corn
Bloating				
Headache				
Joint pain				
Hot flashes				
Your symptom				
Your symptom				

It doesn't matter in which order you choose to reintroduce the foods. I usually tell my patients to reintroduce first the food they miss most. Eat that food at least twice each day for two days, noticing how you feel. On day three, don't eat the food, but continue to observe how you feel. If you have no reaction to the food, you are ready to move on to the next food on day four. If you *do* have a reaction—such as headache, rash, brain fog, fatigue, digestive reaction, or other symptom—write it down in the above table so you don't forget later. **Once you know a particular food isn't good for you, remove it again.** The food reaction should go away within a day or two, but for some people it can take longer. Once that reaction goes away, it is time to try the next food. As an example, if you ate corn and it gave you diarrhea, this means you have a sensitivity to corn, and you should remove the corn again. Once your diarrhea goes away and your bowels are normal again, you can try the next food. But of course you will continue to keep corn out of your diet.

Finding out if you are having a noticeable reaction to gluten is important. If you don't have a reaction and don't have an autoimmune disease, you can add it back into your diet. However, even if you don't react, make sure to remove it again if you have an autoimmune disease.

Be patient—it will take you another two weeks or so to reintroduce all the foods you have eliminated.

Once you've completed this process, you should know whether gluten, dairy, corn, or soy is creating an immune reaction in your body by causing either familiar or new symptoms when you ate them again. If you found that you were sensitive to more than one, that is okay, and it's very common. Personally, I am sensitive to gluten, dairy, corn, and soy. When I eat gluten, my brain is really foggy the next day, which feels like a hangover. When I eat dairy, I experience constipation and sinus congestion. And when I eat corn or soy, my hands swell up the next day. All these symptoms are caused by inflammation that is affecting different parts of my body. Because I have been eating a diet 95 percent free of these foods for more than ten years, my reactions when I do eat them are minor compared to what they once were. But they are still there.

Treatment Program

Once you have determined which foods cause bad reactions in your body and need to be eliminated from your diet, you can begin to eat in a way that best supports your immune system. This is the first step in your treatment program. All of the treatment programs in this book are divided into three tiers. The first tier is treatment with food only, because some people prefer to work only with food, and for others food alone might be all they need. As we've described, changing how you eat is the foundation for every aspect of the functional medicine approach to preventing and treating illness; everyone must include Tier 1 in their program. The three tiers of the treatment program are:

Tier 1: Eating for immune health. Here, we make specific dietary changes that will improve the health of your immune system.

Tier 2: **Additional resources to support a healthy immune system.** In this section, I will discuss mindful eating, and I will also give you a checklist of basic supplements to make sure your immune system is getting the support it needs to be balanced and healthy. There is a complete supplement and herb guide in the appendix with specific product names and how to find them.

Tier 3: **Functional Medicine Options from a Health Care Professional.** It can be very difficult to change the way you eat without the support of a health care professional. If you know that you want to make these changes but feel overwhelmed about doing it on your own, you can get help from an integrative medicine practitioner.

Tier 1: Eating for Immune Health

What does it mean to eat in a way that will support your immune system? This is called an anti-inflammatory diet, and there are four parts to it. First, you must discover what foods you are sensitive to and remove them. We began that process in the self-assessment. Second, you must begin to eat a diet rich in antioxidants (such as fruits and veggies). Third, you must look at the sugar you are eating and focus on eating a low-glycemic-index diet (i.e., one that is low in sugar). And finally, you must focus on eating plenty of good fats because the fat you eat determines the level of inflammation in your body. Here I'll explain each step, and then I am going to give you food lists and menu suggestions for eating this way.

Step 1: Discover Your Food Sensitivities and Remove Those Foods from Your Diet

Now that you have discovered whether gluten, dairy, corn, or soy is causing inflammation in your body, you must remove this food from your diet for at least six months. But just to be clear:

- If you have had a positive test for celiac disease (including anti-gliadin and anti-deamidated gliadin antibodies), your diet should stay gluten free for life.
- If you don't have celiac disease but you have another autoimmune disease and gluten sensitivity, you need to be 100 percent gluten free for now, until you have completely healed your gut and have recovered from your autoimmune disease. After that, you should remain 95 percent gluten free, which means that under normal circumstances you

should live 100 percent gluten free in your daily work and home life, and then on occasion (such as once a month) if you go out to eat or travel, you can go off the wagon. Just remember to get right back on it again when you come home.

Step 2: Eat a Rainbow of Veggies

As our next step, let's focus on something positive: adding color to your diet. Most people do not eat enough fruits and vegetables, which are rich in the micronutrients that your body and immune system need to function at their best, such as antioxidants, B vitamins, and minerals.

What are antioxidants? If you're like most people, you have probably heard the term but you aren't exactly clear about what they are and what they do, so let me explain. Every day your body makes something called free radicals, which are electrically charged molecules released inside your cells during their normal functioning. Unfortunately, these free radicals damage your tissues. Normally your body makes a small amount of these, and their reactivity is "quenched" by antioxidants from your food. Antioxidants act like sponges, which mop up the free radicals in your body. However, when you are exposed to toxins such as mercury or other heavy metals or pesticides, these toxic compounds make more free radicals in your body, and so you need more antioxidants to absorb the free radicals and prevent damage to your tissue. This mopping-up process is really important to protect your DNA and tissues from damage, which can cause autoimmune disease, cancer, and chronic inflammation. We will talk more about toxins causing tissue damage and autoimmune disease in Chapter 11, "Supporting Your Liver."

What is the solution? Nature gave us an abundance of antioxidants in food to help us prevent the buildup of too many free radicals, so you must eat enough of these foods to protect your tissues and cells. This is pretty easy, since fruits and vegetables are bursting with antioxidants! It's also an important change to make, since the standard American diet is typically low in these nutrients.

Some Hints About Adding Antioxidant-Rich Foods to Your Diet

If possible, choose organic fruits and vegetables. Pesticides are chemicals used to keep insects from devouring plants. Because organic fruits and veggies are grown without them, the plants have had to work to fight off the bugs on their own, and they do this by making antioxidants. Therefore, organic produce packs a stronger antioxidant punch than conventionally grown produce, and by eating organic you will reap these benefits.

I know it is not always feasible to go 100 percent organic. If that's the case for you, I suggest you visit the Environmental Working Group's website (www.ewg.org) to see a list called the Dirty Dozen. This includes the twelve fruits and veggies that have been found to have the most pesticide residues and, as a result, really need to be organic when you eat them. The Environmental Working Group also has a list called the Clean 15, the vegetables and fruits that have been found to have the least pesticide residues and do not need to be organic. Both lists are very helpful.

I also recommend using a veggie wash, which can be found in the produce section of most grocery stores, to clean all non-organic fruits and vegetables. This helps remove any harmful pesticide residues.

Here are some suggestions for incorporating into your daily diet more of the foods richest in the antioxidants and minerals that keep your immune system strong and your inflammation low:

- You can eat fruit as a dessert for your meals, as part of a breakfast smoothie, or as a snack.
- Have at least one salad each day made of raw greens and vegetables, either as a main course or as a side dish. (To make it a complete meal, add plenty of protein and healthy fat; see below.)
- For dinner, your plate should be at least half filled with vegetables (steamed or sautéed in olive oil or coconut oil). Most people fill their plate with a huge serving of protein and a big portion of a grain such as rice or pasta or a starchy vegetable such as white potatoes, with little space for vegetables. But you need to change the proportions on your plate and make antioxidant-rich vegetables the centerpiece. The picture of what your plate should look like can be seen in Figure 2.

Step 3: Eat a Low-Sugar Diet

In the medical world, a low-sugar diet is also called a low-glycemic diet, and it is the first step to lowering the amount of sugar floating around in your blood. When your blood sugar is high, it causes inflammation and damages your immune system. There is something called a glycemic index for each food, which is determined by how quickly and severely that food raises your blood sugar level. A high-glycemic diet raises your blood sugar rapidly and puts you at risk for diabetes, high blood pressure, and cardiovascular disease. It also makes you feel tired and depressed.

Figure 2:

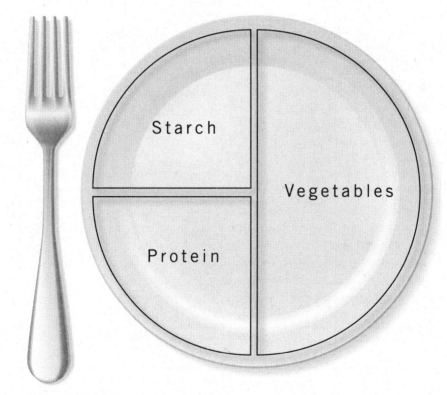

EATING FOR YOUR IMMUNE SYSTEM

Foods Rich in Antioxidants and Immune-Supporting Nutrients			
Antioxidant/ nutrient	Fruit sources	Vegetable sources	Other food sources
Beta-carotene and other carotenoids	Apricots, cantaloupe, mangoes, nectarines, peaches, pink grapefruit, tangerines, watermelon	Asparagus, beets, broccoli, carrots, green peppers, kale, turnip and collard greens, pumpkin, squash, spinach, sweet potatoes, tomatoes	
Vitamin C	Berries, cantaloupe, grapefruit, honeydew, kiwi, mangoes, nectarines, oranges, papayas, strawberries	Broccoli, Brussels sprouts, cauliflower, kale, peppers (red, green, or yellow), snow peas, sweet potatoes, tomatoes	
Vitamin E	Mangoes, papayas	Broccoli, carrots, chard, mustard and turnip greens, pumpkin, red peppers, spinach	Nuts and sunflower seeds
Other antioxidants	Prunes, apples, raisins, all berries, plums, red grapes	Sprouts, onions, eggplant	Beans
Zinc		Peas	Oysters, red meat, poultry, beans, nuts, seafood, whole grains, dairy products

Selenium			Brazil nuts, sunflower seeds, tuna, beef, poultry, grains
EGCG			Green tea

Most important for our purposes, sugar in the blood stimulates your immune cells to actively release inflammatory molecules that travel throughout your body, causing damage and irritation. Instead of eating foods that make your blood sugar skyrocket, eat a low-glycemic diet. The first step in doing so is to eliminate all white flour and processed sugar from your diet. This is one of the most important steps that you can take toward good health (and something you may have done already when following other diet plans).

Watch Out for the White Stuff

White flour, from which most of the fiber, vitamins, and minerals have been removed, is found in all white bread, cakes, cookies, and most other baked goods, which is why all of these have a very high glycemic index. **When I talk about eating too much sugar in your diet, I am also talking about white flour products, since white flour is converted into sugar in your blood.** To avoid these high-glycemic-index foods, choose *whole*-grain breads, muffins, and pasta. Read food labels and look for grain products that have at least 3 grams of fiber per serving, because fiber slows down the absorption of the sugar and reduces the food's glycemic index. How do you know what kind of flour is in the food you are eating? Read the ingredient list and look for the word "whole" when the flour is listed. For example, look for *whole* quinoa, *whole* buckwheat, or *whole* wheat (for those of you who can eat wheat).

When choosing grains, either in bread or crackers or to make as a side dish, move away from wheat (which contains gluten) and corn and try other options such as quinoa, buckwheat, and millet, ancient grains that are delicious and good for you. Eat brown rice instead of white. The recipes in the next chapter are created using these grains so that you can easily begin to bring more healthy diversity (and delicious new flavors) into your diet.

In addition to cutting white flour out of your diet, don't forget about sugar itself. Many people up their sugar intake by consuming it in coffee, soda, juices, cookies, cakes, candy, or other sweets. And you may not have known that alcohol is a high-sugar drink.

Sugar in Your Blood

Sugar-laden foods dump a big dose of glucose into your bloodstream. While you might feel good for thirty minutes when your blood sugar rises, inevitably you feel a crash or energy low when it plummets, which sends you running for more sugar to perk yourself up again. This up-and-down cycle is one of the biggest reasons for fatigue (and weight gain), and simply correcting it gives many of my patients a lot more energy and improves their mood (and often helps them lose a few pounds).

The other thing to keep in mind is that high blood sugar causes inflammation and an emergency release of insulin. Insulin is the hormone that brings down your blood sugar by telling the cells of your body to open up and absorb the sugar to convert it to energy. Usually this is a good thing because this is how your cells get fed. However, when there is *too* much glucose and insulin at once, your body stores the excess glucose as fat. And what happens if you're stressed out on top of this? Your stress hormones direct your body to make belly fat, a metabolically different kind of fat that causes a lot of inflammation (and is hardest to get rid of). Remember, inflammation involves your immune system, so if you have an autoimmune disease or an immune problem, sugar will only make matters worse.

Removing Sugar from Your Diet

Today is the day to stop eating sweets and foods made with white flour. One word of caution: if you have been consuming lots of sugar or having bread, pasta, white potatoes, or white rice with every meal, you might experience sugar withdrawal. **"Withdrawal" may sound like a strange word when talking about food, but for some people sugar truly is a drug and they are addicted.** If you are one of them, your body may have a strong reaction when you eliminate sugar from your diet. I've had patients get headaches and even intense emotional experiences in the first few days of going off sugar. But don't worry, any symptoms and reactions will pass (usually in one to three days), leaving you clearer and more emotionally and energetically stable than you have felt in a long time.

How do you remove all processed sugar from your diet? Here is your guide to foods with the highest hidden or obvious sugar content and ideas for substitutions. Remember to read all the labels on any food boxes or prepackaged containers and avoid those that have more than 15 grams of sugar per serving.

	Best to Eat: Low-Glycemic	Foods to Avoid: High-Glycemic
Sweeteners	Raw unprocessed agave syrup, brown rice syrup, blackstrap molasses, fruit sweetener. These are still sugar, so eat as little as possible. Stevia is the best option: it is non-caloric.	All artificial sweeteners, including aspartame, sucralose (Splenda), and saccharin; high-fructose corn syrup, white or brown sugar, honey, evaporated cane juice, maple syrup
Drinks	Filtered water, decaffeinated herbal teas, seltzer, mineral water. Limit caffeinated coffee or tea to 1 cup per day.	Soda, fruit juices, or other drinks sweetened with sugar or high-fructose corn syrup. Limit caffeine and alcohol.
Bread, grains, and starches	Whole-grain gluten-free bread, pasta, crackers, and wraps*; brown or wild rice, quinoa, whole buckwheat, whole millet, brown rice	White flour, wheat, spelt, barley, kamut, rye flour, corn, white potatoes, white rice
Snacks	Gluten-free whole-grain crackers* with hummus, almond butter, or guacamole; yogurt (coconut, soy, or dairy if it is okay for you), nuts, apples, pears, peaches, plums, all berries	Pretzels, potato chips, corn chips, tortilla chips, popcorn, white-flour crackers; white-flour and white-sugar cookies, cakes, muffins

(continued on next page)

	Best to Eat: Low-Glycemic	Foods to Avoid: High-Glycemic
Condiments	Organic ketchup, mustard, vinegar, all spices and herbs (including salt, pepper, basil, cinnamon, cumin, dill, garlic, ginger, mustard, oregano, parsley, rosemary, tarragon, thyme, turmeric)	Anything with high-fructose corn syrup, corn syrup, or added cane sugar, such as ketchup, barbecue sauce, hot sauce, teriyaki sauce
Desserts	Coconut milk yogurt or ice cream, fruit (fresh or dried), unsweetened dark chocolate, carob, low-sugar dessert recipes in this book: Blueberry Parfait, Chocolate Avocado Pudding, Chocolate Chip Oatmeal Cookies	Frozen yogurt or ice cream, sorbet, cookies, cakes, candy
* See the Pantry Shopping List.		

Here are some suggestions and tips for getting started and sticking with this step of the program:

- Make a list of all the changes you want to make. Decide if you want to remove *all* your sugar and white flour products at once or do it more slowly over time. For some people, it is easier to cut back gradually; for others, quitting cold turkey works best. Either way is fine.
- Choose substitutions from the list above so that you have other choices to satisfy your sweet tooth or snacking needs. Look at some of the dessert recipes in this book.
- Set a start date to begin.
- Plan menus and shop for and prepare foods ahead of time. For example, on Sunday, cut up fruits and vegetables and cook things such as big batches of brown rice and quinoa for the week ahead. Make extra food for dinner every night so that you have leftovers for the next day.

- Make sure you are never hungry, which means planning your meals and snacks ahead of time. Bring snacks to work or anytime you're out of the house for long periods of time, such as when you're running errands or driving long distances.
- If you decide to make gradual changes rather than going cold turkey, make a list and have a plan. Set small manageable goals for yourself. For example, "This week I will stop drinking soda, and if I'm ready, next week I will switch the sugar in my coffee to stevia."
- Perhaps choose a deadline for when you want to have all the sugar out of your diet. And when you get there, give yourself a big pat on the back—you deserve it! Removing sugar and white flour carbs from your diet is one of the hardest things to do for people eating a standard American diet.

Step 4: Eat Lots of Healthy Fat

In the last chapter, I explained how important it is for your immune system to increase the amount of good fats in your diet. These include essential fatty acids, which are fats that our bodies can't produce even though we need them to stay healthy, so we *must* eat them. These are the omega-3 and omega-6 fats that you always hear about. As I described, good food sources of healthy fats include fish, nuts, seeds, and leafy greens—foods typically missing in the standard American diet. The other healthy fats are saturated vegetable fats such as those found in avocado and coconuts.

In addition to eating healthy fat, you must eliminate the bad fats, too. You should avoid trans fats (found in partially hydrogenated vegetable oils) and saturated animal fats (particularly from beef and dairy products).

Trans fats, which are produced when vegetable oils are partially hydrogenated, are most often found in processed foods. Read the labels on all boxes, cans, and packages and look for the words "trans fat" or "partially hydrogenated." If you find them, put the package down and step away from the shelf!

As I mentioned, most of our cattle are fed unhealthy diets filled with corn, which causes their bodies to make more inflammatory saturated fats. When you eat the meat or milk products from these cattle, the fats they contain increase inflammation in your body. If you still want to eat beef and dairy foods, your best bet is to choose organic products from grass-fed cattle if you can find them. (And eat dairy only if it was okay for you when you did the elimination and challenge program.) The meat and dairy that come from grass-fed cattle are filled with healthier fats, and this will transfer health benefits to you when you eat it.

Here is a summary of what kinds of fat to eat and not to eat:

	Good to Eat	Best to Avoid
Animal fats	Fish,* fish oil supplements, grass-fed beef, egg yolks (up to 4/week), ghee (clarified butter)	Cheese, milk fat, beef raised on corn, shortening
Vegetable fats	All cold pressed oils: Olive oil, canola, flax, safflower, sesame, almond, sunflower, walnut, pumpkin. Avocado, coconut oil and milk, palm oil. Nuts, seeds, leafy greens.	Margarine, salad dressings, mayonnaise or other products made with trans fats, hydrogenated or partially hydrogenated oils

* Beware of the high mercury in some fish. I will explain more about this in Chapter 11, but you can find the Seafood Selecter list of the fish that are best at the Environmental Defense Fund website, www.edf.org.

Why Fats Are Important

All of our cell membranes are made of fatty acids, and we make millions of new cells every day. The kinds of fat that build the cell affect how well it functions. If you are eating a diet filled with trans fats or saturated animal fats, your cell membranes and nerve cells are filled with these fats and will not function optimally. For example, our brains are 60 percent fat. These cells are being regenerated all the time, but they need the raw material—healthy fats—to do so.

Tier 2: Additional Resources to Support a Healthy Immune System

Mindful Eating

Because I believe that food is ultimately the best medicine, I want to give you all the tools you need to be able to make good food choices and stick to your best intentions for eating in a healthy way. To do this, **not only**

do you have to learn what to eat, but you also need to learn *how* to eat. Most people eat mindlessly, grabbing the first thing they can get their hands on when they are hungry or inhaling their dinner because they are starving when they get home at night. Think carefully. Do you remember what you ate yesterday or the day before? What did it taste like?

The problem is that mindless eating leads to poor food choices, especially foods high in sugar and bad fat. The other problem with this is that you become disconnected to how your food actually feels in your body when you eat it. Does it make you feel sluggish or energized? Does it feel good going in, as you are chewing and swallowing the food all the way into your stomach? The goal here is to slow down, taste, enjoy, digest, and metabolize all those wonderful nutrients and flavors you are eating. Learning what this feels like and practicing it in your everyday life is so important. To help, I want you to do the following mindful eating exercise, adapted from the Center for Mind-Body Medicine.

Before you begin, read this meditation to yourself before you start, and then see if you can follow the instructions from memory. Another option is for you to record yourself reading it aloud and then play it back while you do this exercise. The latter option allows you to be guided through the exercise by your own voice and you can relax knowing you don't have to remember what comes next. Many phones and computers have recording abilities, so it should be something you can do easily.

Mindful Eating Exercise

Sit in a comfortable chair with a journal or paper and pen nearby. Choose a food to eat for the experiment. It should be one piece or the equivalent of one bite, such as a grape or a raisin, one piece of dark chocolate, or a small bit of any other food with texture and flavor.

If you are doing this without an audio recording, read through the following script, then close your eyes and do the exercise from memory. If you taped it, this is where the recording should begin:

- Place your hands in your lap and close your eyes. Spend a few minutes centering yourself, using your breathing as a guide. Breathe in through your nose and out through your mouth. If your mind wanders, gently bring your attention back to your breathing.
- Most of us eat automatically, without thinking. Now we are going to experiment with eating differently, paying full attention in a nonjudgmental, open way, and staying in the present moment as much as possible.

- Take the piece of food you have chosen and hold it in your hand. Imagine that you are tasting and sensing this object for the very first time.
- Open your eyes. What does it look like? What shape is it? What color? How does it reflect light?
- As you observe this food, think about where it came from. Where was it grown? How many people were part of the supply chain that brought the food to where you bought it? Thank nature for this gift.
- Close your eyes again. Begin to notice how the food feels in your hand. What is its temperature? Its texture? Its density? Perhaps you might also bring it up to your nose. Do you smell anything? Are you salivating? How do you feel about putting this food into your body right now? How does your body feel anticipating eating in this moment?
- Now you are going to put this food into your body. Be aware of your hand moving toward your mouth. Experience the food in your mouth. Chew slowly and completely and focus your full attention on the food's taste and texture. Be aware of any desire you have to rush through so that you can have another bite or piece. Be aware of the intention to swallow before you actually swallow.
- When the food is completely liquefied, you can swallow. Notice how far into your body you can still feel the food.
- Once all the sensations of food are gone, you can open your eyes.
- What did you notice? Pick up your journal or paper and write down anything important that you realized and don't want to forget. This exercise can bring up feelings about almost anything, including powerful insight about your relationship with food. This exercise can be repeated at any time with different foods. I suggest you bring some of this meditative quality to all your meals, every time you eat.

Supplementation with Vitamins and Minerals

Your immune system needs plenty of antioxidants, good fat, vitamin D, vitamin A, selenium, and zinc to be in balance. If you have an autoimmune disease, just replenishing these nutrients is not enough for you to be healed, because we must still find the underlying cause of your immune problem and fix *that*, which is the ultimate goal of *The Immune System Recovery Plan*. Being low in any of these nutrients, especially vitamin D, will make your condition worse, and even interfere with your getting better, so you must include these nutrients in your treatment program. In this section, I will give you a checklist of basic supplementation to make sure your immune system is getting the support it needs to be balanced and healthy.

Antioxidants

If you are eating fruits and vegetables from the list on page 76 at least five times each day, you are off to a good start. If not, I would encourage you to eat more of these antioxidant-rich foods because they will protect your immune system from free radical damage. I recommend that everyone, with or without a concern about their immune system, take a good-quality (I will explain what that means as we go) multivitamin/multimineral supplement that contains the following antioxidants.

Beta-carotene. This is the precursor to vitamin A, meaning when you eat it or take it in a supplement, your body converts it into vitamin A. It is a member of a large family of compounds called carotenes, which are the pigments in yellow and orange fruit and vegetables and in dark leafy greens. If you want to take a supplement, it is best to find a mixed-carotene product that includes alpha- and beta-carotene, lutein, and lycopene. This is one way you will know if a multivitamin is a good quality product: it will contain mixed carotenes and not just one kind. The dose of beta-carotene is 5,000–15,000 international units (IU) of mixed carotenes each day. You can't really take too much. If you take a lot, your palms might turn yellow, which will go away when you cut back on your intake. You can also take preformed vitamin A, but don't take more than 5,000 IU/day. This is because, although studies on vitamin A show mixed results, some have suggested long-term use of higher levels of this nutrient can be harmful to your bones.

Vitamin C. This is such a good antioxidant that it is often used as a food preservative. Ordinary vitamin C (ascorbic acid) tastes sour and can upset your stomach and damage the enamel on your teeth, so be careful not to take effervescent ascorbic acid powder. Instead, choose calcium ascorbate powder or take vitamin C in a capsule or tablet. A good-quality vitamin C product will also contain something called citrus bioflavonoids, which are cousins of vitamin C and help it work better. The dose I usually recommend as a starting point is 1,000 mg per day of vitamin C with bioflavonoids. If you have autoimmune disease, a high toxin load, infections, or other chronic illness, you need more, and I would recommend at least 2,000 mg per day to give your immune cells added protection from free radicals. You can take it all at once or split it into two doses of 1,000 mg each. Buy vitamin C with bioflavonoids, separate from your multivitamin, and take it with food.

Vitamin E. This vitamin is fat soluble (it dissolves in fat), which means that you need to take it with a meal that has fat in it. It also means it is the number one antioxidant that protects all the fat in your body, including cell membranes and your brain. Another bonus is that it prevents your cholesterol from getting damaged and forming plaque in your arteries. Do not choose the synthetic form of vitamin E, dl-alpha-tocopherol. You will know a good-quality vitamin E supplement if it says it contains mixed tocopherols, which means it contains d-alpha, d-beta, d-gamma, and d-delta forms. You may have heard about studies on vitamin E suggesting that it was not good for you. But many of these studies were done using only the synthetic dl-alpha-tocopherol, and this has led to misleading results. The dose to take is 200–400 IU of vitamin E daily as mixed tocopherols.

Selenium. This is a trace mineral that is important for your immune system. Take 200 mcg per day, usually as a capsule. Selenium has also been used to treat anti-thyroid antibodies, and for that I recommend taking 400 mcg per day for three to six months, until the antibodies go away on the repeat blood tests. I will talk about this more in Chapter 14, "Infections and Specific Autoimmune Conditions." You can also eat Brazil nuts—each one has about 100 mcg of selenium.

Essential Fatty Acids

There are two different essential fatty acids that are important for you to take as a supplement. The first is fish oil, which contains EPA and DHA. The second is GLA. I described the benefits of both of these oils in the last chapter. Getting these nutrients by eating plenty of nuts, seeds, fish, and green leafy vegetables is important, but if you have an autoimmune condition, which means you have inflammation in your body, you must supplement as well.

Fish oil. Fish oil contains good fats, such as omega-3 and omega-6 fatty acids, that our bodies can't produce but which we need for our cell membranes to work their best. For rheumatoid or other arthritis I suggest 3,000 mg per day of EPA plus DHA. For general support of your immune system try 1,000–2,000 mg per day. If you are a vegetarian, you can take 1,000–3,000 mg of flaxseed oil, but it isn't as potent as taking fish oil.

GLA. I also suggest taking GLA, which is an omega-6 fatty acid that is very important for your immune system. You can get it from borage oil, evening primrose oil, or black currant seed oil. For rheumatoid arthritis I suggest 450–500 mg per day; for general support of your immune system, take 200–250 mg per day.

Vitamin D

This is one of the most important immunomodulators in the body and very important in the treatment of autoimmune diseases. An immuno-modulator is a nutrient, chemical messenger, or hormone that has an effect on your immune system cells. To measure your vitamin D levels, have your doctor test your 25-OH vitamin D levels. Your level should be over 50 ng/ml. If you aren't sure what your levels are, take 2,000 IU per day of cholecalciferol, or vitamin D_3. Do not take ergocalciferol, which is D_2, because it isn't converted well to D_3 in the body. In my practice, 2000 IU per day is the maintenance dose and doesn't change the blood level very much for most people.

To raise your vitamin D levels, take 4,000–5,000 IU of D_3 per day for three months and then retest your levels. If you start out lower than 30 ng/ml, it will take at least six months to get your levels up above 50 ng/ml. Of course, this is different for everyone and depends on a num-ber of factors, such as how well you are absorbing it. I just want to reas-sure you that you can take these high doses for a long period of time without fear that it will cause an overdose. To be safe, don't go longer than six months without having your levels checked if you are taking a higher dose. I don't recommend the prescription form of vitamin D that is 50,000 IU per week. It is ergocalciferol (D_2) and isn't metabolized well by the body when given that way.

Zinc

This is a very important mineral for your immune system. Fruits and vegetables provide little zinc, so if you cut down on animal products, it is good to take a supplement. I suggest 15 mg of zinc each day unless you are a vegetarian or semi-vegetarian, in which case I suggest 30 mg each day. Often you can find this in a multivitamin/multimineral supplement.

EGCG

This compound is found in green tea and has great anti-oxidant power and a balancing effect on the immune system. I suggest 250 mg of EGCG 1–2 times per day. Drink green tea 1–2 times/day as well for the addi-tional anti-oxidant benefits of the other compounds in the tea like poly-phenols.

• • •

Before we leave this section on supplements for balancing the immune system, I want to tell you about mushroom extracts, such as maitake, and other herbal immune-boosting products such as echinacea and astragalus. Sometimes the mushroom extracts are called AHCC or beta-glucans. I use these products often to help boost the immune system in my patients who have chronic infections or who get sick easily. These compounds can boost your killer T cells directly, which will help your body fight viruses. However, studies have not shown these to be useful or safe for people with autoimmune diseases, and so I do not at this time recommend their use as part of your immune system recovery plan. For people with autoimmune conditions, we are not looking to stimulate the immune system; our goal is to heal and balance it.

Tier 3: Functional Medicine Options from a Health Care Professional

It can be very difficult to change the way you eat without the support of a health care professional. If you know that you want to make these changes but feel overwhelmed about doing it on your own, you can get help from an integrative medicine practitioner.

Health professionals trained in working with elimination, anti-inflammatory, and low-glycemic diets may be physicians, naturopaths, chiropractors, osteopaths, nurse practitioners, physician's assistants, and nutritionists who are trained in functional medicine. Find one at www .functionalmedicine.org. A new certification program is currently being established, and soon there will be a list of certified practitioners. You can also go to one of the functional medicine laboratory websites, such as Genova Diagnostics, www.gdx.net, or Metametrix labs, www.meta metrix.com, and find a practitioner who is regularly using their services. That is a great way to locate someone who is actively practicing functional medicine.

The tests to ask for from your doctor's laboratory:

- 25-OH vitamin D.
- Insulin and hemoglobin A1C. This will tell you if you have been eating too much sugar and if you are at risk for diabetes.
- Cardio CRP and LpPLA2. These will tell you if you have one kind of inflammation specifically important for your heart. Since we don't have tests for every inflammatory molecule your body makes, these tests are a good place to start.

- ESR. The erythrocyte sedimentation rate is another marker for inflammation.
- Zinc and selenium levels in your blood. Your doctor will measure the levels in serum, which isn't best, but it is a good place to start. Red blood cell levels are better but available only from a functional medicine lab.

The tests to ask for from functional medicine laboratories are:
- Urine oxidative stress. This will tell you if you need more antioxidants. More information is available at www.gdx.net.
- Omega-3 index. This will tell you if you are deficient in omega-3 fats. You can get information about this test at www.omegaquant.com.
- Red blood cell mineral levels for zinc and selenium. For information, see www.gdx.net or www.metametrix.com.

Pantry Shopping List

This pantry list was created by our team at Blum Center for Health, with our culinary director, Marti Wolfson, at the helm. In addition to the foods we use in our teaching kitchen, we pooled our favorite choices from our own home pantries.

Grains/Flours

Lundberg—short-grain brown rice, brown basmati rice, brown jasmine rice, brown sushi rice, rice pasta, rice cakes

Texmati—whole grains and rice cakes

Shiloh Farms—quinoa, amaranth, millet, teff, and other less common grains

Harvest Grain—quinoa, quinoa pasta, quinoa flakes

Eden—100 percent buckwheat noodles

Bob's Red Mill—all gluten-free flours and oats

Asian Kitchen—rice and bean thread noodles

Udi's and Food for Life—gluten-free breads

Mary's Gone Crackers—gluten-free crackers

Glutino—gluten-free bread crumbs

Legumes

Westbrae—all canned beans

Eden—all canned beans

Brad's—all canned beans

Shiloh Farms—organic dry beans and lentils

Oils

Zoe—reasonably priced extra-virgin cold-pressed oil
Omega Nutrition—coconut oil (extra-virgin and neutral)
International Harvest—coconut oil
Spectrum—sesame oil, toasted sesame oil, and coconut oil
Purity Farms—ghee

Nut Butters

Once Again—all nut butters
Brad's—almond butter, peanut butter, and tahini

Frozen Berries

Cascadian Farms—blueberries, strawberries, raspberries, blackberries
Woodstock Farms—blueberries, strawberries, raspberries, blackberries

Vinegar and Soy Sauce

Bragg's—apple cider vinegar, liquid aminos
Spectrum—apple cider vinegar
San-J—tamari, shoyu

Non-Dairy Milk

Pacific—organic vanilla and unsweetened rice, almond, soy, and hemp
   milks
Rice Dream—organic rice and soy milks
Whole Foods 365—organic rice and almond milks
Asian Kitchen—canned coconut milk
Edensoy—organic soy milk

Sea Vegetables

Eden—all sea vegetables
Maine Coast—all sea vegetables

Sweeteners

Lundberg—brown rice syrup
Madhava—agave syrup and coconut sugar
Wholesome—Sucanat

Vegetable Stock

Rapunzel—vegan bouillon cubes
Pacific—organic vegetable and chicken stocks

CHAPTER 4

Using Food as Medicine Recipes

My goal in this chapter is to show you that eating gluten-free pasta, grains, and flour can taste good and won't leave you feeling deprived. The recipes in this chapter focus on dishes that you can substitute for your usual gluten-filled muffins, granola bars, pasta, side dishes, and desserts. All of these recipes are also corn, soy, and dairy free, so you can eat them while doing the food elimination challenge in Chapter 3, "Using Food as Medicine Workbook." Marti Wolfson, our culinary director at Blum Center for Health, worked with me to create these recipes, and they are presented as a two-day menu plan so you can get a sense of how to put these dishes together to create tasty, satisfying gluten-, dairy-, soy-, and corn-free meals that are calming to your immune system. Because most of the recipes in this chapter are grain-based (they're all still gluten-free), I suggest checking out the other menus and recipes in Chapter 7, Chapter 10, and Chapter 13 so you can incorporate more salads and protein into your daily meals. (See the appendix for recipe index.)

Recipes
Almond Blueberry Muffins
Almond Butter Granola Bars
Warm Quinoa Cereal with Fruit and Nuts
Asian Soba Noodle Salad
Buddha Rice Bowl with Tahini Dressing
Quinoa Pasta with Peas, Arugula, and Sun-Dried Tomato
Mediterranean Herb-Crusted Salmon
Creamed Spinach
Wild Mushroom Quinoa
Chocolate Chip Oatmeal Cookies

Menu 1

Breakfast
Warm Quinoa Cereal with Fruit and Nuts

Lunch
Asian Soba Noodle Salad

Snack
Almond Blueberry Muffins

Dinner
Buddha Rice Bowl with Tahini Dressing

Dessert
Chocolate Chip Oatmeal Cookies

Menu 2

Breakfast
Almond Butter Granola Bars

Lunch
Quinoa Pasta with Peas, Arugula, and Sun-Dried Tomatoes

Dinner
Mediterranean Herb-Crusted Salmon
Wild Mushroom Quinoa
Creamed Spinach

Almond Blueberry Muffins

These muffins use almond flour instead of wheat or other grain flour, so they are very low in carbohydrates and high in protein, and they are sweetened with honey instead of processed sugar. Chia seeds provide essential fatty acids that our bodies need to reduce inflammation, and they also add a nice crunch. All this makes them a nutritious snack or breakfast. You can change the fruit according to the season, replacing the blueberries with apples in the fall and fresh peaches in the summer.

Makes 12 muffins

Coconut oil (optional for greasing the muffin pan, or you can
    use muffin cup liners)
3 cups almond flour
½ tsp baking soda
¼ tsp salt
1 tsp ground cinnamon
1 tsp ground cardamom
½ tsp vanilla extract
½ cup agave syrup
3 eggs
1 cup fresh or frozen blueberries
1–2 tbsp chia seeds (optional)

1. Preheat the oven to 325 degrees.
2. Line a muffin tin with muffin cup liners or grease the muffin pan well with coconut oil.
3. Mix the almond flour, baking soda, salt, cinnamon, and cardamom in a bowl.
4. In another bowl, combine the vanilla, agave, and eggs and mix well.
5. Add the dry ingredients to the wet and mix until combined.
6. Add the blueberries and mix until combined.
7. Divide batter among the muffin cups.
8. Sprinkle some chia seeds over the top of each muffin.
9. Bake for 18 to 20 minutes or until the tops of the muffins are light brown and slightly firm. Rotate the pan halfway through the baking time.
10. Cool the muffins on a rack.

Almond Butter Granola Bars

Most store-bought granola bars are filled with refined sugars and additives in addition to gluten. These Almond Butter Granola Bars don't contain those unhealthy ingredients, but instead provide you with protein and essential fats from all the nuts and seeds they contain. They're perfect for satisfying a snack craving midmorning or midafternoon and as a quick, easy breakfast. But no matter when you eat them, they offer up important nutrients and taste great. Store them in the freezer and they will stay fresh for three months.

Makes 16 bars

¼ cup almonds, toasted and coarsely chopped
1 cup Bob's Red Mill gluten-free rolled oats
3½ tbsp rice flour
1 scoop (15 grams) protein powder*
¼ cup sunflower seeds
¼ cup dried currants or raisins
½ tsp cinnamon
¼ tsp salt
¼ cup almond butter
½ cup maple syrup
1 tsp vanilla extract
½ cup apple juice
2 tbsp melted coconut oil, plus more for greasing the pan

1. Preheat the oven to 350 degrees.
2. Grease an 8-by-8-inch baking pan using coconut oil.
3. Combine the almonds, oats, flour, protein powder, sunflower seeds, currants, cinnamon, and salt in a medium bowl and stir to combine.
4. Whisk the almond butter, maple syrup, vanilla, and apple juice together in another bowl.
5. Pour the wet ingredients into the dry, stirring until the dry ingredients are thoroughly moistened.

---

* We recommend rice, pea, pumpkin seed, or whey protein (whey is good only if you don't have a dairy sensitivity). Our recipe was tested using pumpkin seed powder. Adding the protein powder is optional but will increase the protein punch in the bar, keeping you satisfied longer.

6. Press the mixture evenly into the prepared baking pan.
7. Bake for 20 minutes.
8. Remove the pan from the oven and cut into 16 bars.
9. Brush the coconut oil over the top of the bars.
10. Return the pan to the oven and bake until golden brown, about another 15–20 minutes.
11. Cool in the pan for about 10 minutes and then remove the bars with a spatula and finish cooling on a rack.

Warm Quinoa Cereal with Fruit and Nuts

Quinoa (pronounced "keen-wah") is actually a seed related to the spinach family, but it cooks up like a grain. Known for its high quality of protein and fiber, it is both delicious and easily digestible. Quinoa is a versatile ingredient, as it works nicely in both sweet and savory dishes. This simple breakfast recipe is a wonderful substitute for oatmeal, since it is gluten free and higher in protein.

Makes 3 servings

½ cup quinoa
1 cup water
1 cup non-dairy milk, such as almond, coconut, or rice milk
½ tsp sea salt
¾ tbsp maple syrup
¼ tsp ground cinnamon
1 tsp vanilla extract
¼ cup raisins or currants
¼ cup slivered almonds or chopped walnuts, toasted
Fresh berries (optional)

1. Rinse the quinoa with cold water in a fine mesh strainer and drain.
2. Put the water, milk, and salt in a pot and bring to a boil.
3. Stir in the quinoa, turn down the heat to medium low, cover the pot, and simmer gently for 15 minutes. Stir the quinoa in the pot.
4. The cereal is done when the quinoa is soft and has the consistency of oatmeal. If more liquid is needed, add more milk and continue to simmer another 5 minutes.

(continued on next page)

5. Remove from the heat and stir in the maple syrup, cinnamon, vanilla, and currants.

6. Transfer to bowls and serve warm or cold with toasted nuts and fresh berries.

Asian Soba Noodle Salad

Despite its name, buckwheat is not wheat. It is a gluten-free grain that contains a good balance of all the B vitamins and is especially high in niacin, folate, and vitamin B_6. This flavorful dish makes a great side salad, or turn it into a complete lunch by adding chicken or tofu. When looking for soba noodles, be aware that not all are created equally. Many brands use a mix of whole wheat and buckwheat flour, so make sure the ingredients list only 100 percent buckwheat flour.

Makes 4–6 servings

1 package 100 percent buckwheat soba noodles
1 red pepper, thinly sliced
½ cup celery, thinly sliced on diagonal
1 cup carrots, cut into thin matchsticks
¼ cup scallions, thinly sliced
1 clove garlic, minced
1 tbsp minced fresh ginger, minced
2 tsp toasted sesame oil
1½ tbsp balsamic vinegar
2 tsp maple syrup
2 tbsp brown rice vinegar
¼ cup sesame oil
Juice of 1 lime
Pinch red pepper flakes
¼ tsp salt
¼ cup finely chopped cilantro
1 tbsp toasted sesame seeds

1. Bring a large pot of water to a boil.

2. Add the soba noodles and cook for 7–9 minutes, stirring occasionally with a fork to prevent sticking. For a quick test to know when the noodles are done, cut a noodle in half; if you see a white dot in the center, they need to cook longer.

3. When they are done, empty the noodles into a colander and quickly run cold water over them to remove all the starch.
4. In a large bowl, combine the noodles, pepper, celery, carrots, and scallions.
5. Whisk together the garlic, ginger, toasted sesame oil, balsamic vinegar, maple syrup, brown rice vinegar, sesame oil, lime juice, red pepper flakes, and salt to create the dressing.
6. Pour the dressing over the salad and toss to combine. Garnish with cilantro and toasted sesame seeds.

Buddha Rice Bowl with Tahini Dressing

This recipe is a staple meal in the teaching kitchen at Blum Center for Health and is enjoyed by students and teachers alike for its nutrition, color, texture, and taste. The "Buddha" comes from the sublime feeling you have after eating this bowl full of colorful vegetables and protein-rich quinoa topped with creamy dressing. For even more protein, add beans, chicken, or tofu. Also, you can change the vegetables according to the season.

Makes 4–6 servings

1 cup short-grain brown rice, rinsed
2 cups water or vegetable stock
Sea salt
4 tbsp extra-virgin olive oil
Freshly ground pepper
2 cups peeled, cubed butternut or kabocha squash
1 medium yellow onion, thinly sliced
6 cups kale, washed, ribs discarded, and leaves chopped
¼ cup tahini
Juice of 1 lemon
1 tsp grated ginger
1½ tsp honey
1½ tsp sea salt
¾ cup hot water
½ cup toasted walnuts or pumpkin seeds
1 avocado, peeled and cubed

(continued on next page)

1. Preheat the oven to 375 degrees.
2. Put the rice, water, and ½ tsp salt in a small pot and bring to a boil. Cover the pot, reduce the heat, and simmer for 40 minutes or until the water is absorbed.
3. Take off the heat, fluff with a fork, cover, and let sit for another 5 minutes.
4. Mix the squash with 2 tbsp oil and add salt and pepper to taste.
5. Spread on a baking tray and roast for 20–25 minutes or until browned and fork tender.
6. Heat a large sauté pan and add 2 tbsp oil. Add the onions and spread them out evenly in the pan. Do not move the onions until they start to brown. Then stir and reduce the heat to low.
7. Continue to let the onions caramelize for 15 minutes, or until they are soft and brown. Remove from the pan and set aside.
8. Add the kale with a pinch of salt into the sauté pan that had the onions and cook until the kale begins to turn bright green and soften slightly. If the kale begins to stick to the pan, add a little water and cover the pan, allowing kale to steam for 1 minute.
9. To make the sauce, mix the tahini, lemon, ginger, honey, and ½ tsp salt. Add the water until you reach a smooth and pourable consistency.
10. Serve in individual bowls with ½ cup brown rice on the bottom topped with caramelized onions, squash, and kale. Put a few cubes of avocado and toasted nuts on top. Drizzle the tahini sauce over the prepared bowls.

Quinoa Pasta with Peas, Arugula, and Sun-Dried Tomatoes

Cutting gluten out of your diet doesn't have to mean you have to give up all types of pasta. Luckily, quinoa pasta is a tasty and healthy alternative. Light and nutty, quinoa pasta can be used in the place of traditional pasta in many of your favorite recipes. You can also use rice pasta if you prefer. The following is a wonderful springtime dish, balanced by sweet peas and bitter arugula. Change the vegetables with the seasons and you can enjoy this dish all year long.

Makes 6 servings

8 oz 100 percent quinoa pasta
2 tbsp extra-virgin olive oil

1 cup diced yellow onion
5 cloves garlic, minced
½ cup sun-dried tomatoes, cut into thin strips
4 cups arugula, roughly chopped
8 oz frozen peas, thawed
Salt
Freshly ground pepper
2 tbsp parsley, finely chopped
1 lemon

1. Bring a large pot of water to a boil.
2. Add the pasta and cook for 8 minutes or until al dente. Drain the pasta and set aside.
3. While the pasta is cooking, heat the oil in a large sauté pan on medium-high heat.
4. Add the onion and cook until golden.
5. Mix in the garlic and sauté for 30 seconds.
6. Add the sun-dried tomatoes, arugula, a pinch of salt, and pepper to taste and sauté just until the arugula is wilted.
7. Combine the pasta, peas, parsley, and another pinch of salt in the pan and mix together until well combined.
8. Add salt and pepper to taste.
9. Add a squeeze of lemon at the very end to brighten the whole dish.

Mediterranean Herb-Crusted Salmon

Wild Alaskan king salmon is one of the best sources of omega-3 fatty acids—an essential fat that is anti-inflammatory and benefits many health problems from heart disease to hormone imbalance. If you ask your fishmonger nicely, he or she will debone the fish, which saves you preparation time. The dill, mint, and parsley in this recipe make it full of flavor. The herbed bread crumb mixture adds a great crunch on top, and the lemons are a nice touch in presentation and flavor.

Makes 6 servings

2 lbs wild Alaskan king or sockeye salmon, boned
4 tbsp prepared mustard

(continued on next page)

½ cup parsley, finely chopped
½ cup mint, finely chopped
½ cup dill, finely chopped
¾ cup gluten-free bread crumbs
4 tbsp extra-virgin olive oil
1 tsp salt
2 lemons, cut into 6–8 wedges each

1. Preheat the oven to 400 degrees.
2. Place the salmon on a baking sheet lined with parchment paper and spread the mustard all over the salmon.
3. Mix the herbs, salt, olive oil, and bread crumbs in a small bowl until well combined.
4. Cover the salmon with the herb mixture, and on the baking sheet line the lemon wedges around the fish snugly, to trap the juices.
5. Roast the fish for about 18 minutes or until cooked through. The time will vary depending on the thickness of the salmon. Garnish with the roasted lemon wedges.

Creamed Spinach

Creamed spinach is one of those comfort side dishes, but the traditional recipe is usually laden with unhealthy saturated fat, flour, and cream. This non-dairy version offers up the same silky, rich satisfaction while providing an array of health benefits that we get from spinach, including vitamins, minerals, antioxidants, and phytonutrients.

Makes 8 servings

2 bunches fresh spinach (about 10 cups)
2 to 3 tbsp extra-virgin olive oil
1 cup chopped yellow onion
2 cloves garlic, chopped
½ cup raw cashews, soaked in water for at least an hour
2 cups water
Pinch red pepper flakes
2 tbsp freshly squeezed lemon juice
Pinch nutmeg
1 tsp salt

1. Chop the spinach and set aside.
2. Heat a large skillet (10 to 12 inches) over medium heat. Add the olive oil, then the onions and garlic.
3. Sauté for about 5 minutes or until the onions soften and begin to change color.
4. Add them to a blender along with the cashews, water, red pepper flakes, lemon juice, nutmeg, and salt and blend until smooth and creamy.
5. Pour the sauce into the skillet and simmer for 5–10 minutes to thicken.
6. Add the spinach to the sauce, stirring until the spinach softens.
7. Season with salt and lemon juice if needed.

Wild Mushroom Quinoa

Mushrooms have long been known for their immune-supportive properties, and in this dish they pack a double punch because they're used both in the cooking broth and chopped up to give the quinoa an earthy flavor. Quinoa is a complete protein, mineral rich, and anti-inflammatory. This makes a wonderful side dish to a main protein such as chicken, beans, or tempeh.

Makes 4 servings

½ oz dried shiitake mushrooms
1 tbsp extra-virgin olive oil
½ cup diced shallots
2 cloves garlic, minced
½ cup quinoa
Salt

1. Soak the mushrooms in 1 cup hot water for 15–20 minutes.
2. Once the mushrooms are softened, drain them and save the soaking liquid. Roughly chop the mushrooms.
3. In a small pot, heat the olive oil on medium-high heat. Add the shallots and garlic and sauté for 2 minutes.
4. Add the quinoa to the garlic and shallots.
5. Then add the mushroom soaking liquid, ¼ cup water, mushrooms, and ½ tsp salt.

(continued on next page)

6. Once the liquid comes to a boil, cover the pot and lower the heat to a simmer. Cook for about 12–15 minutes or until all the liquid is absorbed.
7. Fluff with a fork.

Chocolate Chip Oatmeal Cookies

This is our version of a classic! These cookies have the same taste and texture as the sugar- and gluten-filled kind, so you can still get a satisfying cookie fix. While they do contain sugar, it is less processed, and they are well balanced with healthy fats from seeds and almond butter and fiber from oats, so you can lose the guilt about eating them. Remember to choose gluten-free oats, because oats are often manufactured in the same factory as wheat, which will cause the oats to be contaminated with gluten.

Makes 24 cookies

2 eggs
½ cup almond butter
¾ cup sucanat or rapadura
¾ cup coconut sugar
1 tsp vanilla extract
¼ cup coconut oil
1 tsp baking soda
3½ oz organic dark chocolate, coarsely chopped
½ cup sunflower seeds
3 cups gluten-free oats

1. Preheat oven to 350 degrees.
2. In the bowl of a stand mixer or with a handheld mixer, cream together the eggs, almond butter, sugars, vanilla extract, and coconut oil.
3. Add the baking soda, chocolate, sunflower seeds, and oats and mix until well combined.
4. On baking sheets lined with parchment paper, drop tablespoons of the batter about 2 inches apart.
5. Bake about 12 minutes or until the cookies are brown around the edges and still slightly soft in the middle (they will crisp up as they cool).
6. Cool on a rack.

PART II

Understanding the Stress Connection

Everyone thinks of changing the world, but no one thinks of changing himself.

—Leo Tolstoy

CHAPTER 5

Understanding the Stress Connection

In our go-go-go world, "stress" is a word we use and hear all the time. The phrases "I'm so stressed" and "I'm stressed out" are used like badges of honor, proving that our lives are full and busy. But stress isn't something to take lightly. Although we refer to stress as an emotion, it's much more than that. It actually creates a series of physiological events inside your body, and how often these events occur and how long they last have a huge impact on your health, specifically on autoimmune diseases. To understand this link, it's important to understand a few basic things about stress. Stress describes an experience caused by something called a stressor. Stressors can be emotional or physical. Big-time stressful events include the death of a loved one, a divorce or breakup, or being subjected to physical or emotional abuse or trauma. Less obvious stressors include not sleeping enough, skipping meals, working long hours, overexercising, and taking care of everyone else but yourself. Even positive events such as getting married, landing your dream job, or moving to a new town can be stressors.

Some people are very aware that they're stressed and notice the physical effects in their bodies (such as stomachaches, headaches, or a racing heart) and the emotional effects (such as irritability, fatigue, or cravings for sweet or salty foods) almost immediately. But I've also met many people who have easygoing, happy temperaments and are not aware that their bodies might be suffering or that physical symptoms they're experiencing are related to stress. In fact, many people are so used to living with stress that they don't even notice it. Others seem to thrive on it. Yet, although the specifics can vary greatly, all stressors cause an amazing cascade of events inside your body, called the stress response.

It's important to keep in mind that we all feel stressed at times; I am not suggesting that you can live in a bubble or banish stress from your life completely. This is impossible. What you *can* do is control your reaction to stress. **You can control how stress comes into your body and how it affects your nervous system and your hormones. And you can prevent it from weakening your immune system and making you sick.**

THE STRESS RESPONSE

One critical thing to understand about stress is that your body reacts to it in two major ways. The first is a nervous system response and the second is an activation of hormones, the most important ones being cortisol and adrenaline, both of which are made by the adrenal glands.

The Nervous System's Response to Stress

To understand the nervous system's response to stress, let me give you a little background. Your brain and spinal cord are part of your central nervous system. The rest of the nerves in your body are part of the peripheral nervous system, which has two main parts: the somatic nervous system and the autonomic nervous system. The nerves in the somatic nervous system connect to muscles, and this is the part that you can easily control with your conscious thoughts. For example, this is how you move your hand, lift your leg, or look to the left or right. The autonomic nervous system controls body functions that are viewed as automatic, such as your heart rate, temperature, blood pressure, breathing rate, digestion, and more.

The autonomic nervous system is a critical part of how your body functions, with on and off switches that are supposed to balance each other. The on switch is called the sympathetic nervous system and it fires up when you are stressed. This is one part of your stress response. The off switch is called the parasympathetic nervous system and it acts as the brakes, helping you relax and turn off the stress response. The autonomic nervous system is hardwired, meaning that the stress response starts in your brain and travels down through your nerves stimulating different organs in your body, including your stomach, heart, adrenal glands, and lymphoid organs, where all your T cells are maturing and developing. This hardwiring into your immune system is very important for how your T cells function. See figure 3.

When you're stressed, the sympathetic nervous system initiates something called the fight-or-flight response. One common reaction is that your heart beats faster. This happens for two reasons. First, the sympathetic nerves stimulate your heart directly, and second, the adrenal glands

Figure 3:

A U T O N O M I C   N E R V O U S   S Y S T E M

Parasympathetic   Sympathetic

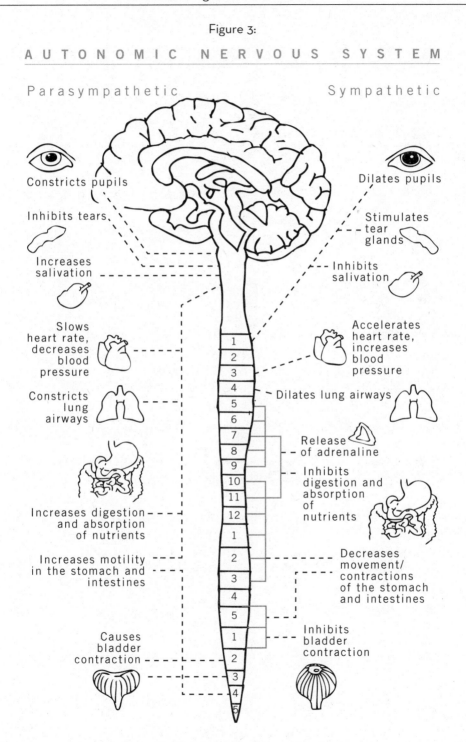

Constricts pupils   Dilates pupils

Inhibits tears   Stimulates tear glands

Increases salivation   Inhibits salivation

Slows heart rate, decreases blood pressure   Accelerates heart rate, increases blood pressure

Constricts lung airways   Dilates lung airways

                                                   Release of adrenaline

                                                   Inhibits digestion and absorption of nutrients

Increases digestion and absorption of nutrients

Increases motility in the stomach and intestines   Decreases movement/ contractions of the stomach and intestines

Causes bladder contraction   Inhibits bladder contraction

Figure 4:

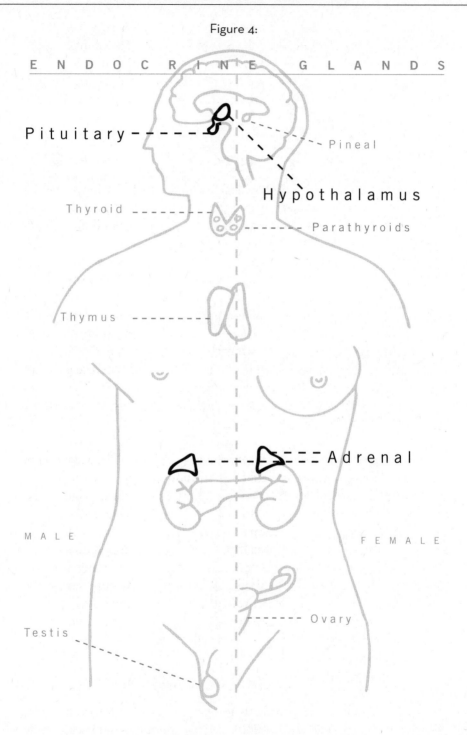

ENDOCRINE GLANDS

Pituitary

Pineal

Hypothalamus

Thyroid

Parathyroids

Thymus

Adrenal

MALE

FEMALE

Ovary

Testis

release the hormone adrenaline, which also increases your heart rate. This double whammy affects all the organs involved in the fight-or-flight response. But your body also has an antidote to this: your parasympathetic nervous system is supposed to kick in to turn off the fight-or-flight response, helping to bring you back into balance so you don't get stuck in overdrive.

THE HORMONE RESPONSE TO STRESS

The second way that your body reacts to stress is by initiating a chain of hormone reactions that start in your brain. This chain reaction begins in the hypothalamus and pituitary gland, two areas of the brain that control your hormone system. Situated side by side, the hypothalamus and pituitary gland are very connected and often thought of as the place where your emotions, thoughts, and feelings are translated into hormone signals. The pituitary gland is the leader of the endocrine orchestra, releasing hormones that in turn stimulate all your endocrine organs, including the thyroid, adrenals, and ovaries or testicles, to make their own hormones (see Figure 3). When the stress response is initiated, the hypothalamus secretes cortisol-releasing hormone (CRH) and then the pituitary secretes a hormone called adrenocorticotropin (ACTH). This causes your adrenal glands to release your main stress hormone, cortisol. In the medical world this hypothalamus-pituitary-adrenal pathway is called the HPA axis and the stress response is said to activate the HPA axis.

Though there are several stress hormones, cortisol is the most potent and has many very important effects in the body. Severe and acute stress leads to high cortisol levels. (See sidebar, "The Effects of High Cortisol.") It raises your blood sugar so you can have the fuel to fight or flee, and it is the main anti-inflammatory hormone in the body, suppressing your immune cells and preparing your body for a potential injury. When you are injured, the inflammation created by immune cells can get in the way during the healing process, and so by suppressing the immune system, cortisol helps prevent it from becoming overactivated and releasing molecules that are damaging to the tissues that need to be healed.

HOW YOU EXPERIENCE THE STRESS RESPONSE

It is crucial to understand these two reactions to stress (the sympathetic fight-or-flight response and the HPA axis cortisol response) because they

THE EFFECTS OF HIGH CORTISOL

1. Increased appetite and food cravings
2. Increased body fat
3. Diminished muscle mass
4. Diminished bone density
5. Increased anxiety
6. Increased depression
7. Mood swings (anger and irritability)
8. Reduced libido
9. Impaired immune system
10. Impaired memory and ability to learn
11. Increase in PMS symptoms, such as water retention and irritability
12. Change in menstrual cycle
13. Increase in menopause symptoms, such as hot flashes and night sweats

have a direct impact on your immune system. But first let's talk about what this stress response *feels* like. You can have an acute reaction to a stressful event, but this reaction may also continue even after the event has passed. For example, if you've ever had a confrontation with a friend or partner or tended to a very ill child or parent, you might have felt your heart racing, found yourself lying awake at night with worry or anxiety, or experienced muscle tension that caused back or neck pain. You can get tension headaches or other types of headaches, stomachaches, and irritable bowel symptoms such as diarrhea and/or constipation. You might have dry eyes, dry mouth, and cold hands and feet. If this goes on too long, you may also find yourself getting sick frequently because now your immune system is not functioning properly.

One of the most common symptoms of chronically high cortisol levels is an expanding waistline. Studies have shown that people who are stressed tend to crave sugar and high-fat foods.[1] These foods stimulate the production of insulin, the hormone that lowers your blood sugar, and this combination of high insulin and high cortisol levels causes fat to settle around your internal organs, resulting in abdominal obesity. Besides making it hard to button your pants, this belly fat is sometimes called "brown fat" because it looks and behaves differently from the other fat in your body, creating a lot of inflammation. And inflammation is a common underlying problem in all autoimmune diseases as well as other conditions such as heart disease, stroke, diabetes, and cancer. (It's also very hard to get rid of this abdominal fat.)

CHRONIC VERSUS ACUTE STRESS

Like many things in life, stress isn't black and white. Not all stress is bad. The fight-or-flight response can be a good thing because the hormones it releases can help you run away from an attacker, get ready to give an important presentation, speak up to your boss, or ski down a black-diamond run. These are examples of acute stress. It has a starting point and an end point. The problem is when your stress system gets stuck in the on position. This is called chronic stress. I once saw a documentary about zebras and lions in their natural habitat. When one of the lions started chasing one of the zebras, it was clear that the zebra was in a fight-or-flight mode as it ran for its life. Finally, when it evaded the lion, its body began to shake wildly. But then an amazing thing happened: this same zebra who had just been running for dear life began quietly grazing in the field like nothing had happened. It had already forgotten about the near-death experience it had just had, and I'm sure that if we measured the stress hormone levels in that grazing zebra, they would have been back to normal. The zebra had a way to turn off the stress response and was now moving on.

Like the zebra's stress system, ours is programmed to find balance. The problem is that, unlike the zebra, we remember the lion. As a result, we ruminate about it and keep reliving the trauma over and over. And because we experience thoughts and images of an event physically and emotionally the same way we do the actual event, we stay in stress mode. In fact, most of us spend more time angsting about the past or worrying about the future than living in the present moment. To get healthy and stay that way, you must learn skills to keep your mind from dwelling on particular thoughts so that you don't damage your body with chronically high levels of cortisol. It is these hormones that are making you sick and keeping you from getting better. And I'm not just talking about autoimmune diseases. Stress is believed to be a contributing factor in an amazing 80 percent of all chronic conditions, including autoimmune disease, heart disease, stroke, diabetes, and cancer.

THE ADRENAL GLANDS

I want to talk a little more about the adrenal glands because they're most responsible for the stress response. If you're not familiar with these glands, you're definitely not alone. When I mention the adrenal glands to my patients, most tell me that they don't know anything about this vital organ. They aren't aware that the adrenal glands and hormones are important both for their health in general and for a properly functioning immune system. When it comes to cortisol, many patients have heard about this stress hormone, but most don't really understand what it does to their bodies. Amazingly, my patients aren't the only ones who haven't paid much attention to the adrenal glands. Conventional medicine has ignored them, too. Why? Because our medical system is primarily focused on looking for disease, and the main diseases of the adrenal glands are extreme situations. They include Cushing's syndrome, which is extremely high levels of cortisol, usually from a tumor, and Addison's disease, an autoimmune condition that destroys the adrenal glands so they fail to make any hormones at all.

But health and disease are not two extremes. It's not black or white; you are not either well or sick. Instead, there is a wide spectrum, including many gray areas where one of your organs might be underfunctioning and on its way to being sick. This is why it is important to see how well your adrenal glands are functioning, something conventional doctors and labs don't think about or have the tools to really look at. They also don't have the training to understand or recognize the symptoms of either overactive or low-functioning adrenal glands. In this chapter I am going to show you how to spot the signs of unhealthy adrenal glands, because this is a critical step to help you restore balance to your immune system.

We all have two adrenal glands, with one sitting on top of each of your kidneys. The outer part of the gland (called the adrenal cortex) produces many compounds. Some of these are hormones and some are pre-hormones. (Pre-hormones are substances that are not quite hormones but help your body to make them.) These include:

- Aldosterone, a hormone that helps regulate blood pressure. If your body makes too much aldosterone, your kidneys retain sodium and the result is rising blood pressure. (This is one possible way that stress causes hypertension.)
- DHEA, a pre-hormone made in the adrenal glands. It can help regulate blood sugar and lipids and helps support your bones. In women, the

adrenals can also make testosterone and estrogen from DHEA, hormones normally made in the ovaries. After menopause, the adrenals take over and make more as the ovarian function declines. Men don't convert DHEA to testosterone as easily, but DHEA has the same direct effects on lipids, sugar, and bones.

- Cortisol, the most potent stress hormone, is considered a primary hormone. This means that if you don't have any, you will die.

When your body experiences the stress response, sometimes all these hormones are released at high levels; at other times it is mostly cortisol that is released. This is different for each person, but the important point is that when you're stressed, the adrenal glands secrete high levels of cortisol and continue to do so until the stressor goes away, you learn to more effectively manage your stress, or your adrenal glands poop out. The last is a condition called adrenal fatigue.

There is no way to predict how long it will take to exhaust your adrenal glands if you exist in a perpetual fight-or-flight state. This depends on how well you are taking care of yourself. The adrenal glands are happiest and healthiest when you're sleeping a minimum of seven but preferably eight or more hours a night, eating balanced meals that contain adequate protein and veggies, limiting sugar and white flour, practicing some form of relaxation, exercising moderately (not too much and not too little), and minimizing your exposure to toxins. (We will discuss toxins in depth in Chapter 11, "Supporting Your Liver.") If you're practicing all these aspects of self-care, your adrenal glands can weather the storm of external stress and trauma more easily. But if your adrenal glands are weakened from bad lifestyle choices, they will fatigue more easily if you are suddenly confronted with a new stressor in your life.

Often the first thing that happens when your adrenal glands get weary is that your DHEA and testosterone levels fall. Why? Because your adrenal glands are focusing all their efforts on making cortisol. DHEA and testosterone are secondary hormones (meaning you might get sick without them but you won't die), and so these hormones are sacrificed to keep the production of cortisol going. This is a big problem because in addition to supporting your sex drive, DHEA and testosterone are also very important for maintaining muscle mass and bone density and regulating your cholesterol and sugar levels, issues that are critical for healthy aging. Often low DHEA is the first thing I notice in blood work, and this tells me the adrenal glands might be in trouble.

If the stress in your life continues and you aren't taking care of yourself, then the adrenal glands get completely fatigued and can no longer produce sufficient cortisol or adrenaline. When your levels of these two crucial hormones begin to plummet, severe exhaustion sets in, often combined with inflammation in the joints or muscles that can cause pain, swelling, or stiffness, especially in the morning, when your cortisol is supposed to be highest. This situation is an issue for your immune system. Studies have shown that stress is a risk factor for autoimmune disease and that people with an insufficient stress response (i.e., low levels of cortisol and the neurotransmitter norepinephrine, which is made by your sympathetic nervous system) have a higher risk of inflammation. Without the ability to respond properly to stress, your body can't control the immune system and inflammation.

There is a way to remedy this damage: you can bring your tired adrenal glands back to life by following the treatment plan in this section along with the other steps in this book that address your diet, physical stress caused by chronic infections, digestive problems, and toxin exposure. This will not only help your immune system recover but also repair and balance your adrenal glands.

HOW STRESS AFFECTS AUTOIMMUNE DISEASE

Much of this information on how your immune system is affected by stress comes from the latest scientific studies and current understanding of how autoimmune diseases begin and persist. Don't worry, I'll keep it simple. But understanding these concepts will help you connect the dots and see how stress is affecting your health, so that you will be motivated to make the changes I am suggesting at the end of this section.

WHAT DO THE STRESS HORMONES ACTUALLY *DO*?

We've talked about what stress is and how it can come into your body and change your hormones and nervous system. But stress does more than affect your cortisol levels: it can change your adrenaline, testosterone, progesterone, and estrogen levels, too. Initially stress causes an increase in all your hormone levels, but if you experience chronic stress, over time these hormone levels begin to fall. This connection between stress and your hormones is one very important way that stress affects the immune system, because all of your hormones are what are called immunomodulators. This is a big word that simply means that the substance can influence the number of immune cells or change their activity, making them weaker or stronger.

In Chapter 2, "Using Food as Medicine," you saw that food can be an immunomodulator because your diet can affect your immune system. The two main stress hormones, cortisol and adrenaline, are also immunomodulators. They greatly influence how your T cells develop and mature, causing imbalances that can influence and even contribute to the cause of your illness. Remember the story of Goldilocks and the three bears? Well, just as Goldilocks didn't want her porridge too hot or too cold, her chair too big or too small, and her bed too soft or too hard, you don't want too much immune activity in your body, which can promote inflammation and cause your immune system to attack your own tissues. You also don't want too little immune activity, which can make you prone to infections. You want it just right. The good news? Your body is resilient, and a stress system that's overactive or underactive can be healed and brought back into balance. I will show you how.

Before doing that, let me back up a bit. We talked about the immune system briefly in Chapter 1, "Autoimmune Disease Basics," but let me give you a quick review because the cells that make up your immune system are greatly affected by stress. Your lymphocytes are the main soldiers in your immune system army. But just like any army, these soldiers don't *all* do the same job. They are divided into groups, and each group has a different responsibility. See figure 5. The soldiers in the army of your immune system include:

Attack Cells

T lymphocyte killer cells. Also called cytotoxic T cells, these lymphocytes work cell to cell, directly attacking any foreigner (such as bacteria, viruses, parasites, or yeast) that gets into your body. These killer cells don't secrete any antibodies.

B lymphocyte antibody cells. When the B cells are activated they make antibodies, which attack the foreigner and cause its destruction.

Control Cells

T helper cells. These cells help accelerate your immune system's response to a foreigner in your body. I think of them as the gas in a car. There are several types of T helper cells, each one doing something different. One can turn on the killer cells (for cell-to-cell combat), another can turn on the B cell antibody production (remember, antibodies are like bullets), and other T helpers cause damaging inflammation.

T regulator cells. These cells suppress or turn off your immune system's response to a foreigner, so I think of them as like the brakes in a car. These cells are very important for preventing and treating autoimmune disease.

When your immune system is healthy, your body makes a balanced amount of T helpers and T regulators. People with autoimmune diseases have too many T helper cells and too few T regulator cells, so the car that is their immune system has too much gas. That means it keeps going and going without the brakes (the T regulator cells) to slow it down.

Another problem for people with autoimmune diseases is that your T helper cells can also be imbalanced. Research has shown that in some autoimmune diseases, the T helper cells create too many killer cells (and these extra cells cause direct damage to your tissues) or too many of the cells that make antibodies (and the extra antibodies cause damage to your tissues). When either the killer cells or the antibody-producing cells are stronger, the other one is weaker. So if you have too many antibodies (a condition called being Th2 dominant), you will have fewer killer cells; when you have too many killer cells (called being Th1 dominant), you have too few antibodies. This imbalance is a big problem and puts your health at risk. Our goal is to figure out how and why this imbalance exists and what we can do about it.

Now that we've gotten into the technical side of things, let me give an example to make this more concrete for you. Let's say you get called into your boss's office and are told you're being laid off. This bad news catches you totally off guard. You're stunned. Just minutes ago you thought things at work were going well—very well, in fact. But now you've been thrown into a sudden state of emotional turmoil, and the psychological stress begins. *How will I tell my spouse? How will I pay my bills? How will I save for my retirement or my child's education? Will I ever get another job?* Your heart starts racing, your breathing gets shallow, and your blood pumps quickly through your body—all signs that your fight-or-flight system has turned on. As a result, your body immediately releases adrenaline, cortisol, and a neurotransmitter called norepinephrine from your nervous system.

For the next two to four hours, this stress also causes an increase in the number of killer cells that float around your body, but this is short-lived. After a few hours, if the stressor doesn't go away, high levels of cortisol

Figure 5:

ADAPTIVE   IMMUNE   SYSTEM

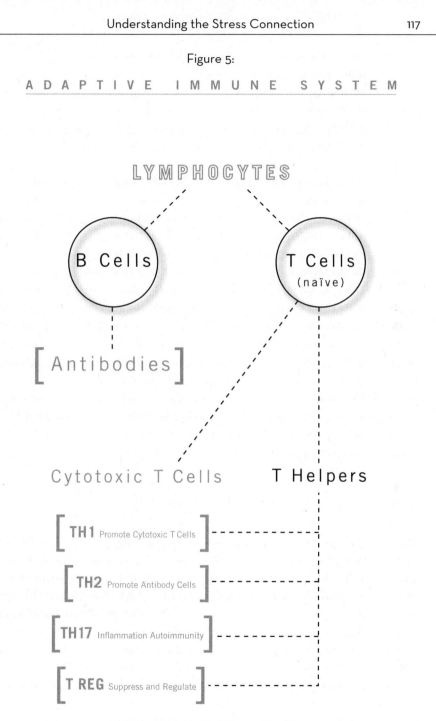

Illustration of the different T cells.

and the activity of your sympathetic fight-or-flight nerves will directly suppress your T killer cells. One study done at Loyola University looked at women's response to getting a breast biopsy for possible breast cancer. The study found that this bad news caused a decrease in the activity of killer cells.[2] Remember, I told you that this immune suppression is imbalanced: while the killers are suppressed, the B cells get turned on and begin making more antibodies. Since the killers are the most important for fighting viruses and infections from bacteria, the first thing you might notice is that you begin to get sick more frequently.

Now back to you and your recent job layoff. Since you're in high-stress mode and your sympathetic nervous system is activated and the adrenaline and cortisol are flooding your body, your immune system cells, which are your first line of defense in fighting infection, aren't working right. This means that if you and a friend who is not under stress are exposed to the same infection, you will have more trouble clearing it out of your body than your friend; you may get sick, but your friend may not have as severe a reaction or may not even get sick at all. Another example of something I see all the time in my practice is infection with the Epstein-Barr virus (EBV), which causes mono. If your immune system is weak from stress, EBV can reactivate, causing severe fatigue and exhaustion. It is really important to keep your immune system strong so that the viruses that are always lurking in your body are kept in check, unable to make you sick.

STRESS RESPONSE:
CORTISOL AND AUTOIMMUNE DISEASE

There are many hormones that influence your immune system. These include the sex hormones estrogen and testosterone, melatonin, and vitamin D (remember, this is actually a hormone). However, cortisol is the major stress hormone and the most potent hormone immunomodulator that you have in your body. So when we're talking stress, we are talking about cortisol.

As I mentioned, your immune cells are made and stored in what is called lymphoid tissue. There is lymphoid tissue in the lungs, bone marrow, thymus, spleen, lymph nodes, and cells just under the lining of the intestines. It's in these tissues that immature T lymphocytes are transformed into the specialized T helper cells or T regulator cells. This maturation needs to go smoothly in order for you to have a healthy immune system. But research shows that a rebel group of immature immune cells can crop up in these organs, too. Rather than maturing into one of the three types of T cells, these rebel cells actually attack your body's own tissue when they should only be attacking outside invaders.[3] As you may remember from Chapter 1, "Autoimmune Disease Basics," this is the start of an autoimmune disorder.

Studies have shown that normally cortisol binds to these rebel cells, which helps weed them out and kill them before too many can emerge, travel through your body, and cause serious damage. This is a good, regulatory process, but there are problems that can arise when cortisol levels get too high or too low. If you have high levels of cortisol, all of the killer cells are suppressed. In the short term this can be good—killer cells send out large amounts of inflammatory molecules when they are activated, so dialing this down can reduce inflammation triggered by things like an infection or injury. For example, if you are in a car accident and your leg is crushed, the tissues are badly damaged from the injury. This is an enormous stressor for the body, and so all the stress hormones are released and the body goes into fight-or-flight mode. High cortisol levels suppress inflammation, so the injury isn't made worse by your own reaction. Once the initial pain and stress of the injury go away, your fight-or-flight response is supposed to shut off; then cortisol levels drop, your parasympathetic nervous system brings balance, and your immune system gets to work, preventing infection caused by microbes that might have penetrated your skin. As you can see, initially the stress response is helpful, but if it goes on for too long, you can end up with a serious infection that can prevent the healing of your leg. The natural course of events for survival therefore is for the immune system to dial down its response after the stress system has been activated, but this suppression is not supposed to go on for long periods of time.

When your killer cells slow down, two things can happen. First, as I mentioned, you have an increased risk of infection. Second, because the suppression of the killer cells is coupled with a shift in which your body produces too many antibodies, this can get out of control, and the antibodies can attack your own tissue. The result is an antibody-dominant autoimmune disease such as lupus.

CHRONIC STRESS AND ADRENAL FATIGUE

Now let's talk about low levels of cortisol. Over time, chronic stress can wear out your adrenal glands. When this happens cortisol levels drop, as do levels of important hormones such as adrenaline and neurotransmitters such as norepinephrine. This is problematic for anyone, even those in good health. But it's a serious issue if you've got an autoimmune disease because this could have been the trigger that started your body's autoimmune response in the first place, and now it is preventing you from getting better. Without enough cortisol to kill off the bad T cells, these cells can turn into the kind that attack your own body. Again, there is a lopsided effect, with the low cortisol levels creating an imbalance between killer cells and antibodies. Killer cells cause inflammation throughout the body, so the more you have, the more inflammation and thus tissue damage you have, too.

How would you feel physically when this happens? When your cortisol is low, resulting in too many killer cells and increased inflammation through the body, you will experience nonspecific symptoms such as puffiness, stiffness and achiness in the joints and muscles, and general exhaustion. But if you develop an autoimmune disease in a specific organ—such as your joints, for example, which is what happens in rheumatoid arthritis—then your main symptoms might be pain, swelling, and even deformity in your joints. In fact, most autoimmune diseases have this kind of imbalance: an excess of killer cells attacking your own tissue. This is definitely a problem and is why it is crucial for people with autoimmune conditions to restore the function of their adrenal glands and stress system. In fact, research reveals that if you have low-functioning adrenal glands, you have an increased risk of developing an autoimmune disease, especially autoimmune thyroid disease, rheumatoid arthritis, lupus, and Sjögren's syndrome.

One important study published by the Mount Sinai School of Medicine focused on a patient who had developed Graves' disease, a condition in which the body makes antibodies that stimulate the thyroid to produce high levels of thyroid hormones, which are very important for metabolism and energy, among other things. But you need just the right amounts of this hormone, and if the levels get too high, you can have palpitations, weight loss, and insomnia, among other symptoms. This can be very dangerous for your heart. The seventy-one-year-old woman in this study was found to have extremely low levels of cortisol. Researchers gave her cortisol in a pill form, just enough to replace what her adrenal glands would naturally produce on their own if they were healthy. After one month her thyroid hormone levels were normal, and two years later her Graves' disease was completely gone.[4] Even though this was a very small case study, it highlights the connection between cortisol and autoimmune disease. It also underlines the importance of helping your adrenal glands recover and make more cortisol if they are low. I very rarely use prescription cortisol in my medical practice, but I do use herbs and other supplements to help nourish the adrenal glands and boost cortisol levels, and I will show you how to do this in the workbook chapter that follows.

DO YOU HAVE ADRENAL FATIGUE?

Exhaustion and fatigue are the most common complaints that I hear from new patients. Often they have seen many different specialists, trying to identify the cause of their lack of energy and to get treatment that will make them feel better. After finding no relief, many people begin scouring the Internet for ideas and solutions and learn about this condition called adrenal fatigue. And then they come find me, or another functional medicine or integrative medicine practitioner, to help them get diagnosed and treated, because poorly functioning adrenal glands usually are not evaluated by conventional doctors.

There are many reasons you might be exhausted, and adrenal fatigue is just one of them. I begin to suspect the cause is your adrenal glands if you have a history of a lot of stress and not taking very good care of yourself. The five self-care steps to healthy adrenal glands are: getting a good night's sleep, exercising regularly, practicing some form of relaxation daily, eating a whole-foods diet like the one I described in Chapter 2, "Using Food as Medicine," and living a low-toxin lifestyle, which I will explain in Chapter 11. If your stress has been high for several years, you aren't sleeping or exercising, you are eating a diet high in sugar and bad fats, you don't ever slow down and relax, and you have a high toxic load (which can be mercury in your fish, pesticides in your food, or other exposure to environmental chemicals; again, see Chapter 11, "Supporting Your Liver"), your adrenal glands may be exhausted.

The first clue for me is your story: stress and self-care. The next clue is your pattern of energy during the day. If you wake up tired, feel best during the middle of the day, crash and need a nap in the late afternoon, and then get a second wind at night, you have the classic pattern of tired adrenal glands. Keep in mind that there are other reasons you might be tired, such as eating too much sugar, nutritional deficiencies, low thyroid hormones, too many toxins in your body, and chronic viral infections. But if your story fits the pattern that I describe above, your adrenal glands are likely the problem.

In the workbook chapter that follows, I will provide you with self-assessments to help you identify how your story and your symptoms can lead to a diagnosis. There is also testing available, which I will share with you, too.

OTHER IMPORTANT ADRENAL HORMONES

Before we finish up this section on adrenal fatigue, I want to tell you something about DHEA, which is a very important hormone made in the adrenal glands. On its own, DHEA has been shown to help reduce cholesterol and balance blood sugar in both men and women. In women, DHEA can be converted into testosterone in many tissues of the body, including the adrenal glands. So while DHEA isn't a hormone like testosterone, it can increase hormonal activity in your body.

The specific hormones that DHEA activates are called androgens. Androgens help us build bone and muscle, which is particularly important as we age because androgens prevent osteoporosis and loss of muscle mass. For women, making sure the adrenal glands are healthy and producing plenty of DHEA will also be good for your testosterone levels. This is different for men, because they make all their testosterone in their testicles, but they still need DHEA from the adrenal glands, too. When you experience sustained stress, your DHEA is the first adrenal hormone to get depleted, even before your cortisol levels start falling. Chronic stress also causes your testosterone levels to fall, both because your DHEA production has dropped and because your stress has turned on the enzyme aromatase, which converts testosterone to estrogen.

Low levels of DHEA and testosterone have been found in patients with rheumatoid arthritis and lupus. This isn't good, because DHEA suppresses the release of inflammatory molecules from T cells and testosterone has been shown to help kill off activated immune cells, thus keeping them from getting out of control. To examine this further, researchers at the Johns Hopkins School of Medicine gave a group of lupus patients 200 mg of DHEA daily for three months. At the end of that time, all the patients saw their symptoms improve and 53 percent were able to decrease their dose of the medication prednisone. Study participants who had the worst symptoms and were on the highest amount of medication had the greatest success with this approach.[5]

And this isn't the only study showing the beneficial effects of raising DHEA or testosterone levels in people with autoimmune diseases. At the University Hospital in Utrecht, the Netherlands, researchers found that a group of women with rheumatoid arthritis had low DHEA levels before and after their diagnosis of this disease. After giving these women testosterone, researchers found that all of them had less pain and were less disabled by their disease.[6]

Not only is there good evidence for this kind of treatment in the literature, but I have seen the benefits of this in my practice. I always evaluate DHEA and testosterone levels in all my patients, and when they are low, we use stress management and supplementation to help remedy this. Keep in mind that fixing your adrenal foundation and managing stress are primary, and this will help support your DHEA and testosterone levels, even if you decide to take supplements. Stay tuned—I will show you how to supplement DHEA in the workbook in the next chapter.

So what is the solution to all the stress around you? While you can't live in a bubble and get rid of all the stress in your life, you must learn to manage it better. You must learn how to control the way it's coming into your body and making you sick. You must learn tools to be more mindful and aware of when you are feeling stress in your body so that you can take a deep breath and relax, preventing the stress response from turning on and staying stuck in the on position. This will help you balance your stress hormones. I will show you how in the next chapter, which is our assessment and treatment workbook.

STRESS AND INFECTIONS

I will talk more about how infections can cause autoimmune disease in Chapter 14, "Infections and Specific Autoimmune Conditions." But in this section, I want to point out how stress *plus* an infection can snowball into an autoimmune problem. Amazingly, every viral disease that you've ever had leaves some residual viral particles in your body. These include cold sores, chicken pox, shingles, hepatitis, Epstein-Barr, and more. All of these viruses can be reactivated when stress hormones or neurotransmitters suppress your immune system, making it harder for it to fight off infection. How does this happen? It is believed that severe stress causes suppression of cellular immunity (this part you know already—these are the cytotoxic T cells), which allows the virus to establish itself inside the tissues in your body. Because there is evidence that many autoimmune diseases might be triggered by infections, allowing viruses to thrive in your body is another way that stress can cause an autoimmune disease or make an existing one worse. And as we've discussed, this includes both emotional stress as well as the severe physical stress that results from an unhealthy lifestyle of smoking, drinking, and bad food choices. Keeping the immune system strong will help keep these viral particles in remission.

STRESS, GUT HEALTH, AND THE IMMUNE SYSTEM

Your whole gastrointestinal system is often called your "gut," a slang term that includes your stomach, small intestine, and large intestine. In Part III, "Healing Your Gut," we will detail the importance of having a healthy gut. But here I want to mention that studies show that stress changes the environment inside your stomach and intestines.

More and more research shows that various types of stress have a major impact on the physiology of your intestines. For example, there is a clear link between stress and conditions such as irritable bowel syndrome and inflammatory bowel disease. But for now I want to focus on the stress-related gut changes that impact your immune system. Seventy percent of your immune system is located in your digestive tract, so it's easy to see why it's critical to keep this area healthy, which is best accomplished in two ways. The first way to maintain the health of your digestive system is to make sure you have the right amount of good bacteria in your digestive tract. The second is making sure that the cells that line your entire digestive tract and form a barrier that regulates what can pass into your bloodstream are healthy. If you don't have enough good bacteria in your gut, or if the cellular barrier lining the digestive tract is weak or permeable, your immune system is compromised.

Research has found that stress can lower the number of good bacteria (specifically those called lactobacilli and bifidobacteria) and promote an overgrowth of bad bacteria in the small bowel. It does this in a few different ways. First, stress can directly suppress an immune molecule (called secretory IgA) that helps keep the good bacteria strong and growing and the bad bacteria and yeast out. In addition, studies have shown that stress causes the release of substances such as adrenaline and norepinephrine into the gut, which can lead directly to an overgrowth of bad bacteria.[7] Stress also makes the lining of your digestive tract more permeable, so bad bacteria and bacterial antigens (the "name tag" from the bacteria that the immune system reads) can seep into the body.[8] This weaker barrier (a.k.a. leaky gut) also allows things such as proteins from food to get into the bloodstream, where they stimulate the immune system, causing inflammation and the possibility of new food allergies or sensitivities.

We described this in Chapter 2, "Using Food as Medicine," but now you know exactly how chronic stress might have played a role in how you developed a food allergy or sensitivity.

THE MIND-BODY CONNECTION

Now that we've talked about all the damage stress can do, it's time to do something about the level of stress in your life. It's time to learn ways to engage your relaxation system and turn off the hormones and neurotransmitters that are causing the bad health effects of chronic stress. These hormones and neurotransmitters will be there when you need them, but when you don't, they should remain on standby. So how do you engage your relaxation system? For a long time we believed that our autonomic nervous system was automatic. Then, beginning in the 1930s, Hans Selye studied mice and detailed the mechanisms of the stress response, and we found out that the response to stress and the effect on your autonomic nervous system can be influenced by aspects of the environment, including food and living conditions.[9] His studies helped us understand what we already knew about monks living in caves in the Himalayan Mountains who could regulate their body temperature with meditation. They were able to do so because meditation causes blood vessels to relax and dilate; as a result, more blood could flow through their bodies, making them feel warm. The fact that you can actually control body functions such as blood pressure, heart rate, temperature, and your immune system is a shocking realization for many people, but it's true.

This is part of mind-body medicine, a branch of integrative medicine (functional medicine is also a branch of integrative medicine). It looks at how your thoughts, feelings, and emotions affect your physical health and how your physical health affects your spiritual and emotional well-being. When practiced regularly, mind-body techniques such as meditation, guided relaxation, and guided imagery can have a powerful positive effect on you and your health. There are two main benefits you will gain by beginning a mind-body practice. First, your body can actually learn to have a different kind of response to a situation so that you don't turn on the damaging hormones and instead maintain a balanced inner world that will help you prevent and reverse any chronic illness you may have, especially one involving the immune system. But equally as important, these techniques will help you begin to understand the amount of stress that is coming into your body, and this awareness will help you see what changes need to be made in how you are living your life and how certain things you are doing may be hurting you. Mind-body medicine offers the tools for this sort of exploration and for regaining balance.

You might be wondering if these skills are hard to learn. But I promise that they are not. I have taught them to people from all walks of life. For example, in 2012 I went to Haiti with faculty from the Center for Mind-Body Medicine to teach mind-body skills to the very stressed population around Jacmel, an area hit hard by the 2010 earthquake. The Haitian people are among the poorest in the world and experience serious stress in their daily lives in a way many of us can't even comprehend. They struggle to simply meet their everyday needs and survive. Of the 130 people who came to this training program, I had the opportunity to personally work with a group of ten. In eight 2-hour sessions, I taught them skills such as deep "soft belly" breathing, guided relaxation, and imagery. They also did drawing and writing exercises to learn more about themselves. They were all sponges for this information, going home every night to practice.

My group included Haitians with higher education, those with very little education, and people whose education levels fell somewhere in between. Some of these people were leaders in the community; others were everyday folk. But despite these differences, everyone, without exception, was able to learn skills that lowered their blood pressure, relieved headaches, and improved sleep. Additionally, they came to understand the changes they needed to make in their lives that would allow them to be happier, less angry, and less frustrated. And they left the training with tools to continue this practice and figure out what they needed to be healthy in body, mind, and spirit. I had gone to Haiti to help teach the people of Jacmel; what I didn't realize was how much the people of Jacmel would teach *me*. Not only did they touch me deeply with their warmth, kindness, and appreciation, but the experience helped prove to me how these mind-body skills are universal in their appeal and that everyone can do them. As you continue through this section, I will give you the information and instruction to learn them at home. And you can learn more about the Center for Mind-Body Medicine at www.cmbm.org, where you can find information on their programs in the United States and around the world, and resources that might be helpful for you, too.

OTHER BENEFITS OF MIND-BODY TECHNIQUES

It turns out that when you begin to learn these mind-body skills something interesting happens: you start feeling better immediately. Why? Because you are doing something for yourself. You are taking care of you (rather than just taking care of those around you). You are being proactive about your health. This helps you move from a position of hopelessness to one of power and control. Many, many studies have shown that self-care is healing in and of itself, even without the added benefit of balancing the autonomic nervous system. These techniques work because of the reaction in your nervous system. Realizing that you are the only one who can "fix" you is a cornerstone of why you will get better.

Another benefit of these techniques is the chance they give you to learn about and understand yourself better. Using words, drawings, movement, meditation, and visualization helps you become aware of your burdens and stresses and bring them to the surface so you can do something about them. Knowledge is power, and self-knowledge will guide and anchor you as you explore and understand your body and how it may be responding to different stressors around you. This is very exciting, because it shows that *you* have the power to improve your health.

In Chapter 6, "Understanding the Stress Connection Workbook," I will help you assess your stressors and find out if some of your symptoms are related to stress. Then the treatment program will provide do-it-yourself exercises for you to try at home and resources to find outside help.

MY PERSONAL JOURNEY

I began practicing these mind-body skills and looking inside myself after my first training with the Center for Mind-Body Medicine many years ago, when I was going through a difficult time. I was unhappy but not sure why. I had three children under the age of ten and some financial stress at home that was difficult but manageable. For some reason I couldn't figure out why everything felt dark. Was it my husband? (It's so easy to blame those closest to us, especially when everything feels crummy.) Was it taking time off from work to be a full-time mom? I wasn't sure. So I found a therapist and spent eighteen months on the couch trying to discover what was wrong.

Then one day I received a brochure for a nine-day professional training course in mind-body medicine. I'd never been away from my husband and kids for that long. But a voice inside told me that I needed to go.

Thank goodness I listened, because it was the most transformative experience of my life. That's where I met James Gordon, M.D., who for years, along with others at the Center for Mind-Body Medicine, has been teaching health professionals how to use mind-body techniques for themselves and their patients. For those nine days, I immersed myself in learning active and quiet meditation techniques, guided imagery, biofeedback, and how to use drawings and writing for self-awareness. What I particularly loved was the guided imagery and the active meditations.

At that nine-day training, I learned more about myself than I had in eighteen months of therapy. It was amazing. I realized that my unhappiness was inside *me* and had nothing to do with anyone else. I needed to find myself. I needed to figure out who I was and what I wanted to do with my life. I also needed to determine my own path to happiness and my own answers as to how to make the changes I needed to make. I shared my revelations with my therapist, and he was amazed. We wrapped up our sessions and I haven't gone back since.

Ultimately, I learned that feeling lost about my life's work was causing my problems and that my happiness was going to be found outside conventional medicine. I needed to find a path into a more holistic type of medicine. This has been my most transformative life experience, and I still practice those mind-body techniques today. They have helped me find my way to my current medical practice, which is focused on functional medicine and mind-body medicine.

At Blum Center for Health, we offer mind-body skills groups following this model. I have had the great joy of watching many people undergo a transformation in their body, mind, spirit, and ultimately their lives, just as I did. Seeing the healing my patients experience on every level gives me such a deep sense of satisfaction that's hard to describe in words. It's why I do what I do and why I wrote this book. *You* can do this, too. Let me show you how.

CHAPTER 6

Understanding the Stress Connection Workbook

By now you know that your stress system is the physiological response of your body to stress, which includes stress hormones and your autonomic nervous system. This system can cause an imbalance in your immune system and cause or worsen an autoimmune disease. You don't want your stress system to be either always on high or always on low; you want it to turn on when you need it and then turn off when you don't. Most people, by the time I see them, have low-functioning adrenal glands with low levels of cortisol and adrenaline because they have been stressed for so long, not only from their life experiences but also from the emotional and physical stress of their disease. Maybe you feel that way too, and you're just worn out. The goal is to fix your stress response system so that it regains its resiliency and flexibility. The first step to fixing it is to determine how badly it is broken. The self-assessments in this section will help you determine exactly how impaired your stress system is and what you can do to fix it.

But first let me tell you about Monica, a fifty-five-year-old woman who came to see me because she was completely exhausted and had gained ten pounds a year for the past seven years. Four months prior to meeting with me, Monica's doctor told her she had rheumatoid arthritis. His solution was a pile of prescriptions, but fearing the side effects and wanting to see if there was another way, she came to me.

It turns out that Monica has a history of autoimmune diseases. She's had Hashimoto's thyroiditis (the same condition I had) for twenty years and the skin condition vitiligo, which runs in her family, for fifteen years. Vitiligo is an autoimmune disease that involves loss of pigment in the skin. It's pretty easy to spot, so when I saw blotchy white patches on Monica's arms and neck, I knew exactly what it was before she told me. What I found fascinating was the story she told me about how her skin disease "happened overnight" when she had a traumatic experience in her life.

She called this the "big boom" because she had lost her husband, her home, and all her money in the course of a few weeks. Obviously, her stress level was through the roof. Within days, she said, she started seeing white areas cropping up all over her skin. Because her aunt and mother had vitiligo, she knew what it was and was convinced all this stress had triggered it.

And her stress didn't stop there. For the next ten years, she lived hand to mouth in a state of perpetual worry and anxiety. But like so many of my patients with autoimmune diseases, Monica never thought that her stress level was a huge part of why she was now so sick.

She had terrible food reactions and many digestive complaints, such as gas and bloating in her abdomen, feeling like she was six months pregnant after eating any food at all. Clearly, there were other things that we needed to work on, in addition to her stress and hormones. But I started with a thorough stress history, just like the one you'll find in this chapter. After you take the test, I will tell you more about Monica's assessment, what I learned, and how I treated her.

ANALYZING THE INFLUENCE OF STRESS IN YOUR LIFE

Maybe you have realized, at least to some degree, that stress is a piece of your puzzle, and perhaps you've even noticed how it causes your symptoms to flare up. But thinking back to when you first got sick, could stress have played a part, as it did for Monica? Maybe it wasn't sudden or seemingly overnight the way it was for her, but even a difficult time over the course of a few years can be a problem. Keep in mind that stressors aren't always bad—stress can come from moving, getting married, or speeding up the corporate ladder, which often involves changing your job. A study done at the University of Athens School of Medicine found that women who had recently experienced three or more stressful events had an increased rate of relapse from multiple sclerosis.[1] This is a good reminder of how a really stressful event or series of events or changes could have been a trigger for you—something I've certainly seen in my practice.

However, it is also clear that to balance your immune system, you need to fix everything that is pushing it in the wrong direction. This includes learning how to manage your stress, so that we can heal your adrenal glands, cortisol levels, and sympathetic nervous system. As I've said, I've helped hundreds, maybe thousands, of people to do this, even in places such as Haiti, so I know you can do it, too.

Self-Assessments

Where is your stress system right now? Is it overactive, balanced, or fatigued? The following self-assessments will help you figure it out, and then I will show you what to do with the results. When it comes to evaluating how stress is influencing the health of my patients, I look at the following categories of issues and add them up: past stressors, current stressors, self-care, and adrenal fatigue. I have divided the self-assessments that follow into four sections based on these categories. After you answer the questions in all four sections, you will add it all up for a grand total and we'll explore your results together. **The following gives you an overview of the four categories of questions that I will ask you in the assessments in this chapter.**

Self-Assessment 1: Past Stressors

Have you suffered from past trauma, severe difficulties in your life? Could these experiences still be affecting you now?
Many people suffer extraordinary stress and trauma in their families (or because of their lack of a family), and your stress system can be damaged in these early years as a result. This is very important because it might be influencing your stress system now. Included in this category are stressful events in the past. Because I live in the New York area, I have seen many people affected by the 9/11 attacks on the World Trade Center. Recently I had a new patient whose husband died in one of the towers of the World Trade Center. A decade had passed and she had remarried, but within five minutes of sitting down in my office, I asked a question that opened this up for her, and she started crying about this loss and the trauma that followed for her and her children. Clearly, she was still carrying heavy emotions about what had happened to her. You, too, may be bearing the burden of emotions or experiences that happened a while ago.

While this 9/11 widow could easily identify the past as a stressful time, she didn't realize that the bottled-up emotions still activated her stress system and were making her sick. I have also seen many people who are able to let their feelings stream through them. It doesn't mean these people don't get emotional when they think of past trauma; rather, they are able to express and then release the feelings instead of letting them get stuck inside. It is the stuck feelings that activate and put pressure on the stress system, and so learning mind-body techniques such as meditation and imagery are powerful tools that can help these feelings and stressful emotions move up and out.

Self-Assessment 2: Current Stressors

What is going on in your life right now? Are you experiencing stress at work or in any of your relationships? Have any of your loved ones been sick recently? Have you lost a loved one recently?
This is extremely common. Everyone experiences loss at one time or another. Most people accept this as a normal part of life, but if added to your loss is trouble at work or a difficult spouse at home, your stress system might be in overload. I bet you will be surprised when you see how many items you can check in this portion of the assessment, and I hope you will give yourself a big dose of compassion when you see how much you are dealing with.

Self-Assessment 3: Self-Care

How are you taking care of yourself?
This is where I will ask you all about your sleep, eating habits, exercise, and stress management (relaxation) habits. If you have good self-care, you might score low on this section, which is a positive thing. Taking care of yourself builds resiliency in your system and can prevent some of what you have gone through in the past and some of the stressors you are experiencing now from making you sick. If you score high here, chin up—there is plenty you can do, and I will show you how.

Self-Assessment 4: Adrenal Fatigue Symptoms

Are you already having physical effects of stress?
Sometimes I hear stories of such difficult lives that I am amazed at how well the person in front of me has handled it, somehow not getting really sick from it. If you have an easygoing nature, it protects you just a bit from the events around you, so that they might not be making you as sick compared to a friend who gets emotionally stressed, worried, and anxious. If you are that person who gets stressed easily, small things might turn on your system. Because everyone has a different temperament and

different amounts of trauma and stress, the point is to know where you stand with your stress *right now*. To determine this, I am going to ask you questions about physical symptoms so that I can diagnose you with an overactive, balanced, or fatigued stress system. So it's not enough just to know about your stressors—I need to know about *you*.

Self-Assessment 1: Past Stressors

In this section, I want you to think about your life prior to the past two years (which we will address in the next section, on current stressors). Have you had any of the following things happen to you? For each question, if you *have not* had that experience, circle 0. If you *have*, circle the number that represents the intensity of the experience.

	No	Mild	Moderate	Severe
Did you experience death or illness of a spouse?	0	1	2	3
Did you experience death or illness of a child?	0	1	2	3
Did you experience physical or emotional abuse in childhood?	0	1	2	3
Did you witness any kind of abuse or trauma in the past?	0	1	2	3
Was there alcohol abuse in your house growing up?	0	1	2	3
Have you been in difficult or abusive relationships as an adult?	0	1	2	3
Have you experienced financial hardship?	0	1	2	3
Have you been ill for more than two years?	0	1	2	3
Did you experience a divorce?	0	1	2	3
Have you ever been fired or let go from a job?	0	1	2	3
Total				

Add the numbers you circled above. Then write your total on the appropriate line below:

_____1–10: Mild past stress
_____11–20: Moderate past stress
_____21–30: Severe past stress

When Monica took this assessment, she scored a 21. She grew up in a difficult household with lots of stress. After her divorce, Monica was homeless for many years. For the past ten years, she's had severe fatigue that has made it very difficult for her to function. She has also experienced pain in her muscles and joints. This important information gave me a sense of how damaged her stress system was in the years prior to her illness. **In other words, what happened in the past created a foundation that changed her immune system, and made her susceptible to getting sick from the *triggering* events that came next.** Her score of 21 out of 30 told me that she suffered from chronic, severe stress for a long time, so her immune system had to be really out of balance even before that last trauma put her over the top and crashed her system completely.

If you scored:

1–10: Your levels of past stress were mild, so you came into your current health crisis with a good foundation.

11–30: Your levels of past stress were moderate or severe. This puts you at a higher risk for a low-functioning stress system because it might be pooped out from working so hard for so long.

Self-Assessment 2: Current Stressors

Now it is time to think about what has been going on in your life for the past two years. The instructions are the same as those for Section 1. Have you had any of the following things happen to you? For each question, if you *have not* had that experience, circle 0. If you *have*, circle the number that represents the intensity of the experience.

Stressors	Never	Mild	Moderate	Severe
Did you experience death or illness of a spouse or child?	0	1	2	3
Did you get separated or divorced?	0	1	2	3
Did you lose your home or experience financial hardship?	0	1	2	3
Did you or your partner unexpectedly lose a job?	0	1	2	3

Are you depressed or anxious?	0	1	2	3
Any difficulties with children?	0	1	2	3
Do you have trouble handling the stress in your life?	0	1	2	3
Do you have family stress with your siblings or parents?	0	1	2	3
Are you having problems with your spouse or partner?	0	1	2	3
Have you had a major life change, such as marriage, moving to a new community, or a new job?	0	1	2	3
Total				

Write in your total on the appropriate line below:

_____1–10: Mild current stress

_____11–20: Moderate current stress

_____21–30: Severe current stress

When Monica took this assessment, she scored a 14. This shows me that she was experiencing fewer external stressors now than she did in the past. But her illness was still causing her severe stress that she really couldn't handle. She was depressed and anxious, despite the fact that she had remarried a loving and supportive man years after her divorce and their financial situation was okay. I think the fact that her life was a bit more stable was the reason she was ready to make the changes she needed to make in order to get better.

If you scored:

1–10: Your current external stressors are mild. This means that you are in good position to use the tools I will give you and get quick results.

11–30: You have moderate to severe stress around you. Therefore, it's more likely that your stress system is sick and contributing to your illness. It is really important that you develop healthy ways to turn off the inner stress switch as well as look around you and figure out a way to calm your stressful environment. We will talk more about that later.

Self-Assessment 3: Self-Care

Now we'll look at how well you take care of yourself and your lifestyle choices. For each question, circle the number that best represents your current lifestyle.

Self-Care	All the Time	Most of the Time	Sometimes	Hardly Ever
Do you sleep through the night?	0	1	2	3
Do you go to sleep before 11:00 p.m.?	0	1	2	3
Do you get at least seven hours of sleep a night?	0	1	2	3
Do you meditate, do yoga, or practice another relaxation exercise?	0	1	2	3
Do you eat breakfast?	0	1	2	3
Do you eat frequent meals and snacks during the day? (This means you don't skip meals.)	0	1	2	3
Do you exercise three times per week or more?	0	1	2	3
Do you have any hobbies that help you relax, such as knitting, hiking, or painting?	0	1	2	3
Do you get acupuncture, massage, or other body treatments?	0	1	2	3
Do you find time to see your friends at least weekly?	0	1	2	3
Total				

Write in your total on the appropriate line below:

_____1–10: Your self-care is great.

_____11–20: Your self-care is not ideal.

_____21–30: Your self-care is terrible, a problem that is very likely harming your health.

When Monica took this assessment, she scored a 22. Just before taking it, she had been eating a healthier diet, but she was going to sleep after midnight and then not sleeping well. She wasn't practicing any relaxation, seeing friends, or exercising, and she didn't have any hobbies that helped her relax. She wanted to exercise but was too tired, which is an issue I come across all the time.

In order to have healthy adrenal glands, you must score under 10 on this assessment. Go back and look at what needs to improve. I will be giving you instructions on how to sleep better and start a relaxation program or find a hobby. But for now, the most important thing to realize is that if you scored high on this assessment, self-care is something you need to work on; you *must* improve this score in order to get better. These are things you can change, and I will help you do that.

Self-Assessment 4: Adrenal Fatigue

In this section, we will look at your physical symptoms and help you determine if you have adrenal exhaustion. Keep in mind that when you have stress, the first stage is a high cortisol level and then your adrenal glands eventually get tired and your cortisol and adrenaline levels drop. Depending on where you are in this process, your symptoms might be mild because you are just beginning to be fatigued or you are still in a high cortisol state. If you score high on the test below, that means you have progressed to exhaustion with low levels of cortisol. This is important for us to know because your immune system can't recover until your adrenal glands are healthy. After you take the test, I will explain how to interpret the results.

Symptoms of Adrenal Fatigue and Low Cortisol Levels	Never	Sometimes	Often	All the Time
Do you feel tired when you wake up, even if you slept seven hours or more?	0	1	2	3
Do you feel exhausted in the afternoon?	0	1	2	3
Do you get a burst of energy at night?	0	1	2	3

(*continued on next page*)

Symptoms of Adrenal Fatigue and Low Cortisol levels	Never	Sometimes	Often	All the Time
Do you get dizzy, irritable, or sleepy if you go without food for four to five hours?	0	1	2	3
Do you crave salty food?	0	1	2	3
Are you having pain and/or inflammation in your muscles or joints?	0	1	2	3
How often do you get sick or catch colds or the flu?	0	1	2	3
How often is your sex drive lower than you would like it to be?	0	1	2	3
Do you have trouble handling even small stresses?	0	1	2	3
Are you depressed, feeling no energy to do anything?	0	1	2	3
Total				

Write in your total on the appropriate line below:

_____1–10: Your adrenal glands are not fatigued.

_____11–20: You probably have moderate adrenal fatigue.

_____21–30: Your adrenal glands are exhausted.

When Monica took this assessment, she circled 3 for nine of the questions and 1 for one question, for a total score of 28. This told me that her adrenal glands were pretty shot, something that was confirmed by lab testing. (More on that later.) If you scored high on this test and your adrenal glands are exhausted, follow the treatment plan for adrenal fatigue in the next section. If you still aren't sure, in the next section I will help you bring in the results of the other sections so you understand where you are.

PUTTING IT ALL TOGETHER

Because you cannot change your past and the stress history that's a part of it, your total score on the first section of the assessment will not be counted as part of the total number we are adding up below. This total number is more about what is happening right now. However, learning the stress management techniques I will teach you in the next chapter will help you release the stored feelings from the old stressors, and this is important for you if you scored high on this first section.

Now we want to focus on understanding your results and how to choose the right treatment program. Please fill in your results.

SECTION	SCORE	GOAL
Section 2: Current stressors		< 10
Section 3: Self-care		< 10
Section 4: Adrenal fatigue symptoms		< 10
Total score:		< 30

First, let's look at your total.

1. If your total was less than 30, congratulations. Your stress system is probably in good shape.
2. If your total was greater than 60, your adrenal glands are most likely fatigued, your stressors are out of control, and you need to improve your self-care. If this is you, then you have what I call the "bathtub drain problem." Your adrenal glands are pooped, but when you try to fix them, it is like filling a bathtub with water when the drain is open. All your efforts are for nothing because your life is still filled with stress and you aren't taking care of yourself. Figuring out how to close that drain by learning self-care and finding ways to reduce the stress in your environment are going to be key for your recovery. You will need to follow all three parts of our treatment program in the next section.
3. If your total was 30–60, then we need to look closely at your results in each section of the self-assessment to understand what is going on.

I have organized the possible results into different patterns because I want to help you identify where you need to focus your treatment. These are the patterns I see in my office every day. If you have pattern 1, you need to focus your efforts on reducing the stress around you. If you have pattern 2, you need to focus on treating adrenal fatigue. If you have pattern 3, you need to focus on your self-care. If you have pattern 4, you need to focus on both your stressors and your self-care.

• • •

Pattern 1: Your adrenal symptoms aren't bad, but you have lots of stress and are not taking care of yourself.

SECTION	SCORE	GOAL
Current stressors (Section 2)	20–30	< 10
Self-care (Section 3)	10–20	< 10
Adrenal fatigue symptoms (Section 4)	0–10	< 10
Total	30–60	< 30

If this is your pattern, your stress system is still working in overdrive because you have so many stressors in your life. The good news is that you haven't become completely exhausted yet. But you are on your way. The bad news is that you most likely have high cortisol and high adrenaline, which aren't good for your immune system either and have plenty of their own health consequences (see pages 109–14). So for you the focus needs to be on reducing all the stressors in your life so your adrenal glands don't poop out.

Using the bathtub analogy, your bathtub drain is wide open but the water is running so fast (high cortisol) that it has been keeping the bathtub filled with water. This means that your adrenal glands are still okay. But eventually the faucet will dry up and the bathtub will empty. How long will that take? That depends on how high your numbers were for self-care and current stressors and if you are having any signs of adrenal fatigue yet. The higher the numbers, the quicker this will happen.

Pattern 2: Your adrenal glands are shot, but you don't have many stressors and you have been doing better taking care of yourself.

SECTION	SCORE	GOAL
Current stressors (Section 2)	1–10	< 10
Self-care (Section 3)	10–20	< 10
Adrenal fatigue symptoms (Section 4)	20–30	< 10
Total	30–60	< 30

This pattern shows someone who has an empty bathtub with a drain that is closed. Why isn't the bathtub filling with water? Why aren't your adrenal glands bouncing back? If you started your self-care and stress management programs only within the past year, my guess is that it just

hasn't been long enough. You should still focus on the treatment suggestions in the following section, but pay extra attention to the herbs
and supplements that can help your adrenal glands recover. Perhaps they
need a little extra boost.

Keep in mind that stress isn't the only thing that strains your adrenal
glands. You might have other systems in your body that are not functioning properly, such as your detox system or gut. Or you're eating foods
that are causing stress for your system and keeping your adrenal glands
from recovering or making them sick. Make sure you look at all the sections in this book and fix these systems, too, because they might be the
key to healing your adrenal glands.

Pattern 3: You have minimal stressors around you, but your adrenal glands are moderately tired. In this instance, the issue is that you
aren't taking care of yourself and lifestyle factors are affecting your stress
system.

SECTION	SCORE	GOAL
Current stressors (Section 2)	1–10	< 10
Self-care (Section 3)	20–30	< 10
Adrenal fatigue symptoms (Section 4)	10–20	< 10
Total	30–60	< 30

It is important to keep in mind that your adrenal glands can be tired
even if you aren't aware of the stressors around you or don't have the
feeling of being stressed. If you aren't taking care of yourself by doing
the things mentioned in the checklist in section 3, your lifestyle is hurting you. In order to get better, you must improve your self-care levels. You will need to focus on this in the treatment chapter, coming up
next.

Pattern 4: None of your scores showed severe problems, but your score
in one or more categories was between 10 and 20. This means that your
current stressors, self-care, or the health of your adrenal glands is not as
good as it should be.

SECTION	SCORE	GOAL
Current stressors (Section 2)	**10–20**	< 10
Self-care (Section 3)	**10–20**	< 10
Adrenal fatigue symptoms (Section 4)	10–20	< 10
Total	30–60	< 30

Here is an example of someone with moderate amounts of daily stress who isn't doing great with self-care, and whose adrenal glands are just hanging in there. If this is you, beware, because this is the danger pattern—you are living on the edge. A lack of signs of severe imbalance can lull you into believing all is going well in your stress system. You should focus on improving your current stressors and self-care, because if this doesn't change, your adrenal glands are at risk for pooping out. Read all of the treatment plans, and make at least Tier 1 changes in all categories.

Treatment Program

Here are the steps to treating (and preventing) adrenal fatigue and balancing your stress system. I have based the following programs on the patterns that you discovered when you put your self-assessments together. However, if you had a very high score for any one of the self-assessments, you should pay extra attention to it, in addition to following the suggestions for that pattern.

1. **How to manage your stressful life.** This treatment plan will show you how to remove or reduce your stressful life, including reducing outside stressors and learning to manage them better. If your results fit into patterns 1 or 4, you should include this treatment plan in your program. If you scored very high (20–30) on self-assessment 2, pay extra attention to this program.
2. **Improve all aspects of self-care.** This treatment plan will show you how to improve your self-care, including sleep, food, and exercise. If your results fit into patterns 1, 2, 3, or 4, you should include this treatment plan in your program. Clearly, self-care is important for every-

one. If you scored very high (20–30) on self-assessment 3, pay extra attention to this program.

3. **How to treat your tired adrenal glands.** This treatment plan will show you how to treat your adrenal glands with food and supplements. If you have adrenal fatigue, this will be critical for your recovery. If your results fit into patterns 2, 3, or 4, you should include this treatment plan in your program. If you scored very high (20–30) on self-assessment 4, pay extra attention to this program.

Understanding the Stress Treatment Program

How to Manage Your Stressful Life: Treatment Plan for Self-Assessment 2

If your score on the assessment of your current life stressors is above a 10, no matter what you scored on the other sections, you must start looking around and noticing how you can make your life easier. The first step is awareness. Now that you have taken the test and seen all the things you are dealing with, it will help you understand yourself better. After giving yourself a healthy dose of compassion and understanding for what you've been going through, you need to move on to do two things. First, look around and see what you can change. Second, for those things you can't change, you need to learn tools to protect yourself, so that the stressors don't make you sick. I will teach you these tools in this chapter.

You are probably thinking it is easy for me to tell you to change your circumstances, while you feel stuck and unsure how to do this. You are right. I can't tell you what to do. I am only interested in helping you see clearly what you are dealing with, to help you know that it is just too much and it is affecting your health. Then my goal is to give you tools to discover what to do next.

Tools for Taking Charge of the Stress in Your Life

Honestly, you might need a coach, counselor, therapist, or other professional to support and help guide you through these life changes I'm suggesting. I have found professional support to be helpful personally, and I recommend this for many of my patients, as I did with Monica. In our first meeting together, she made it clear that she knew how much stress was involved in her illness. She did not need more awareness about this connection. But she *did* need to learn how to relax.

I taught her a simple technique, called "soft belly" breathing, a tool I learned from my friend and mentor, James Gordon, M.D., founder and director of the Center for Mind-Body Medicine and clinical professor of psychiatry and family medicine at Georgetown University School of Medicine, who recently served as chairman of the White House Commission on Complementary and Alternative Medicine Policy. Monica started practicing this at home every day and it became an important part of her recovery.

The answer to managing stress will be different for each person. The point is that you can use meditation, imagery, drawings, and journaling for self-awareness so that you can get these answers, too. I have shared how relaxation exercises and therapies are great for learning more about yourself. But they are so much more than that. These tools are a foundational part of your self-care and will help you balance and heal your stress system. It is the single most important way that you will prevent the stressors in your life from making you sick.

Tier 1: Change Your Stress Environment on Your Own

What should you change? How should you or could you change it? The simplest way to get these answers is to start a journal. Get a notebook and begin to write down your thoughts and ideas. This is much like talking to yourself, but if you choose a quiet, contemplative time of day and location to do this, you can tap into your inner self to get some answers. Make a list of the biggest stressors in your life. Identify the one you feel has the most impact on your stress levels and your health. Write all about this one thing. For example, Monica had terrible work stress. I had her write a whole story of how she felt at work, why it was stressful, and what details about it made her unhappy.

Next make a list of all the possible ways this situation can be changed. Is there something you can do? What needs to happen? Write down all your thoughts on this. Monica was so sick and exhausted, but her job required her to be on her feet all day. She came to the conclusion that she would have to ask to change to a desk position or find a different job that wasn't so demanding. The first step was talking to her employer, which she did. Monica used the writing exercise to help her realize it was her work that was her biggest stressor and also to help her know the first step toward making a change.

Find simple ways to relax and make time for yourself every day. Take a bath, spend time with friends, learn to garden, or get outside for a leisurely walk. Consider starting a new hobby such as knitting or join a book club. These are all things that you can enjoy and that will rest your mind and body from the constant pressure of the switched-on stress system. You need to find time every day to be in the off mode so that your body and mind can relax. Even if you can't see the way to change a bad situation right now, you *can* choose to add something positive to your day and your life. This one change often has tremendous, powerful results because you are moving to a place of taking care of yourself, which in itself is empowering and feels good.

Tier 2: Change Your Stress Environment with Additional Resources

I believe we all need a teacher to help us learn mind-body skills, such as different types of meditation and guided imagery (also called visualization). Yet it isn't always possible to find a "teacher" in your area, or one who is affordable, so I recommend bringing a teacher home with you. The best way to do this is to purchase a CD or a book with a CD, or to directly download or watch recordings online.

Today, I am going to teach you the simplest breathing exercise I use in my office and the one I taught Monica. It is called "soft belly" breathing. Practice this every morning when you wake up for ten minutes. You can also do this at your desk during lunch, while waiting in the car at school, or before bed if you have trouble falling asleep. The nice thing about breathing exercises is that you can do them anywhere!

Soft Belly Breathing

Adapted from James Gordon, M.D.

This is a relaxation exercise that works in several ways.

1. It helps expand the base of your lungs, which helps bring extra oxygen to your brain. This lowers anxiety and induces greater relaxation.
2. The words "soft belly" create an image of a soft belly in your mind, which increases the effectiveness of the relaxation response.
3. The exercise is a simple relaxation technique that turns off the sympathetic nervous system and turns on the parasympathetic nervous system, lowering the blood pressure, slowing the heart rate, enabling deeper breathing, and inducing a state of calmness.

4. Focusing on your soft belly will give your mind a rest from the constant chatter and thinking. This will help you feel more relaxed and also help you focus and concentrate better during the day.

You can read these instructions first, and then close your eyes and begin. Or you can record the instructions on your phone or computer and play them back to guide you the first few times you do it.

- Sit up in a chair or bed, as erect as possible. Get comfortable and close your eyes. Loosen any clothing that feels restrictive.
- (If you are recording, start here.) Breathe deeply, in through your nose, and out through your mouth. In through your nose . . . out through your mouth.
- Now, imagine your belly is soft. This will deepen the breath and improve the exchange of oxygen, even as it relaxes your muscles. Say to yourself in your mind "soft" as you breathe in and "belly" as you breathe out. Soft . . . breathing in . . . belly . . . breathing out. As you breathe in, imagine your belly puffing out. As you breathe out, imagine your belly flattening in. Soft . . . breathing in and your belly puffs out . . . "belly". . . . breathing out and your belly flattens.
- Sit quietly and practice "soft belly" breathing for five minutes.

If you notice your mind wandering away, just come back to "soft . . . belly." Over time and with practice, this will happen less and less.

While learning the technique, you can put your hand on your belly to help you feel it expanding out and flattening in. The belly acts like a bellows, and when expanded out, it allows the diaphragm to drop down into the abdomen more fully, bringing oxygen to the base of the lungs.

Do this exercise for five minutes two or three times a day—though not right after meals, or you may fall asleep. You can do it at bedtime if you are having trouble falling asleep, or right before the journaling exercise I shared with you in Tier 1. Choose a time when you won't be preoccupied with how long you've been doing it or how long you have left. Soon you'll find that in times of stress you can take a few deep breaths and say "Soft . . . belly" and relaxation will come.

There are many, many options for purchasing other guided exercises like this one:

- Our website, www.immuneprogram.com, offers a Learn to Relax Kit, and individual CDs for you to get started on your own at home.

- The Center for Mind-Body Medicine website, www.cmbm.org, offers the Best of Stress Management Kit for you to learn mind-body skills on your own.
- The book *Unstuck*, by James Gordon, M.D., offers many resources and is especially useful if you are also depressed or anxious.

Other resources can be found in the appendix for:

- Great websites that offer many options, such as CDs for stress, depression, anxiety, trauma, or self-awareness.
- Recommendations of my favorite CDs for specific goals, like guided imagery to go inside to ask for guidance with a problem, or if you just want to learn how to meditate.

Remember, these are tools that need to be practiced. Commit to daily (or at least five days per week) practice for two months. Like any new muscle, it needs exercise to grow stronger. While you might struggle at the beginning—for example, if your mind won't seem to quiet down or you aren't getting an image in a visualization exercise—try not to be hard on yourself. And don't give up. Keep practicing and you will notice your body and mind will begin to respond and you will feel the benefits of the practice.

Tier 3: Lifestyle Change with Professional Help

If you are struggling in your life and making any kind of change feels overwhelming, you might benefit from seeking outside help. Help can come in the form of a religious counselor, social worker, therapist, life coach, or other health care provider. It needs to be someone with whom you feel comfortable and trust to keep your confidence.

If you have followed the steps in Tiers 1 and 2—you've made your lists and tried some new exercises from audio teachers at home—and you are still struggling to learn your new skills, it is time for a teacher in the flesh. I learned to meditate from my cousin, but also from meditation classes and retreats that I attended. There are many options for workshops around the country and I will give you resources in the appendix. But my first suggestion is to look around where you live, because a meditation teacher might be right next door.

Look for a yoga, tai chi, or qi gong class if you want something active. These classes are very mindful and meditative and will help quiet your mind so you can hear the messages from your heart.

Consider having massages, acupuncture, or other bodywork such as craniosacral therapy. It is wonderful to let someone else help you relax. I call these body-mind therapies, since they start with the body and then your mind quiets down, too. Some people, especially those who are very anxious and wound up, really need an outside person to help calm down their nervous system. In these moments of being in a quiet and relaxed state, you can go beyond the noise of your everyday life to listen deeply to your heart's desire, and to get answers to your most difficult problems.

Look for meditation classes, sometimes held at the local Y or yoga studio, or for a mind-body skills group taught by a health professional trained by the Center for Mind-Body Medicine. You can go to www .cmbm.org to find someone certified in your community. Joining a mind-body group is a great way to learn these skills in a supportive group environment. There are often therapists who work with guided imagery and visualization with their clients. See if you can find one. Some of the people trained by the Center for Mind-Body Medicine do individual consults. What always amazes me is that once you start looking, the right person shows up. This is called synchronicity. Open your eyes and look around.

How to Improve Your Self-Care: Treatment Plan for Self-Assessment 3

Self-care is the heart of all health care. Statistics prove that good self-care helps prevent diseases, and it is necessary for you to recover from and reverse chronic illness. You measured your self-care in Self-Assessment 3. The higher your score, the more you really need to focus on this section because your bathtub drain is seriously wide open. In other words, if your adrenal glands aren't pooped yet, they will be soon. You really want your score to be less than 10. Let's take a look at your self-care checklist and see how I can help. You have learned how to manage your stress better by adopting new mind-body techniques and ways to relax; now we will look at the rest of the self-care checklist.

Sleep

A good night's sleep is critical for your self-care routine and is an important part of keeping your stress system in balance.

Tier 1: Tips for Sleeping Better That You Can Do on Your Own

Are you going to sleep after midnight? It turns out that going to bed by 10:00 p.m. or even 11:00 p.m. gives your body the best rest. That's because 10:00 p.m. until midnight are key hours for your adrenal glands to get recharged for the next day. So your first step is to make a new bedtime. Ask yourself why you are going to sleep so late. I find that most people do so because they're enjoying solitude after spending a long day taking care of others. If this rings true for you, it is important to acknowledge it and find some time for yourself earlier in the day. If you're going to bed late because of others, perhaps a partner or spouse is keeping you awake, I encourage you to address this directly and work out a compromise. And finally, if you are staying up too late because you don't think you can fall asleep any earlier, then our suggestions below should really help.

To set the stage for a good night's sleep, do the following:

- **Four hours before bedtime:** Complete any strenuous exercise. Exercise elevates your body temperature, which can make it harder to sleep. Regular exercise earlier in the day, however, promotes healthy sleep. If you're eating a heavy dinner, finish now so that it is fully digested before you go to bed. Stop drinking any caffeinated beverages. This is a general rule so that the caffeine doesn't disturb your sleep. However, some people find that they need to stop drinking these as early as midday or that they need to quit drinking them completely. Though caffeine may not keep you from falling asleep, it can be a cause of disturbed sleep later on in the night. This is especially true if you are going through menopause and waking up in the middle of the night has become a problem for you.
- **Three hours before bedtime:** If you're eating a lighter dinner, finish it now. Also, stop drinking any alcohol-containing drinks. It may seem like alcohol will make it easier to fall asleep, but it can actually cause you to wake up several times throughout the night. Limiting or eliminating alcohol completely is important for healing your adrenal glands. If you are drinking every day, cut back to the weekends only. Or consider eliminating it completely for two weeks to see if it has contributed to your sleep problem. This is especially true if you are waking up during the night with hot flashes or night sweats from menopause.
- **One hour before bedtime:** Turn off all electronics. This includes your TV, computer, phone, iPad, etc. Both the light from the screen and the

stimulation from what you're watching keep your brain in the on position. Start to wind down with a nightly routine that includes soothing activities such as a warm (not hot) bath or shower, soothing music, lighting a scented candle, and/or reading an uplifting book.

- **At bedtime:** Go to bed at the same time every night, even on weekends. This helps to regulate your body's internal clock. For the same reason, it's also important to keep a steady wake-up time in the morning, even on weekends. Be sure your bed is comfortable. The life of a standard mattress is about ten years. Keep your bedroom cool, dark, and quiet and reserve the bed for sex and sleep only. Watching television and even reading in bed can increase tension and anxiety and wake the brain.
- **Relax into sleep:** Meditation, progressive relaxation, breathing awareness, and guided imagery can all help the body and mind prepare for sleep. You can also try the soft belly exercise in this book (page 145) and see if that does the trick.

If none of the above help you sleep better, move on to Tier 2 treatment.

Special note if you are taking sleep medication: Follow the guidelines for better sleep in this section and then see if you can fall asleep on your own. If you can't fall asleep within thirty minutes, take your sleep aid as usual. When you are ready to discontinue your sleep aid, we suggest you taper off slowly, which might mean taking it at a lower dose and/or taking it every other day. If you have any concerns about tapering off a medication that you have been prescribed by your doctor, make sure to call him or her with any questions before changing anything.

Tier 2: Supplements and CDs

These are the supplements I prefer to use and recommend to resolve sleep issues. Keep in mind that you might need to try a few to find what works best for you.

- **Theanine.** This is a very safe compound extracted from green tea. It is especially good for people who are a bit anxious or have a noisy mind preventing them from falling asleep. I suggest 100 mg at bedtime. You can also take 100 mg in the middle of the night if you wake up and can't fall back to sleep. I've recommended this supplement for many years and have rarely seen it cause a morning hangover.
- **Herbal blends with valerian and passionflower.** These herbs have been around for centuries and are both relaxing and sleep inducing. With my

patients, I use a brand called Mycocalm PM, which will help you fall asleep and stay asleep.

- **5-HTP.** 5-hydroxytryptophan is the precursor for serotonin, one of the brain chemicals that help regulate your body's sleep and wake cycles, and I often recommend this for sleep in my patients who are also depressed or feeling in low spirits. If you are taking an antidepressant, consult with your doctor before taking this supplement. I typically recommend 100 mg at bedtime, which will help you stay asleep, though not fall asleep.

These supplements have fewer side effects (such as morning drowsiness, dizziness, and headaches) the next morning than prescription sleep medications.

Mind-body exercises to help you fall asleep:

- Choose a sleep CD from the resource list on page 325.
- Try journaling thirty minutes before bed. First, close your eyes and focus on your breath for a few minutes, or focus on "soft belly" breathing. Then write down everything that is on your mind. I call this downloading your thoughts before bed so they don't wake you during the night. You can also ask yourself a question and then write down the answer, for example: "What is on my mind?" or "How do I feel right now?" Most people find this very helpful. There are some great books that can guide you, and you can find my suggestions in the resource list on page 325.

Tier 3: Getting Professional Help

There are many professionals who can help you figure out how to sleep better at night. Some options include:

- Find a functional medicine practitioner at www.functionalmedicine .org.
- You can go to a naturopath or chiropractor who is skilled in using nutritional supplements to guide you.
- If you are in perimenopause or menopause and hot flashes are waking you up, you can try acupuncture or homeopathy, or go to a functional medicine practitioner, to balance your hormones.

Continue working through this book to fix your other foundations, because inflammation from food, digestive issues, or too many toxins can stimulate the body, making it hard to sleep.

Eating without Stress

In Chapter 2, "Using Food as Medicine," I focused on what to eat for a healthy immune system. In Chapter 3, "Using Food as Medicine Workbook," I gave you a mindful eating exercise to help you notice what you feel when you eat. Here I will add another important nutritional piece: *how* you eat is just as important as *what* you eat.

Tiers 1 and 2: Tips for Stress-Free Eating You Can Do on Your Own

- Eat breakfast, lunch, a snack, and dinner every day. Going more than four hours without eating activates your stress system. Have a mid-morning snack if your lunch is more than four hours after breakfast.
- On the weekend, plan your food for the upcoming week so you can go shopping and have everything you need.
- If you work outside your home, bring your lunch and snacks with you, planning and packing them up the night before.
- Have the majority of your calories before 3:00 p.m. Your fire burns brightest with the sun, so the morning and lunchtime are when your metabolism is at its peak. People who don't eat all day are often ravenous at night and crave all sorts of food since their body is missing the nutrients it needs.

Tier 3: Getting Help

Consider going to a functional medicine practitioner, nutritionist, or health coach to help you figure out the right food plan for you. Sometimes even the best intentions aren't enough, and finding the right person to help you get organized and to be your coach and cheerleader really helps.

Exercise

This is a big topic and largely outside the scope of this book. There are many studies looking at exercise and the effects it has on everything from the immune system to diabetes and cancer, but we won't review all that information here. Exercise is really good for making healthy T cells and killer cells, in addition to the positive effects it has on your adrenal glands. Exercise also helps close the bathtub drain; it is an important part of self-care, and you must make a plan for moving your body and keeping it active. For my patients with extreme fatigue, this is often the last thing we focus on, waiting until the fatigue lessens and their energy is on the way up, before getting started. If you are very tired, you can put this last on your list and work on the other sections of the book first. But don't forget to come back!

When you are ready to get going, these are the tips:

Tier 1: Exercise on Your Own

If you are overweight and new to exercise, it is always good to have your primary care physician give you the okay to exercise before beginning any program. Once you are cleared, on your own, you can begin to walk outside if the weather (and your knees) permit. I generally recommend two hours per week of something aerobic. Aerobic means you have mild difficulty talking while you are exercising. So pick up the pace if you are out for a stroll; you should feel warm and slightly out of breath. Of course, this is the minimum to reap the health benefits we are looking for, and you can increase the pace or the time you spend if you want to increase your fitness level.

Tier 2: Exercise Resources You Can Buy

When you are ready to go beyond walking on your own, the next thing to add is upper-body weight-bearing exercises to prevent osteoporosis. And while walking is good for your heart and hips, you need to strengthen your spine with other exercises. You can join a gym and go to yoga or other strength-training classes, or you can buy a video or watch online classes or trainers give you instructions.

Tier 3: Exercise Help on the Way

I often recommend that my patients get a personal trainer for several sessions, either at the gym or with someone who will come to their home. A trainer can design an exercise program for you that you can then do on your own. After the initial investment, you will have a personalized program that takes into account your personal physical limitations and health concerns. A physical therapist can also design a home program, and may actually be covered by your insurance.

How to Treat Your Tired Adrenal Glands:
Treatment Plan for Self-Assessment 4

If you scored high on this section, you have tired adrenal glands; if you scored over a 20, they are really exhausted. In order to heal your immune system and reverse your autoimmune disease, you need to treat your adrenal fatigue.

Tier 1: Using Food as Medicine:
Foods That Support Your Adrenal Glands

In general, the adrenal glands are happiest when your blood sugar stays nice and even all day. This means no wild ups and downs. How to do this? Eliminate all white flour and white sugar. Eat only breads and baked goods that are whole-grain and high in fiber, limiting yourself to one to two servings of gluten-free grains per day. (We talked about gluten in Chapter 3, "Using Food as Medicine Workbook.") Stop drinking soft drinks and adding sugar to your tea and coffee.

Eat protein with all your meals and snacks, as this will stabilize your blood sugar. I recommend plant protein from nuts, seeds, organic non-GM soy (in moderation), and legumes, in addition to free-range organic chicken and grass-fed beef. Adrenaline is made from the amino acid tyrosine, so you want to eat plenty of tyrosine to support this important energy hormone. Tyrosine is found in almonds, dairy products, lima beans, and pumpkin and sesame seeds.

While I find dairy causes nausea, reflux, gas, bloating, sinus congestion, postnasal drip, acne, or joint pain in most of my patients, if you did the elimination diet in Chapter 3 and found dairy did not cause any of these symptoms, then feel free to eat organic yogurt as part of your program. It is the healthiest dairy option. But honestly, I find 90 percent of my patients feel better without dairy in their lives. Remember, there is plenty of calcium in other foods, so you don't need to eat dairy for healthy bones.

Also, include healthy fats from avocado, coconut, fish, nuts, or seeds with every meal. Cortisol and other adrenal hormones are made from cholesterol, so it isn't good to let your cholesterol get lower than 140. Eating healthy fat is good for lowering inflammation as well. Tyrosine is also found in avocados, another good reason to eat them.

In addition to tyrosine and healthy fat, your adrenal glands need B vitamins, especially B_5, which is otherwise known as pantothenic acid, and B_6, a key vitamin for the production of adrenaline and many other critical functions in the body. Remember, vitamin levels decrease dramatically when the foods are frozen or canned. The vitamins will best be retained if you lightly cook the foods or eat them raw. Excellent sources of vitamin B_5 include cremini and shiitake mushrooms, calf's liver, yogurt, eggs, cauliflower, cucumbers, avocados, asparagus, broccoli, celery, turnip greens, tomatoes, sweet potatoes, collard greens, chard, and bell peppers.

Excellent sources of vitamin B_6 include summer and winter squash, bell peppers, turnip greens, shiitake and cremini mushrooms, spinach, cauliflower, mustard greens, cabbage, asparagus, broccoli, kale, collard greens, Brussels sprouts, green beans, leeks, tomatoes, garlic, tuna, cod, chard, calf's liver, turkey, and salmon.

In the next chapter, "Understanding the Stress Connection Recipes," you'll find ten delicious dishes that use these ingredients. Have fun experimenting!

Tier 2: Supplements for Adrenal Support

There are four kinds of supplements for your adrenal glands. Adaptogens are a class of herbs that increase your body's resistance to physical, chemical, and biological stressors. They help you adapt and function well under different conditions. Think of them like a nourishing balancer of stress hormones and also of the immune, nervous, and cardiovascular systems. There are three classic herbs that are adaptogens for the adrenal glands. They can be taken as individual supplements, but they are often blended together in an adrenal support formula. Keep in mind that the doses of each one can be lower when you buy the blended formulas. You can find the latest information about these products on our website, www.immuneprogram.com. In general, I usually recommend starting with one in the morning and one with lunch.

- Eleuthero (Siberian ginseng) or Asian ginseng, herbs that originated in Russia and China, are traditionally used during times of high stress to support adrenal function. The typical dose is 100–200 mg of ginseng, standardized to contain 4 to 5 percent ginsenosides.
- Rhodiola is a very popular herb to support the adrenal glands. The typical dose is 100–200 mg per day of a *Rhodiola rosea* extract standardized to contain 2–3 percent rosavins and 0.8–1.0 percent salidroside.

- Ashwagandha has been used in Ayurvedic medicine in India for hundreds of years. If taken alone, a typical dose of ashwagandha is 500 mg once a day.

B vitamins are very important. Take 300–1,000 mg per day of B_5 and 30–100 mg per day of B_6.

Licorice is a great herb for people with inflammation, especially arthritis or muscle tenderness. But don't take more than 500 mg per day of licorice unless you are under the guidance of a professional or if you have high blood pressure. A good starting dose is 50–100 mg per day.

DHEA is also important, especially for people with autoimmune diseases such as lupus or Sjögren's, but it should be taken under the guidance of a professional (see Tier 3). I will also talk more about this in detail in Chapter 14, "Infections and Specific Autoimmune Conditions."

Tier 3: Getting Professional Help

If you aren't sure what to do, or if you have severe adrenal fatigue and are just too overwhelmed to try this on your own, you can get help from an integrative medicine practitioner. Find a physician, naturopath, chiropractor, or osteopath who is trained in functional medicine at www.functionalmedicine.org. A new certification program is currently being established, and soon there will be a list of certified practitioners. You can also go to one of the functional medicine laboratory websites, such as Genova Diagnostics, www.gdx.net, or Metametrix labs, www.metametrix.com, and find a practitioner who is regularly using their services. That is a great way to locate someone who is actively practicing functional medicine.

Practitioners trained in acupuncture, herbal medicine, homeopathy, and naturopathy (naturopathic doctors) are all able to treat adrenal fatigue. You can integrate these approaches with functional medicine or use them alone if there are no functional medicine options where you live.

Make sure the practitioner you see gives you the following tests:

- Adrenal saliva test to evaluate the twenty-four-hour pattern in your adrenal glands. It isn't enough to be high or low in one measurement, as this doesn't give us the complete picture.
- Blood work to measure DHEA, an important hormone made by the adrenal glands. Since this level drops with age, there is no one good number for everyone. However, if you are under sixty and your level is

under 60 mcg/dl, it is a sign of tired adrenal glands. Your DHEA level will slowly increase as you do all the treatment steps in this chapter. You can also take a DHEA supplement under the guidance of a health practitioner, because your blood levels need to be checked every six months. The usual starting dose in my office is 25 mg/day.

- Blood work to measure testosterone levels. In my lab, the range for total testosterone is 5–45 ng/dl for women, 200–800 ng/dl for men. I have found that both men and women feel best when their numbers are in the top half of the range. Under the supervision of a doctor, women should increase testosterone by taking DHEA, fixing their adrenal glands (by following this chapter), and adding 1–2 tablespoons of ground flaxseeds to the daily diet. Flaxseeds will block the enzyme that drops testosterone by converting it to estrogen. For men, stress management and ground flaxseeds are the first step. If after reading this book and doing all the steps your testosterone levels haven't come up, ask your doctor for topical testosterone cream or gel.

CHAPTER 7

Understanding the Stress Connection Recipes

By now you know that there are many different kinds of stressors—emotional and physical events or situations that cause reactions from your nervous system and adrenal glands. In terms of food, stressors come from a diet that contains too much processed sugar and caffeine and too little protein. Going for longer than four hours without eating is also a dietary stressor. If you keep eating this way for more than a year, you're creating chronic stress, which can damage both your adrenal glands and your immune system. But you *can* change the way you are eating to nourish your adrenal glands.

This is how we use food as medicine: eat plenty of protein, especially the amino acid tyrosine, which makes adrenaline; healthy fats, because cortisol is made from cholesterol (yes, you *need* some cholesterol); and foods high in vitamins B_5 and B_6, the specific B vitamins that help the adrenal glands. Our culinary director, Marti Wolfson, created recipes for me that include avocados and almonds, foods rich in the amino acid tyrosine and the good fats, omega-3s and monounsaturated fatty acids. The recipes in this chapter are also high in protein, a nutrient that helps you feel full longer and gives you sustained energy for several hours after you eat. Protein keeps your blood sugar level nice and even throughout the day, preventing the ups and downs that make you feel tired and cranky. It is a big stressor for your body when your blood sugar plummets, so eating protein regularly throughout the day will help stabilize it and take the pressure off your adrenal glands. Though some recipes contain chicken and salmon, there are many with terrific vegetarian sources of protein, such as beans, soy, and quinoa.

Recipes
Pesto Scrambled Eggs
Weekend Frittata

Spicy Black Bean Quinoa Salad
Ginger Bok Choy
Lemony Kale and Avocado Salad
Cinnamon Mashed Sweet Potatoes
Mushroom Tempeh "Scaloppine"
Mediterranean Chickpea Patties with Red Bell Pepper Sauce
Cod with Puttanesca Sauce
Coconut Chicken with Almond Lime Sauce
Chocolate Avocado Pudding

Menu 1

Breakfast
Pesto Scrambled Eggs

Lunch
Mediterranean Chickpea Patties with Red Bell Pepper Sauce

Dinner
Coconut Chicken with Almond Lime Sauce
Cinnamon Mashed Sweet Potatoes
Ginger Bok Choy

Dessert
Chocolate Avocado Pudding

Menu 2

Breakfast
Weekend Frittata

Lunch
Mushroom Tempeh "Scaloppine"
Spicy Black Bean Quinoa Salad

Dinner
Cod with Puttanesca Sauce
Lemony Kale and Avocado Salad

Pesto Scrambled Eggs

Eggs are an excellent source of protein. Plus the yolk contains essential minerals and vitamins as well as healthy fats. Just make sure to look for free-range, organic, or cage-free eggs since these have the highest amount of omega-3 fats, which support the health of your adrenal glands. The pesto adds more color and nutrition to same old scrambled eggs and is something that can be made all year by using seasonal greens, including basil, arugula, kale, or parsley. Store it in the freezer in small containers or an ice cube tray so you can defrost just what you need.

Makes 2 servings

4 eggs
2 cups basil
½ cup toasted walnuts
1 tbsp white or yellow miso paste*
Juice of ½ lemon
1 clove garlic, minced
Salt
¼–½ cup extra-virgin olive oil

1. Whisk eggs in a medium bowl and set aside.
2. In a food processor, combine basil, walnuts, miso, lemon juice, garlic, and a generous pinch of salt. As the food processor is running, slowly drizzle in the olive oil until a smooth consistency is reached. Add salt and additional lemon juice to taste.
3. Heat 1 tbsp olive oil in a medium nonstick pan over medium heat. Add the eggs to the pan along with 1 heaping tablespoon of pesto.
4. Mix the pesto into the eggs as you move the eggs around in the pan continuously.
5. As soon as the eggs are cooked through, remove from the heat.

Weekend Frittata

A frittata is a cross between an omelet and a quiche. It's an omelet that's finished in the oven and doesn't have the unhealthy pastry crust of a

---

*Miso gives this recipe a cheesy Parmesan-like taste. But if you prefer not to eat soy, you can skip the miso altogether and add an extra pinch of salt.

quiche. Frittatas are also an easy way to create a beautiful and nutritious dish for friends and family, so it's ideal for Sunday brunches or other get-togethers at home. We add greens to this weekend frittata for color and to boost the detox benefits for your liver. Here we make it with Swiss chard, but you can try it with any of your favorite greens, such as spinach, broccoli, and kale, since they are rich in B vitamins, antioxidants, and phytonutrients, all good nutrients for the adrenal glands.

Makes 8 servings

5 tbsp extra-virgin olive oil
1 medium onion, thinly sliced
2 cups sliced mushrooms
2 cups Swiss chard, washed and trimmed of stems, cut into ribbons
8 eggs
1 cup Parmesan or goat cheese (optional)
¼ cup chopped parsley
Salt
Freshly ground black pepper

1. Preheat oven to 400 degrees.
2. Heat a large 10–12-inch nonstick pan on medium-high heat. Add 2 tbsp oil to the pan.
3. Add the onions, spreading them out evenly. Let them brown for about 7 minutes.
4. Turn the heat down to medium and continue to let the onions caramelize, moving them around to release some moisture, about 8 minutes more.
5. Then add the mushrooms and sauté together until they have released their moisture and are cooked through, about 5 minutes.
6. When the mushrooms are nearly done, add the Swiss chard and sauté until barely wilted. Remove the mixture from the pan and set aside.
7. Clean out the pan and set it back on the heat. Add 3 tbsp oil.
8. In a large bowl, beat the eggs with a little water. Add a generous pinch of salt and pepper.
9. Add the herbs, cheese, and vegetables to the eggs.
10. Pour the egg and vegetable mixture into the skillet and then turn the heat down to medium-low. Cook, undisturbed, until the mixture firms up on the bottom, then transfer it to the oven.
11. Bake until the top is cooked, about 10 minutes.

Spicy Black Bean Quinoa Salad

Some foods go really well together, and one great example is quinoa and beans. Together, they pack a big protein punch. It's no wonder people in South America have been eating this combination for centuries. This salad takes on the wonderful Latin flavors of cumin, jalapeño, and lime to create a nice lunchtime salad or side dish.

Makes 4–6 servings

1 cup quinoa
1¾ cups water
Salt
Juice of 1½ limes
1 tsp cumin
3 tbsp olive oil
1½ cups cooked black beans
2 scallions, thinly sliced
2 small cloves garlic, minced
1 red bell pepper, diced small
½ cucumber, peeled, seeded, and diced small
1 small jalapeño, minced
2 tbsp chopped cilantro

1. Rinse the quinoa in a fine mesh strainer under cool water. Place the drained quinoa in a pot on medium-high heat, and cook for 2–3 minutes or until the water is absorbed and the quinoa releases a nutty aroma. We use this stovetop technique, sometimes called toasting, to quickly release the flavor of a nut or seed before boiling.
2. Add the water and a generous pinch of salt and bring to a boil.
3. Cover the pot, lower the heat, and simmer for 15 minutes or until all of the water is absorbed.
4. Fluff the quinoa with a fork into a medium bowl and let it cool.
5. Mix the lime juice, cumin, oil, and salt until well combined.
6. Pour over the quinoa and toss with a fork.
7. Add the black beans, scallions, garlic, red pepper, cucumber, jalapeño, and cilantro and toss again. Add additional salt and lime juice to taste.

Ginger Bok Choy

Bok choy is a common ingredient in Asian cooking and marries well with more intense flavors such as ginger, tamari, and sesame oil. Bok choy is a vegetable that's rich in antioxidants, vitamin C, and vitamin B_6, all of which are necessary for healthy adrenal glands. The ginger aids in digestion and inflammation, which is good for immune health.

Makes 6 servings

1 pound baby bok choy
2 tbsp light sesame oil
1 shallot, thinly sliced
2 tbsp minced fresh ginger
1 tbsp mirin
1½ tbsp balsamic vinegar
Juice of ½ lime
Salt
¼ tsp toasted sesame oil

1. Trim off the bases of the bok choy and discard.
2. Cut each piece in half lengthwise.
3. Heat the light sesame oil in a wok or large sauté pan over medium-high heat, then add the shallot and ginger and sauté for 30 seconds.
4. Add the bok choy, mirin, and balsamic vinegar and sauté for about 3 minutes or until the leaves are wilted and the stems have a nice crunch.
5. Turn off the heat and add lime juice, a generous pinch of salt, and the toasted sesame oil.

Lemony Kale and Avocado Salad

Kale has stepped into the culinary spotlight, and for good reason—kale is rich in iron and one of the most nutrient-dense vegetables available. It is high in beta-carotene, vitamin K, vitamin C, calcium, and phytonutrients. For your adrenal glands, kale provides lots of B_6, and for your liver, it offers lots of antioxidants for incredible additional support for your detox pathways. Think of this salad like ceviche in that the lemon helps to tenderize the kale. Another bonus: kale salads are wonderful because

(continued on next page)

they hold up for at least five days in the refrigerator, so you can make a big bowl and enjoy it throughout the whole week.

Makes 4–6 servings

Juice of 1 or 2 lemons (depending on the size of the bunch of kale)
¼ cup olive oil
½ tsp salt
1 bunch kale, either curly or Tuscan, center rib discarded and leaves chopped
¼ cup peeled carrot, shredded
1 avocado, cubed
¼ cup raisins (optional)
¼ cup toasted sunflower seeds

1. Mix the lemon juice, olive oil, and salt.
2. Pour over kale and carrots and let it sit for at least an hour.
3. Then add the raisins, avocado, and sunflower seeds.
4. This can be made and refrigerated overnight.

Cinnamon Mashed Sweet Potatoes

Sweet potatoes are a delicious and satisfying substitute for high-sugar and high-carb side dishes such as white potatoes, corn, and white rice. They are an excellent source of beta-carotene and potassium. We oven-roast them to bring out their natural sweetness. Ghee adds a velvety texture and is naturally healing to the gut. With just a touch of ginger, cinnamon, and maple syrup, this flavorful side dish is sure to please the entire family.

Makes 6 servings

2 lbs sweet potatoes, peeled and cut into 1-inch cubes
2 tbsp extra-virgin olive oil
¼ tsp ground cinnamon
½ tsp ground ginger or 1 tsp freshly grated ginger
Salt
Freshly ground pepper
1 tsp maple syrup

1 tbsp ghee*
½ cup vegetable stock
Squeeze of lemon juice (optional)

1. Preheat oven to 375 degrees.
2. Line a baking sheet with parchment paper.
3. Toss the potatoes with the oil, cinnamon, ginger, ½ tsp salt, and ¼ tsp pepper until well coated. Spread out on the baking sheet.
4. Roast for 25–30 minutes or until soft and tender.
5. While the potatoes are roasting, heat the stock in a small saucepan until steaming.
6. Transfer the potatoes to a food processor; add the maple syrup, ghee, stock, and a pinch of salt and process until smooth.
7. If you feel it needs a little brightness in flavor, add a squeeze of lemon juice.

Mushroom Tempeh "Scaloppine"

This is an elegant vegetarian version of scaloppine with savory notes from the garlic, wine, and mushrooms. Tempeh is a fermented soy protein, originally from Indonesia. It is meatier in texture than tofu, and because it is fermented it is considered a probiotic food like yogurt. The cremini mushrooms are very high in pantothenic acid, vitamin B_5, which is a critical vitamin for your adrenal glands.

Makes 4 servings

1 package tempeh†
1 egg, beaten
¼ cup gluten-free bread crumbs
¼ cup almond flour
Salt
Freshly ground pepper

* Ghee is clarified butter, which means that the milk proteins are gone, leaving behind the clear oil that is good for your gut. You can have ghee if you are dairy sensitive because it has no milk proteins or sugar. To buy ghee, see our Pantry Shopping List at the end of Chapter 3.
† If you're avoiding soy, simply substitute boneless chicken breasts. Pound out the chicken until it's ⅛-inch thick. Skip steps 1 and 2 and proceed with the other directions.

(continued on next page)

1 tbsp extra-virgin olive oil
½ cup vegetable broth
¼ cup cooking wine
1 cup cremini mushrooms, sliced
1 tsp dried crushed oregano
1 tbsp ghee
Lemon wedges
2 tbsp minced parsley

1. Fit a steamer basket in a medium pot with just enough water in the bottom to not come through the basket. Place the tempeh in the pot, cover, and bring to a boil. Steam the tempeh for 10 minutes.
2. Remove the tempeh from the pot and set to the side to cool.
3. While the tempeh cools, beat the egg and set aside. Mix the bread crumbs, almond flour, and generous pinches of salt and pepper together in a shallow dish.
4. Cut ¼-inch-thick slices of the tempeh crosswise on an angle in order to get wide slices.
5. Dredge the tempeh in egg and then dip the tempeh into the bread crumb mixture and coat both sides well, shaking off any excess.
6. Heat the oil in a medium sauté pan over medium-high heat.
7. Add the tempeh and cook about 3–4 minutes on each side or until golden.
8. Remove from the pan and set aside. Clean out the pan and then add the broth and wine on medium-high heat. Bring to a simmer.
9. Add the mushrooms, a pinch of salt, and the oregano.
10. Simmer for about 10 minutes or until the sauce reduces and thickens.
11. Once the sauce thickens, whisk in the ghee.
12. Add salt and a squeeze of lemon to taste.
13. Add the tempeh and parsley to the sauce and heat for another minute.

Mediterranean Chickpea Patties with Red Bell Pepper Sauce

Chickpeas or garbanzo beans are an excellent source of protein as well as thiamin and vitamin B_6, two essential B vitamins that convert food into energy. These chickpea burgers get an extra boost from anti-inflammatory spices such as cumin and paprika and a silky, spicy sauce made with roasted red peppers and tahini, which is high in zinc, another nutrient critical for a healthy immune system. You can reap the most nutrition from these beans by cooking them yourself, as they lose some of their nutrients when they come in a can.

Makes 6 servings

2½ cups cooked chickpeas
4 tbsp extra-virgin olive oil
½ cup chopped onion
½ cup chopped celery
2 tbsp gluten-free flour
2 tbsp chopped parsley
1 tbsp paprika
¼ tsp ground mustard
Pinch red pepper flakes
1 tsp salt
1 tsp ground cumin
Red Bell Pepper Sauce (recipe follows)
½ cup toasted slivered almonds, for garnish

1. Put the chickpeas in a food processor with the metal blade and process until ground.
2. In a sauté pan, heat 2 tbsp olive oil over medium heat. Add the onion and celery and sauté until softened, about 5 minutes.
3. Transfer the chickpeas to a large bowl and add the sautéed vegetables, flour, parsley, paprika, mustard, red pepper flakes, salt, and cumin.
4. Add a bit of water if the mixture seems too dry and crumbly and doesn't stick together.
5. Using your hands, form the mixture into 6 patties about 3 inches in diameter and 1 inch thick.
6. Heat 2 tbsp olive oil in a sauté pan on medium high heat and cook until golden brown, about 4 minutes per side.
7. To serve, pour ½ cup of Red Bell Pepper Sauce onto each plate. Place a warm cake in the center and sprinkle with slivered almonds.

Red Bell Pepper Sauce

Makes about 1 cup

2 roasted red bell peppers
2 tbsp tahini (amount may vary if you have a drier or more
    liquid tahini)
Pinch of salt
1 small clove garlic, minced
Pinch of cayenne
Juice of ½ lemon
1 tbsp parsley
¼ tsp ground cumin

1. Place all ingredients in a blender and blend until smooth and
   creamy.
2. If using a drier tahini, you may need to add a little water or olive oil
   to achieve the desired consistency.

Cod with Puttanesca Sauce

Puttanesca is one of those sauces that anyone can make in no time and
produce an elegant, flavorful dish. And it elevates mild, omega-3-rich
cod to another level. At the end of a staff meeting on a warm spring day,
my team enjoyed this light dish. Serve with Lemony Kale and Avocado
Salad for a complete meal.

Makes 4 servings

1 lb cod fillet
Salt
Freshly ground pepper
2 tbsp extra-virgin olive oil
½ medium onion, sliced
3 cloves garlic, finely chopped
¼ cup pitted Kalamata olives
1 tbsp capers, drained
⅓ cup dry white wine
14-oz can Italian plum tomatoes, partially drained
1 tbsp chopped fresh parsley

1. Preheat the oven to 375 degrees.
2. Season the fish on both sides with salt and pepper and place on a lightly oiled baking sheet.
3. Place in the oven and cook for 10 to 12 minutes, or until the fish starts to flake. Time will depend on the thickness of the fillet. Once the fish is done, remove from the oven and keep warm.
4. While the fish cooks, heat the oil in a large pan over medium-high heat. Add the onion and cook for 3 to 5 minutes until the onion is translucent.
5. Add the chopped garlic and continue cooking until softened and fragrant.
6. Add the olives and capers and cook for 2 more minutes, until heated through.
7. Add the wine, tomatoes, and parsley. Increase the heat and bring the mixture to a boil. Cook for 4 to 5 minutes, breaking the tomatoes up as they cook, until the sauce has thickened and the excess liquid has evaporated.
8. Taste for seasoning and adjust if necessary.
9. Place the fish on a plate and spoon some sauce over the top. Transfer the remainder of the sauce to a bowl and serve with the fish.

Coconut Chicken with Almond Lime Sauce

Chicken is a great source of protein for an adrenal-friendly diet. Look for organic free-range chicken, since the hormones and antibiotics in conventional chicken can put more stress on already fatigued adrenal glands. These moist chicken tenders get a nice crunch by being coated in shredded coconut and gluten-free bread crumbs. If you can't find gluten-free bread crumbs, you can easily make your own from gluten-free bread or crackers.

Makes 4–6 servings

½ cup almond flour
½ cup coconut flakes, unsweetened
½ cup gluten-free bread crumbs
½ teaspoon salt
¼ teaspoon pepper
1 egg
1 lb chicken tenders
Almond Lime Sauce (recipe follows)   (continued on next page)

1. Preheat oven to 400 degrees.
2. Mix the almond meal, coconut flakes, bread crumbs, salt, and pepper in a shallow bowl.
3. Beat the egg in a separate bowl.
4. Coat one piece of chicken in egg and then dredge in the almond flour mixture, shaking off any excess.
5. Place chicken on a baking sheet lined with parchment paper and bake approximately 20 minutes or until chicken is cooked and the outside is slightly crispy. Baking time will depend on the thickness of the chicken tenders.
6. Serve with Almond Lime Sauce.

Almond Lime Sauce

This delicious dipping sauce is rich in tyrosine, the amino acid that helps make both adrenaline and thyroid hormones. My sixteen-year-old son thought this tasted like Thousand Island dressing, which was just about the best news I had heard in a long time! (If you have teenagers, you know what I mean.) He couldn't get enough of the coconut chicken, either.

Makes 1 cup

¼ cup almond butter
Juice of ½ lime
½ tbsp maple syrup
½ tsp toasted sesame oil
½ tbsp balsamic vinegar
Pinch red pepper flakes
2 tbsp water

1. Place all the ingredients in a blender and blend until smooth and creamy.
2. Depending on the almond butter, more water might be necessary.

Chocolate Avocado Pudding

Remember the commercial in which people exclaimed, "I can't believe it's not butter"? This pudding will have your tasters saying, "I can't believe it's avocado!" Avocado gives this raw pudding a smooth and fluffy texture, not to mention healthy fats and the amino acid tyrosine, which is important for hormone regulation as well as metabolism and memory. Best of all, this is rich and filling, so you won't have to eat much to satisfy your sweet tooth.

Makes 4 servings

½ medium very ripe avocado
3 tbsp unsweetened cocoa powder
2½ tbsp honey
Pinch salt
2½ tbsp coconut milk or almond milk
½ cup fresh raspberries (optional)

1. Blend all ingredients except raspberries together until smooth and creamy.
2. Chill for at least 1 hour and serve with raspberries.

PART III

Healing Your Gut

And the day came when the risk it took to remain tight inside the bud was more painful than the risk it took to blossom.

—Anaïs Nin

CHAPTER 8

Healing Your Gut

You've probably heard and even used the expression "trust your gut" or said that you had a "gut feeling," "gut instinct," or "gut reaction" to or about a situation in your life. These expressions refer to an instinctive feeling or intuition that you have deep within your core. "Gut" is also a slang term that includes your whole digestive tract, including your stomach, small intestine, and large intestine. The gut is literally at the center of your body and plays a central role in your health, just as your "gut feeling" plays a central role in your instinct. But before I go into detail about the gut and its impact on your health, let me first explain its crucial link to your immune system.

WHAT'S GUT GOT TO DO WITH IT?

Every day you expose your body to things that may cause infections or illness, such as viruses, bacteria, mold, parasites, and foreign proteins in food. These outside agents are typically brought into the body through your mouth and nose. As your first line of defense, the immune system in your gut is faced with the task of clearing out the bad agents while keeping what your body requires to stay nourished and healthy. It also has the job of repairing any damage caused by these foreign substances and any reactions they've caused in your body, such as inflammation or infection.

To carry out these important tasks, the immune system is divided into two systems. Each one plays a role in protecting you from the invaders that come into your body every day. The first is called the *innate immune system*, which is the front line of defense. These cells are always alert and ready for action and need no priming or prep time. Antigen presenting cells are one type of cell from the front line, and here's how these cells get their name: an antigen is a substance, like a bad bacteria, yeast, parasite, or virus, that is recognized as foreign when it meets up with these cells. To simplify, I often call the bad bacteria, yeasts, parasites, and viruses "invaders" or "foreigners." An important type of antigen presenting cell that makes its home in your gut are the dendritic cells, which live right under the surface of your intestinal lining in large numbers. There they lie in wait, their cell surface filled with receptors like antennae, ready to touch and then react to any foreigners that come their way. If the dendritic cells touch something they see as foreign, their job is to spread the word to the cells that make up your immune system's second line of defense. As you can see, the two important roles of your immune system's front line of defense are to recognize what is foreign and then to sound an alarm by telling other cells in the immune system to react.

The group of cells that make the second line of defense is formally known as the *adaptive immune system*, because they are cells that adapt to the alarm that's been sounded. In the gut, the dendritic cells sound the alarm and activate your immune cells (more formally known as lymphocytes), which include your T cells and B cells. Both groups of immune cells live within and underneath the lining of your intestines. While the dendritic cells respond immediately, it takes a bit of time, anywhere from hours to days, for the lymphocytes to mobilize to either make more killer cells or to make antibodies to attack the foreigner.

When this process goes smoothly, there are signals and messages sent between the dendritic cells and T cells that keep the immune system in balance. T regulator cells help turn the alarm off when the immune system's job is done. For example, let's say that there was salmonella, a type of bacteria, in something you ate for dinner last night. If things are working correctly, your dendritic cells recognize the salmonella as foreign and sound an alarm to the T cells and B cells, which then attack the bacteria and clear it out of your system. But if the T regulator cells are not working correctly, the killer cells and/or antibody-producing cells can get stuck in overdrive and become confused about what is foreign and what is not. This confusion can then cause autoimmune diseases. All of the steps in this book are aimed at balancing your killer cells and your antibody-producing cells, and to do so we must focus on fixing your T regulator cell function.

So now you can see that your digestive system has a lot of influence on your immune system. **In fact, 70 percent of your immune system lives in your gut.** Yes, you read that correctly: 70 percent. It sounds surprising at first, but it actually makes sense if you think about it. After all, you bring the outside world into your body through your mouth every day, so your front line of defense *needs* to be in your gut. Because so much of your immune system is in your gut, it's critical to keep your gastrointestinal system healthy and in balance. It is also one reason why in functional medicine we look at the gut first when it comes to any chronic disease. These immune cells release many, many inflammatory molecules when they are activated, traveling around the body and causing inflammation in your joints, hands, blood vessels, brain—you name it! Since there is always inflammation at the root of all chronic disease, the gut is the place to start.

The immune system within your gastrointestinal system is called the gut-associated lymphoid tissue, or GALT for short, and this is one of the places in your body where new immune cells are constantly growing and maturing. A lot of research is now focused on understanding what influences the maturation of T cells in the GALT because abnormal balances in these cells is an underlying problem in all autoimmune diseases.[1]

THE ROLE OF INTESTINAL BACTERIA

The good bacteria that live in your intestines have the most important influence on the function of the T cells that are located there. Besides immune cells, the gut is also home to an estimated 70 to 100 trillion beneficial bacteria of various species. Though the word "bacteria" typically has a negative connotation, flora are a natural part of us and are critical for so many of your body's functions. You may recognize the names of some of these good bacteria, like *Lactobacillus acidophilus* and bifidobacteria, because in recent years their presence in certain things such as yogurts and probiotic supplements has been highly marketed. Experts are conducting ongoing research to understand the differences between the various species of these beneficial bacteria and the importance of each one. But for the purposes of this book, we'll discuss the good bacteria in general (rather than differentiating between the various kinds) and detail the health benefits they offer, especially when it comes to the development and maintenance of your immune system.

As I have mentioned, there is an epidemic of autoimmune diseases today. **It is believed that imbalances in gut flora are a big part of the problem, causing both autoimmunity and making your symptoms and antibodies worse if you already have a diagnosed autoimmune dis-**

ease.[2,3,4,5] How does the gut flora get out of balance? One theory is called the hygiene hypothesis, and it suggests that we have been so focused on fighting germs—with things like antibiotics, antibacterial wipes, cleansers, hand sanitizers, and more—that we've sterilized our environments *too* much.[6] Many children today live in concrete jungles instead of being surrounded by dirt, trees, and grass, the way most children were generations ago. As a result, they are not exposed to the bacteria, parasites, and molds that they would naturally encounter if they played outside all day, every day. Because of this city living and our culture's obsession with banishing germs, our children live in worlds that are too clean, and without enough germs to fight, their immune systems don't develop properly. After all, it is exposure to germs when you are young that helps teach your immune cells what is bad and what is not. Then when you get older, your immune system remembers and recognizes the dangerous germs and reacts against them. Exposure to germs also brings in many good bacteria, and the gut immune system has to learn how to live with these trillions of bacteria and not attack them. Learning the difference between good and bad bacteria is called tolerance, and this tolerance is something that develops in your body when you are very young. Tolerance is very, very important because without it your immune cells get confused and begin to overreact and attack your own good flora and your tissues, which is exactly what happens in autoimmune diseases.

When you are born, your body is sterile, meaning your skin, lungs, and intestines don't contain any bacteria at all. When you pass through your mother's birth canal, you are exposed to bacteria from the outside world and your gut begins a harmonious and beneficial relationship with more than a thousand strains of good bacteria. The point is that after you are born, you need to be exposed to the many bacteria that will later live within you. In fact, the hygiene hypothesis has recently been renamed the "old friends hypothesis," with the "old friends" being the good intestinal bacteria. The most widely used approach is to rebalance the gut with herbs and probiotics (also called healthy flora supplements), which we will do in the next chapter, "Healing Your Gut Workbook," but first it is important to understand what's going on in your gut and why the bacteria that live there, or should be living there, are so crucial for a strong immune system and robust health in general.

For a healthy immune system, your body is dependent on a good relationship with the beneficial bacteria that live in your digestive tract. Although there is much evidence that other things such as toxins, stress, infections, and food trigger autoimmune diseases, the epidemic rise in autoimmune diseases in the last few decades suggests that something *inside* our bodies has changed. One of these recent changes is the balance of good bacteria. Whether you have had an imbalance of good bacteria since childhood or whether it happened later in your life from things like taking too many antibiotics and antacids, drinking too much alcohol, or experiencing too much stress, we need to focus on what we can do now, *today,* to bring your gut back into balance. A huge part of this healing includes making sure you have enough beneficial bacteria. But first let's talk about what these good bacteria are actually doing inside you.

HEALTHY FLORA AND THE IMMUNE SYSTEM

There is a lot of research looking at the bacteria that live in the gut and how they grow, develop, and help our immune systems function properly. As I mentioned before, it appears that gut flora play a huge role in early infancy in helping your immune cells develop properly and in the right balance. Beneficial bacteria also seem to help the immune system learn the difference between your own tissue and a foreign substance. Thus, the immune cells develop tolerance to these good bacteria rather than try to kill them.

Good bacteria are key players in the relationship between your immune system cells in both the first line of defense and the second. Changes in your good bacteria can have a significant influence on your body's T helper cells that, as we discussed in "Understanding the Stress Connection," help accelerate your immune system's response to a foreigner. However, these cells can get stuck in overdrive, keeping your immune response going on and on without stopping. Sometimes they get stuck making more killer cells (which, as I described earlier, is called Th1 dominance). Sometimes they get stuck making more B cells and antibodies (which is called Th2 dominance). Good bacteria help regulate this balance and help the T regulator cells work better. Ideally, we want them all to be working in balance.

Beneficial bacteria also stimulate the production of a protective antibody that's one of the main defenses in your gut. It's called immunoglobulin A, a compound made by the immune system to fight off foreign substances. (This compound is so important that one way to tell if your gut immune system is working properly is to have the levels of this antibody measured in your blood, stool, and saliva.)

Good bacteria make something called short-chain fatty acids, which feed and strengthen all the cells that line your digestive tract, keeping them healthy. They also help form your intestinal lining, the protective barrier that helps keep the food you eat and the outside world in your intestines and not in the rest of your body when you eat. Creating this barrier is no small task considering that the surface area of your intestines, if opened up and spread out, would be greater than that of a tennis court. These good bacteria interact with your immune cells to directly protect you from harmful infections and maintain the function of that barrier so that unwanted foreign proteins and infectious agents can't seep into the bloodstream. If this barrier is compromised, you can develop what is called leaky gut syndrome, a condition that can lead to autoimmune diseases. (More on that later in this chapter.)

We are constantly exposed to toxins from cleaning products, pesticides, and additives in the food we eat and the air we breathe. Our good bacteria help us begin the process of metabolizing these toxins, which means changing their form to make them less harmful. They also make enzymes that improve digestion. In particular, they help the body break down gluten, a protein found in wheat, barley, spelt, and kamut. As we discussed in Chapter 2, "Using Food as Medicine," gluten is a very toxic protein that often causes an allergic reaction or other immune response and is a big problem for people with autoimmune diseases. Properly digesting and breaking down gluten decreases the chance that your immune system will react when you eat it. **It is entirely possible that**

So what does it feel like when you don't have enough good bacteria in your gut? You can have:

- Constipation
- Diarrhea
- Gas
- Bloating after eating
- Abdominal cramping or discomfort
- Upper stomach problems such as reflux and indigestion

Fixing the bacteria imbalance is critical not only to alleviate all these gut symptoms but also for you to heal your immune system, and we will do that in the next chapter, "Healing Your Gut Workbook."

impaired digestion and a leaky gut due to a lack of beneficial gut flora are the reasons some people develop gluten issues in the first place. Lastly, good bacteria also help the body process vitamins such as B_{12} and K so they can be better utilized and absorbed by the body. **The bottom line is that having enough friendly flora in your gut reduces the incidence of allergies and autoimmune diseases,** and restoring and balancing these flora in the gut can treat and reverse these conditions as well (something else we'll discuss later in this chapter).

BELLY OUT OF BALANCE

Before we move on to healing your gut, let's look at all the things that can go wrong in the gut that harm your immune system. We will start at the top with your stomach.

YOUR DIGESTIVE POWER

I like to describe the entire digestive tract as a river. The stomach is at the top of that river and has a major influence on what the balance of good bacteria, and thus your immune health, will be downstream. The contents of the stomach empty into the small intestine, which flows into the large intestine and then out of the body. As the river flows, the stomach secretes acid and the enzyme pepsin, which begins the digestion of protein. It also secretes messengers that tell the pancreas and gallbladder to release enzymes and bile to continue the digestion process. Without adequate amounts of these acids and enzymes, food doesn't break down properly, so it sits in your stomach, refusing to leave. This poor digestion can cause reflux or heartburn.

THE IMPORTANCE OF ACID

Speaking of heartburn, another important part of your stomach is the acid it contains. If you think back to high school chemistry, you may remember that pH is a measure of how acidic or alkaline something is. There is a pH scale that goes from 0 to 14. Anything less than 7.0 is acidic, anything more than 7.0 is alkaline, and 7.0 is neutral. Many people take antacids to reduce the acid in their stomachs, yet the pH of your stomach *needs* to be 1.5, a very acid pH, for several important reasons. First, a pH of 1.5 kills any viruses and bacteria that you might ingest and prevents unwanted infections from coming into your body and stressing your immune system. (Think of it as your own personal food sterilizer.) An acid pH also helps the food in your stomach digest quickly and move forward instead of refluxing backward into your esophagus. Good bacteria are very tolerant of acid, while unfriendly flora and yeast are not, and so an acid pH will help the bacterial balance in your small intestine, which is downstream from your stomach, stay in favor of good bacteria.

The right pH is also necessary for the digestion and absorption of many vitamins and minerals, which is key because certain vitamin deficiencies can cause an array of health problems. For example, a B_{12} deficiency can harm your ability to make red blood cells, which you need to bring oxygen to tissues throughout your body. This is a condition called anemia, where you tend to feel very tired. Calcium and magnesium deficiencies can contribute to osteoporosis, a disease in which your bones become very porous and at risk for fracturing. In fact, many studies link antacids to an increase in fractures, believed to be caused by the poor absorption of minerals such as calcium and magnesium in an alkaline pH. The absorption of other minerals such as zinc, which is a key player in the immune system, is also affected. Low stomach acid can really impair your digestion of protein, which provides the body with amino acids that are critical for the creation of new tissue, especially immune cells. To have enough amino acids for a healthy immune system, you need to be eating enough protein. But you also need to digest protein properly so it can be absorbed; stomach acid helps activate your digestive enzymes so this can happen. After leaving the stomach, the food you eat moves into the upper part of the small intestine, called the duodenum. This area is where the enzymes from your pancreas and the bile from your gallbladder meet up with the food to further digest proteins, carbohydrates, and fats. These enzymes need a low pH to work well. If your stomach acid or digestive enzymes aren't doing their best, they don't finish their job, and partially digested food makes its way further down into the intestines. To have these particles traveling where they don't belong adds to the problem of leaky gut syndrome (an issue we'll discuss shortly) and increases the risk of food sensitivities and autoimmune reactions. In fact, studies have shown that people who take antacids and proton pump inhibitors have an increased risk of developing food sensitivities.

Now you can see why antacids, which many people think *help* their stomach, actually do the opposite and harm your immune system.[7] So if you regularly pop them, we need to get you off them. But don't worry.

You don't have to choose between having heartburn and your stomach having the right pH. There are other ways to treat heartburn.

What's commonly known as heartburn is caused by a stomach lining (which is called the mucosa) that has worn away, making it raw and sensitive to the amount of acid that *should* be in your stomach. As we discussed, this acidic environment is normal; it's the worn stomach lining that is not. Many things can cause this lining to wear away, including stress, alcohol, stomach bacteria called *H. pylori* that cause infections, aspirin, and medications. Once the lining is damaged, you feel the acid that it is normal to have in your stomach, but which you wouldn't feel if your lining were strong, thick, and healthy. Because acid is so important, the answer is not to get rid of it. The answer is to heal the lining, something we will do in the next chapter.

Surprisingly, many people with reflux or heartburn actually have too *little* stomach acid, a condition called hypochlorhydria. Acid is made in special cells in your stomach called parietal cells. If your stomach lining is constantly irritated, these cells can become damaged and produce less acid. It is also possible to develop antibodies to these stomach cells, a fairly common condition called autoimmune gastritis that affects up to 2 percent of the population and is even more common among those living with autoimmune diseases. For example, researchers at the University of Antwerp in Belgium found that people with type 1 diabetes and autoimmune thyroid disease were three to five times more likely to have autoimmune gastritis than those who did not have either of these conditions. Low stomach acid is also caused by *H. pylori* infection, getting older (acid levels decrease as you age), and chronic stress-related gastritis.[8] But whatever the cause, low stomach acid has been associated with many autoimmune diseases, including Addison's disease, lupus, myasthenia gravis, celiac disease, dermatitis herpetiformis, Graves' disease, pernicious anemia, rheumatoid arthritis, Sjögren's syndrome, and vitiligo.

Let me give you an example from my practice. My patient Linda, a forty-year-old African American woman, came to see me four years after she was diagnosed with Sjögren's syndrome. Sjögren's is an autoimmune condition in which antibodies attack and damage your salivary glands and tear ducts. Linda had a classic case of Sjögren's syndrome, with the common symptoms of dry mouth and eyes and joint pain. (Most patients have some sort of inflammation, usually arthritis or muscle tenderness.) Linda had also been living with constipation and abdominal pain that she said had been going on "forever," probably since her mid-twenties. She also had a persistent cough and reflux that she remembers began when her aunt died five years prior. Twelve months before she came to see me, an endoscopy revealed signs of a chronically irritated stomach lining and inflammation in her stomach. Her doctor prescribed a proton pump inhibitor (PPI), which is a medication that reduces the amount of acid in the stomach and is commonly used to treat acid reflux and heartburn. But she didn't want to stay on the medication because she was worried about developing osteoporosis and the risk of fracturing a bone, because as I mentioned earlier, numerous studies link PPIs to an increased risk of fracture. She also wanted to get off the medication because her persistent, bothersome cough, which is one of the medication's possible side effects, still lingered. As a result, she came to see me for help with her digestive issues.

One of the first things I did was to put Linda on the elimination diet that we discussed in Chapter 3, "Using Food as Medicine Workbook," removing gluten, dairy, soy, and corn for three weeks. Almost immediately, the joint pain she'd been living with for four years disappeared, a result that is pretty typical. (When we talk about leaky gut syndrome later in this chapter, I will explain how some of the foods you eat can cause inflammation in your joints.) However, we needed to go further because a stool test showed an overgrowth of yeast and bad bacteria and a lack of good bacteria in her gut. (A stool test is when a sample of your stool is sent to a laboratory for analysis.) After treating Linda's gut with herbs such as berberine and oregano and with probiotics, which are live bacterial cultures that help balance the flora in the gut, her abdominal pain and constipation were gone.

However, Linda still had reflux and, although she was free of any physical symptoms of Sjögren's syndrome (dry eyes and mouth), a blood test showed that her antibody levels for this condition were still high. So I decided to focus on her stomach and her digestive power and added two supplements to her regimen. One was a digestive enzyme and the other was something called betaine hydrochloride, which is stomach acid in a pill form. Just two weeks after she started taking these supplements, the reflux Linda had lived with for five years was finally gone. Making her stomach more acidic so that the pH was close to 1.5 activated the digestive enzymes. Linda was finally able to properly digest the foods she ate. The fact that these enzymes and extra stomach acid worked showed me that Linda's reflux was caused by poor digestion, a poor production of stomach acid, and a chronically irritated stomach lining due to stress.

Note that there are foods you can eat instead of taking supplements to boost your enzymes and stomach acid, such as apple cider vinegar and umeboshi plums; you will learn more about these foods in Chapter 9, "Healing Your Gut Workbook."

Six months after her first appointment, Linda repeated her initial lab tests. There was no sign of Sjögren's syndrome and her antibody levels were now normal. For her, all the answers to changing her health (and thus her life) sat right in her gut! The same could be true for you, as it often is for those with autoimmune conditions, which is why this part of *your immune system recovery plan* is so important.

DYSBIOSIS:
AN IMBALANCE IN YOUR GUT'S GOOD BACTERIA

When the amount of healthy bacteria in your gut is too low, a condition called dysbiosis occurs. Sometimes you might also have an overgrowth of harmful bacteria, yeast, or parasites, and this makes the dysbiosis more severe. The severity of dysbiosis can cause a lot of intestinal symptoms, and as I mentioned before, many people are given a diagnosis of irritable bowel syndrome because they have chronic constipation, diarrhea, gas, bloating, abdominal cramps, or nausea after they eat, and sometimes they also don't feel good after they eat any food at all. In addition to your digestive symptoms, these changes in your gut flora have profound effects on both your immune system's first and second lines of defense, and so it is not surprising that an imbalance has been linked to autoimmune diseases.

Researchers at the University of Arizona College of Medicine recently reviewed the literature on this topic and found good evidence that dysbiosis plays a role in rheumatoid arthritis and, in animal studies, multiple sclerosis. Because we are just now beginning to understand this relationship, research in this area should really explode in the years to come.

There are five types of dysbiosis. Unfortunately, you can have more than one kind of dysbiosis at the same time.

The mildest form of dysbiosis is *insufficient good bacteria*. Here you have a lack of the beneficial bacteria needed to balance the gut.

Next is *small intestinal bacterial overgrowth (SIBO)*, which occurs in the upper part of the small intestine when bacteria from the colon grow in the wrong place. People with SIBO might also have stomach symptoms such as heartburn and reflux.

The third type is *immunosuppressive dysbiosis*. Here toxins from harmful bacteria, yeast, or a parasite lower your levels of good bacteria and give off toxins that weaken or break down the gut lining and cause leaky gut syndrome. People often get this form of dysbiosis when they have an overgrowth of yeast in the body, which is what happened to Linda. I discovered this after seeing the results of her stool test. Though a stool test is helpful, you do not need to do one to diagnose yourself. I'll show how using the self-assessment in the next chapter. People with this kind of dysbiosis often have sensitivities to many different foods, feel tired and puffy, and have difficulty concentrating right after eating or even the next day.

A fourth type is *inflammatory dysbiosis*, which is when the body has an exaggerated response to your body's imbalance of good bacteria. Physical symptoms of this type of dysbiosis include muscle and joint pain in addition to digestive symptoms such as gas and bloating. This form of dysbiosis is often seen in autoimmune diseases.

The last type is *parasites*, which can infect the digestive tract and put stress on the population of good bacteria. Parasites often cause diarrhea, cramping, and bloating. But they can also be silent, causing no obvious gut issues but resulting in hives for no clear reason or food and environmental allergies that you have never had before. The only way to diagnose a parasite is to do a stool test.

All types of dysbiosis except the first one require the removal of bad bacteria, yeast, or parasites. And all of them can be thought of as infections that aren't detected by routine medical tests or procedures. Dysbiosis can be caused by an overuse of antibiotics and antacids, including proton pump inhibitors, which lower the production of acid in the stomach; gastrointestinal infections; gastrointestinal surgery; chronic digestion problems, because undigested foods wreak havoc in the intestines; chronic constipation; eating the standard American diet, which is very low in the fiber that your beneficial flora need to thrive and be healthy; and eating foods that your body's immune system is reacting to. A good example of this is gluten, which causes many different kinds of reactions in the body, one of which is celiac disease, as we discussed in detail in Chapter 2, "Using Food as Medicine." Chronic stress, which can lower the levels of the friendly flora in your gut, can also cause dysbiosis.[9]

What's really important to note is that even a small disruptive event in your gut—for example, taking a short course of antibiotics for a sinus infection—can create a severe or chronic condition such as yeast overgrowth or small intestinal bacterial overgrowth. That said, a relatively minor change—if carefully conceived—can sometimes restore that balance and, as a result, your gut health. For example, simply taking a daily probiotic supplement can create or stimulate major changes in your good bacteria and ultimately decrease an allergic reaction or other symptoms that you may be having.

The bottom line is that dysbiosis can trigger or promote an auto-immune disease because the lack of healthy flora and the influence of harmful flora cause the immune system to malfunction. Dysbiosis can also lead to leaky gut syndrome, a problem on its own that we'll discuss shortly. My point here is that finding out if you have dysbiosis and treating it is a foundational part of how I work with patients in my office and in the program I'm sharing in this book. Research shows that restoring healthy flora to the gut helps improve immune function, and I am continually amazed at how balancing the good bacteria in the gut helps almost everyone feel better.[10,11,12]

WHAT IS LEAKY GUT SYNDROME?

I've mentioned leaky gut syndrome a few times already, so let me finally explain it in some detail. Normally, the cells that line your intestines stick tightly together and form a protective barrier that is hard to penetrate. Sitting on top of this cell lining is a layer of mucus that is also an important part of the barrier. This barrier's job is to regulate everything that passes between your intestine and the rest of your body. Together with the immune cells located in your gut, the barrier helps control how your immune system reacts to anything foreign. When this barrier is weak or compromised, you have a condition called leaky gut syndrome. The problems caused by this condition are easier to understand if you imagine the barrier to be like a brick wall made of intestinal cells and what is called intercellular tight junctions, which are the "mortar" that holds these cells together. When the "mortar" breaks down, there are cracks in between the cells that allow food particles and bacteria to leak into your bloodstream (hence the name "leaky gut syndrome"). Researchers at the University of Maryland School of Medicine recently identified a molecule called zonulin that is part of this "mortar." They found that when the zonulin is damaged, the result is leaky gut syndrome.[13]

Leaky gut allows anything that is inside your intestines—such as food proteins, good bacteria, harmful bacteria, yeast, and parasites—to be "seen" by the immune system that is lying beneath your intestinal lining. When this exposure is chronic, meaning that it goes on and on for months, the immune reaction over time begins to malfunction, putting you at risk for an autoimmune disease. The researchers who identified zonulin found that in people who have a genetic predisposition to auto-immune disease, damaging zonulin and the rest of the "mortar" that holds the cells together caused them to develop an autoimmune disease more often than people who had a normal intestinal barrier.

This "mortar" in between the cells gets damaged by things such as dysbiosis from yeast, parasites, or bad bacteria; severe stress; alcohol; certain medications; a viral infection; or chemotherapy. When this happens, you are also likely to develop food sensitivities. These food sensitivities can happen not only in childhood but later in life, too, something that comes as a surprise to most people, especially if they had no food sensitivities or allergies as children. Maintaining a strong barrier is the best way to keep your immune system healthy, which, as I have said, means that it knows when to turn on and off, knows the difference between self and not self and has tolerance of the good bacteria lining the digestive tract.

Some things that can cause leaky gut syndrome include:

- Antibiotic use. Typically this means taking antibiotics multiple times over multiple years, but taking them only one time can also be an issue.
- Acute emotional or physical trauma, such as surgery or food poisoning.
- Chronic stress.
- Infections or exposures that were never resolved, such as traveler's diarrhea or a parasite.
- Chronic dysbiosis. Bad bacteria can secrete enzymes that destroy the "mortar" between the cells.
- Non-steroidal anti-inflammatory drugs (NSAIDs), medications such as ibuprofen and other prescriptions.
- Toxins, such as those secreted by the yeast candida. These can bind to part of the protective barrier, breaking it down. They also can create pores across the membranes of the barrier.
- Alcoholism.

WHAT DOES LEAKY GUT FEEL LIKE?

People with leaky gut syndrome often have digestive symptoms such as constipation or gas and bloating after they eat. But it is also possible to have leaky gut syndrome and have absolutely *no* digestive symptoms at all. Instead, you might feel your hands and feet swell up after you eat, your muscles are tight and stiff in the morning, and you have brain fog and difficulty thinking after eating certain foods. These symptoms are a result of what's called systemic inflammation, which simply means that there are irritating molecules running around your body after you eat certain foods. Sometimes it is hard to know which food is the culprit because it seems like you react to so many. I hear this story very often from my patients with bad leaky gut syndrome. Also, when you get symptoms that are nowhere near your stomach, such as joint pain or headaches, you may not realize they are even related to your diet.

HOW DOES LEAKY GUT CAUSE AUTOIMMUNE DISEASE?

Let's go into a bit more detail about how you can get autoimmune disease from leaky gut syndrome. The latest research on leaky gut syndrome and autoimmune disease shows that almost everyone with an autoimmune disease has leaky gut syndrome, even if there are no gut symptoms.[14, 15] This lack of symptoms is why, with all my patients, I do a comprehensive digestive stool analysis to make sure their gut flora is healthy.

As we discussed, when your intestinal barrier is weak or broken down, partially digested food or antigens from bacteria and yeast can seep into your body, bump into the lymphoid tissue and immune cells in your gut, and then also get into your bloodstream. Your immune cells react by making lots of T helper cells, which are directly in charge of revving up the killer cells and antibody-producing cells to attack anything they don't recognize as an invader. However, problems can occur when your body starts producing an abundance of T helper cells, especially if the T regulator cells don't do their job to turn this attack off. These extra T helper cells can:

- Rev up the killer T cells too much, prompting them to mistake your own tissues for foreign invaders.
- Tell the killer cells to make inflammatory molecules that are sent out all over your body, causing inflammation and pain at distant places.
- Tell immune cells, called B cells, to make antibodies that bind to the foreigner and form something called an immune complex. These immune complexes can circulate throughout the body and build up in tissues, causing irritation, inflammation, and swelling. Since food is a big trigger for these kinds of reactions when you have leaky gut syndrome, I always recommend eliminating gluten, dairy, soy, corn, and eggs from your diet. (I haven't told you to eliminate and test your sensitivity to eggs yet, but don't worry, it's coming.) This can really improve symp-

toms dramatically. While you will still have a leaky gut when you are on an elimination diet, you are no longer eating the foods that trigger inflammation and worsen symptoms, so you begin to feel better immediately. Once you fix the leaky gut, you will be able to eat those foods again, but this will take at least six months. (I will show you how to heal your gut in the next chapter.)

- Tell the B cells to make antibodies to the foreigner. These antibodies can make a mistake and attack your own tissue instead, which is called "molecular mimicry" and is believed to be one of the ways that a viral infection and a food such as gluten can trigger autoimmune disease.
- Get stuck in the on position, and so the immune response keeps going without stopping.

In order to reverse your immune disease or illness and have the healthiest immune system possible, we need to find what is causing your T cell imbalance, so that we can turn off your revved-up T helper cells and calm down the killer cells or the antibody-producing cells. Helping your T regulator cells work better is important to help this balance.

In order to fully heal and balance your immune system, we must heal your intestinal lining and make sure you have a good, intact barrier. Otherwise, your immune imbalance and your reactions to food and other antigens will not be cured and will come back again and again. The first step is to treat the cause, which is usually dysbiosis or impaired digestion.

Now you can see why it is so important to figure out what's going in your gut and heal your dysbiosis and/or leaky gut syndrome if you have them. To do so, let's move on to the next chapter, where you will find self-assessments for these conditions and a treatment plan based on the results. Just think: you're getting closer and closer to healing your gut and feeling better.

CHAPTER 9

Healing Your Gut Workbook

As I described in the introduction, Sidney Baker, M.D., one of the fathers of functional medicine, famously said, "If you are sitting on a tack, the answer is not to treat the pain. The solution is to find the tack and remove it." This is exactly what we're doing to balance your immune system. One by one, we are finding the tacks that are impacting your health. We already found your food tacks in Chapter 2, "Using Food as Medicine," and your stress hormone tacks in Chapter 5, "Understanding the Stress Connection." Now we need to look for and remove the tacks in your gut.

Our first step toward removing them—that is, balancing your gut—is to find out if there is anything irritating you inside. Discovering what's going on inside your body takes the detective work of functional medicine. With my patients at Blum Center for Health, the approach I take to understand and repair the digestive system is a three-step gut restoration plan. Here I will explain the basic principles and you will complete the self-assessments. Your scores on those assessments will help you identify the treatment plan that is best for you.

CAROL'S STORY

But first let me introduce you to my patient Carol, a fifty-eight-year-old teacher. Four months before she arrived at my office, Carol had gone to see her primary care physician complaining of exhaustion, weight gain, and feeling puffy. If these symptoms weren't enough, Carol's fingers were stiff, swollen, and painful most mornings when she woke up.

After a basic blood test, Carol's doctor diagnosed her with rheumatoid arthritis, an autoimmune disease that causes inflammation of joints such as wrists, fingers, knees, feet, and ankles and surrounding tissue. Typically, rheumatoid arthritis requires treatment with steroid medications or other biological medications that shut off the immune system, which is exactly what Carol's doctor prescribed. Even worse, the doctor told her it was highly likely that she would have to take these medications for the rest of her life. This remark from her doctor didn't surprise me, as it is something I hear from patients all the time. Traditional medicine believes that this condition (and many other autoimmune diseases) can only be managed but not cured. Previously an upbeat, energetic, and productive woman, Carol was fed up with the moody, negative person she had become. Her chronic symptoms were greatly affecting the quality of her life, and the weight gain of about twenty pounds on her five-foot-four-inch frame left her feeling lethargic and depressed. Plus she was wary of the serious side effects of the rheumatoid arthritis medications, including more weight gain, fatigue, osteoporosis, and hair loss, among others. On the advice of a co-worker who had been my patient for several years, Carol came to see me.

Carol stood up slowly when I greeted her in the waiting room. She had a weary expression on her face and carried herself as if the weight of the world was on her shoulders. Like many of my patients, Carol arrived at my office with a diagnosis, a folder bursting with medical tests and papers, and a sense of hopelessness. In order to help her, I knew I needed to look beyond the papers and diagnosis she brought with her. I had to take a deeper look at her symptoms, her life, and her history. After a lengthy discussion, I gave Carol the assessments that you will take in this chapter. They revealed that she had symptoms that had been part of her life so long that she was used to them. In fact, she didn't even realize they were symptoms or remember what life was like without them until we did the assessments. These included severe bloating and gas pains every time she ate, three to four loose stools (bordering on diarrhea) per day, and severe bouts of exhaustion almost daily. She found herself waking in the middle of the night and gasping for air because of a chronic sleep disorder called sleep apnea, and as a result she suffered disrupted, not restful, sleep. Carol also had serious reactions to eating fast food, including heart palpitations and quick and shallow breathing, but had been told she could eat anything she wanted because previous food allergy testing done by an allergist had been negative. In addition, Carol had a history of taking antibiotics, often for long periods of time.

The assessments I did on Carol's first visit revealed that she had dysbiosis, the imbalance of the normal flora of the intestines and leaky gut syndrome. Because of her dysbiosis, I immediately started her on the Tier 2 dysbiosis treatment plan. On this plan, she would take herbs to scrub the bad bacteria and yeast from her gut, probiotics to supply her gut with the good bacteria, and a glutamine powder blend to begin to strengthen her intestinal lining. I also sent Carol home with instructions to follow an elimination diet for three weeks. You will do this complete elimination diet in Chapter 12, "Supporting Your Liver Workbook." It involves the removal of gluten, dairy, corn, soy, eggs, peanuts, beef, shellfish, caffeine, and alcohol. Because she had arthritis, I also told her to remove nightshade vegetables (tomatoes, potatoes, eggplant, and peppers) because they can trigger arthritis symptoms. This list of foods is part of the complete elimination diet because numerous studies have shown that these are the most common triggers of immune reactions in the body. Because blood tests are limited in their ability to measure the different reactions possible from food (digestive problems, arthritis, and headaches, for example), I have come to rely on this elimination diet to identify foods that might be causing some of my patients' chronic symptoms and/or contributing to the development of their autoimmune diseases. It is the most inexpensive way of assessing food sensitivities and, best of all, can be done simply and easily by anyone at home.

Four weeks later, Carol returned to my office. Before she said a word, her body language told me that she felt better—*much* better. In fact, she was ecstatic. She had dropped two clothing sizes and the swelling and pain in her legs and fingers was gone. She was sleeping through the night without waking and gasping for air, so she felt more rested. Her gas and bloating were gone and her energy level had skyrocketed. And these positive results were just the beginning.

During her second appointment, Carol and I discussed the results of her blood work. It did *not* show that she had rheumatoid arthritis. What she *did* have was a positive result on the anti-nuclear antibody (ANA) test. This positive result is something traditional doctors often look for as the first screening test for autoimmune diseases such as lupus, rheumatoid arthritis, Sjögren's syndrome, and scleroderma. However, being positive for ANA doesn't tell you if you have one of these specific diseases, just that you *might*, and so you need to do further testing to check. Carol had a positive ANA, and even though she had joint pain and swelling, the additional rheumatoid arthritis tests (called rheumatoid factor and anti-CCP) were negative or normal. Her previous doctor had interpreted these results to mean that she was in the early stages of rheumatoid arthritis and that the test results would become positive later. I told Carol that if we did nothing, they very well *could* end up positive in the years to come. But my goal was to work with her toward a normal anti-nuclear antibody level so we could prevent this serious disease. Her blood tests also revealed that she had a mild version of Hashimoto's thyroiditis. The good news is that treating the foundations of the immune system treats all autoimmune diseases at the same time, so our treatment plan also targeted her thyroid.

As a result of the elimination diet, most of Carol's original symptoms were gone and for the first time in ten years she was losing weight easily. She was stunned and elated. But I wasn't surprised. Weight loss is actually very common when you remove foods that cause inflammation in the body. That's because this inflammatory reaction interferes with fat metabolism, making it difficult to shed pounds. Removing these foods and thus the inflammation leads to easy weight loss. Carol left my office that day with a plan to continue the elimination diet and finish the three months of the leaky gut treatment program. After that, she would return to see me to discuss how she felt and follow up with repeat testing of her thyroid hormones and antibody levels.

Since we began two treatments—the food elimination diet and the gut treatment plan—at once, it is hard to know which one had the biggest impact. For this reason, I don't always do them at the same time for all of my patients. Still, because of my experience and training, I know that there is a link between immune function, gut health, and food, so I am confident that both are important and need to be addressed.

In the first year of treating any autoimmune condition, my goal is to improve or completely resolve all symptoms without the medication typically offered by Western medicine. If patients are already on medication, my goal is to help them feel well enough to ask their rheumatologist (or other prescribing specialist) to taper off and stop the prescription. While the symptoms can resolve rather quickly (Carol's did in just one month), the laboratory results may take longer to show improvements, and so my expectation was that Carol's ANA level would stop being positive as we continued to work together, but that this might take six months to a year after her symptoms were resolved. In fact, that is exactly what happened. She returned to my office three months later and her blood work revealed that her Hashimoto's thyroiditis antibody levels had become normal. So we knew we were on the right track even though her other antibody level, ANA, was still positive.

One year after she first entered my office, Carol had lost forty-five pounds and was maintaining a diet free of gluten, dairy, soy, corn, and tomatoes because those were the foods that caused her swollen joints, sleep apnea, gas, and bloating to come back. At one year, her ANA was almost normal and she was completely symptom-free. She had great energy and was very happy. Moreover, she was confident and said she felt good about herself for the first time in years. In another six months we redid the lab testing, and at that point all her antibodies were gone.

Now that I've shared Carol's experience of healing, it is your turn to start your journey toward better health. Take the following self-assessments and score each one. After that, you will be directed toward your treatment plan and the first steps toward better gut health. Get excited! You're about to make a huge difference in your health *and* your life.

Self-Assessments

Your gut health is determined by whether you have dysbiosis, how well you are digesting your food, and whether you have leaky gut syndrome. In this section, I am going to help you assess all three of these issues, and then offer you a three-tiered treatment plan to repair each one.

Self-Assessment 1: Do You Have Dysbiosis?

As we've discussed, dysbiosis is an imbalance in the normal flora of the intestines caused by too little beneficial bacteria or an overgrowth of harmful bacteria, yeast, or parasites. The following self-assessment will help determine if you need to restore the proper balance of beneficial bacteria in your gut.

Give yourself one point for each question you answer with a yes.

Do you get "stomach bugs" a lot?	
Do you have chronic diarrhea?	
Do you have cramps, urgency, or mucus and blood in your stool at least once a week?	
Do you have chronic constipation?	
Do you notice that you have decreased cognitive function or brain fog most days?	
Do you have gas, bloating, and abdominal discomfort most days?	

(continued on next page)

Do you notice that you have intolerance to carbohydrates, especially beans and fiber?	
Do you have fatigue and/or low energy most days?	
Do you feel depressed or anxious most days?	
Do you have chronic sinus congestion?	
Do you have itching in the vagina, anus, or other mucosal membranes most days?	
Do you have chronic bad breath?	
Have you used antacids daily for more than thirty days in the past two years?	
Have you taken antibiotics more than three times in the past year?	
Do you have a history of traveler's diarrhea during foreign travel?	
Have you been diagnosed with a vitamin D deficiency?	
Do you have any food sensitivities?	
Have you been diagnosed with an autoimmune disease or condition?	
Have you been diagnosed with arthritis or fibromyalgia?	
Do you experience severe chronic stress?	
Have you been diagnosed with reflux, heartburn or a hiatal hernia?	
Total points	

SCORING

0 to 7 points: Good news! Your low score means that you probably have good amounts of the beneficial flora and either no or low amounts of harmful bacteria, yeast, or parasites in your intestines. While a low score doesn't guarantee this, chances are that if you do have dysbiosis at all, it is very mild.

8 to 14 points: Your score tells me that you definitely have a mild to moderate case of dysbiosis. This means that you have an overgrowth of harmful bacteria, yeast, or parasites, which is causing your symptoms. Your intestinal flora must be fixed for you to get better.

15 to 20 points: Your score tells me that you have severe dysbiosis. I am concerned that your intestinal flora are causing big problems for you, and the overgrowth of harmful bacteria, yeast or parasites is significant. We will have to work hard to balance and correct your gut flora.

Self-Assessment 2: Are You Having Problems with Digestion?

As you know, there are three parts to a healthy digestion: pancreatic enzymes, bile acids, and additional stomach acid. In this self-assessment, we will test each of these three things. Food needs to be completely digested to prevent unwanted pieces of partially digested food from traveling across the leaky gut barrier and into the bloodstream. Besides the fact that poor digestive power can cause reflux, abdominal gas, and bloating, it can also cause poor absorption of nutrients.

Self-Test for Pancreatic Enzymes

These are enzymes made by the pancreas to aid in digestion. They are released as soon as food leaves your stomach and then they break down fat (lipase), carbohydrates (amylase), and protein (protease). If your pancreas is not secreting enzymes as it should, you may experience the symptoms below.

Give yourself one point for each question you answer with a yes.

Do you have indigestion/fullness two to four hours after a meal?	
Do you have stomach distension, bloating, or flatulence two to four hours after a meal?	
Do you have undigested food in your stool?	
Do you have chronic constipation?	
Were you ever told you have a B_{12} deficiency (often discovered as a cause of anemia)?	
Do you have swelling in the ankles?	
Do you bruise easily? (This can be a sign of a vitamin K deficiency.)	
Have you been diagnosed with glucose intolerance?	
Do you have pale, foul-smelling, or bulky stool?	
Total points	

SCORING

0 to 3 points: No enzymes are needed as part of your regimen.

4 or more points: We need to add enzymes to your regimen.

Self-Test for Bile Acids

Your liver makes bile, which is then stored in your gallbladder. When you eat fat, it travels into your stomach and then a message is sent to your gallbladder telling it to contract and squeeze the bile into an area at the top of your small intestines where the stomach empties, called the duodenum. The bile then helps emulsify the fats so that they can be digested and absorbed by the body. Inadequate bile prevents the absorption of fat and fat-soluble vitamins.

Give yourself one point for each question you answer with a yes.

Have you had your gallbladder removed?	
Has blood work ever revealed that you were low in vitamin A, E, or K?	
Do you have chronic diarrhea?	
Total points	

SCORING

0 or 1 point: Your bile flow is probably okay, so there is no need to add a supplement.

2 or more points: You need a supplement to help your body produce more bile.

Self-Test for Stomach Acid

Give yourself one point for each question you answer with a yes.

Do you experience bloating or belching immediately following most meals?	
Do you have a sense of fullness or nausea after eating?	
Do you often have itching around your rectum?	
Are your fingernails weak, peeling, and/or cracked?	
Do you have acne (and you're no longer an adolescent)?	
Do you have undigested food in your stool?	
Do you have dilated capillaries on your face or been diagnosed with rosacea?	

Do you have an iron deficiency?	
Do you have chronic intestinal infections such as candida or parasites?	
Do you have a history of multiple food allergies?	
Do you have flatulence with your bloating?	
Have you been diagnosed with reflux or gastroesophageal reflux disease (GERD)?	
Do you have a history of taking proton pump inhibitors, acid blockers, or antacids?	
Total points	

SCORING

0 to 4 points: We don't need to include stomach acid supplements in your treatment plan.

5 points or more: You have low stomach acid. Chances are that if you have gastroesophageal reflux disease (GERD), you probably have either hypochlorhydria, which is a condition where you don't have enough stomach acid and have low digestive enzymes, or dysbiosis further down in the intestines. These problems impair the functioning of the stomach and prevent food from moving out of the stomach. Instead of your digestive river moving downstream, it gets dammed up in the stomach and refluxes up into the throat. If you scored a 5 or above, we will treat you for hypochlorhydria and get your river flowing in the right direction.

You're almost there! One more self-assessment for leaky gut, and then I will show you how to replace pancreatic enzymes, bile acids, and/or stomach acid as part of your healing your gut treatment program.

Self-Assessment 3: Do You Have a Leaky Gut?

As we've discussed, leaky gut syndrome is a condition when the barrier function of the intestinal wall isn't working properly and undigested particles of food can get into the bloodstream, causing an immune and inflammatory reaction throughout the body.

Give yourself one point for each question you answer with a yes.

Did you uncover more than one food sensitivity from the elimination diet in Chapter 3?	
Did you score over a 10 on the stress scale in Chapter 6?	
Did the dysbiosis self-assessment above reveal that you have dysbiosis?	
Have you been diagnosed with an autoimmune disease?	
Total points	

SCORING

0 or 1 point: You probably do not have leaky gut syndrome, because you don't have the conditions that are known to cause it, like severe ongoing stress and dysbiosis. You also don't have conditions that are associated with it, like food sensitivities and autoimmune disease.

2 or more points: It is very likely that you have leaky gut syndrome. This means that your intestinal barrier is not working properly and needs to be fixed so that your immune system can be repaired.

Healing Your Gut Treatment Program

Now it is time to move on to your personalized treatment program. But first let me explain how this will work. The treatment programs, just like the self-assessments, are divided into three parts: treatment for dysbiosis, treatment for improving digestion, and treatment for leaky gut syndrome. Keep in mind that you might not need treatment for all of these conditions; this is determined by your score on the self-assessments.

Each of these programs is divided into three tiers, and again, your score from the self-assessment will determine which tier you will follow. Here are the general definitions for each tier:

Tier 1: Using Food as Medicine

Here we make specific dietary changes that can treat symptoms if you have them and improve your general immune and digestive health. Everyone starts here. If you don't have any digestive symptoms and all the assessment tests are normal, you should still follow this program to ensure that you are eating the right foods for you. The good news is that for some of you, this treatment is all you need to guarantee good gut health. However, if you scored positive for any of the self-assessments, add Tier 2 to your treatment plan.

Tier 2: Nutritional Supplements

Here you will add nutritional supplements and herbs to the dietary changes you have made in Tier 1, which should do the trick for most of you. However, if your digestive symptoms remain after completing Tier 1 and Tier 2 for three months, move on to Tier 3. There is a complete Supplement and Herb Guide in the appendix with specific product names and how to find them.

Tier 3: Laboratory Testing and Functional Medicine Evaluation

You need further testing to reveal the "tack" in your system and to get the treatment you need. Here I'll provide the resources for this laboratory testing and treatment.

TREATMENT FOR DYSBIOSIS
Your score on Self-Assessment 1: Do You Have Dysbiosis? (page 195)

0 to 7 points: Good news! You don't need the dysbiosis treatment program. However, you should take a probiotic daily to protect and support your digestive health and immune system and follow the Tier 1 dysbiosis diet to promote the friendly flora in your digestive system. See below for instructions on taking probiotics.

8 to 14 points: You have mild to moderate dysbiosis. To remedy this condition, follow Tier 1 and complete the supplement program in Tier 2 for two weeks.

15 to 20 points: You have severe dysbiosis. To remedy this condition, follow Tier 1 and complete the supplement program in Tier 2 for four weeks.

Tier 1: Restoring and Maintaining Healthy Gut Flora with Food

Here we will focus on foods that support digestion, restore flora, and heal the gut.

First, you need to **remove all white sugar and white flour from your diet.** This includes white bread, cookies, cakes, ice cream, candy, soda, chips, pretzels, and crackers. Yeast and many harmful bacteria love sugar because it gives them a growth spurt and causes them to give off toxins and gas as they ferment the sugar. Starving these bad guys of their food is the first step. Some people actually feel symptoms such as moodiness, mild headache, and fatigue when they first remove sugar from their diets. It is almost like a detox reaction, something you will read more about in Part IV of this book, "Supporting Your Liver." However, these symptoms usually last no more than two to three days.

Eat only breads and crackers made from whole grains. Look for the word "whole" high up in the ingredient list, or make sure bread and crackers have at least 3 grams of fiber per serving. If you are reading this book because you have an autoimmune disease, make sure the whole-grain foods are gluten free. **Whether or not you have diagnosed yourself with dysbiosis on the self-assessment, you should follow this program because it will help maintain the healthy flora in your gut. It can also help you achieve and maintain a healthy weight and prevent diabetes and heart disease.**

If you have dysbiosis, also take 1 tablespoon coconut oil (organic and unrefined if possible) twice daily as part of your treatment plan. It contains lauric and capric acids, compounds that discourage viruses and yeast, so it's also a great food to maintain your intestinal health once your treatment is finished. You can add coconut oil to hot cereal or use it to stir-fry vegetables. Another idea is to use coconut milk in your gluten-free granola or in your smoothies, sprinkle coconut in your granola, or cook with it. My favorite is cultured coconut milk kefir and yogurt. Though coconut has a reputation for being high in calories, the body metabolizes this oil quickly, so as part of a balanced diet (meaning a serving of coconut milk or a few tablespoons of coconut oil), it will not make you gain weight. Coconut oil also contains medium-chain triglycerides, which support immune system function in your gut.

You also need to restore or maintain the friendly flora in your gut, something that is important for *everyone* no matter how you scored for dysbiosis. This nutritional approach will help to support your beneficial bacteria, which is especially important for people with any immune imbalance, as we discussed previously. First, you need to **include pre-biotics in your diet.** Prebiotics are non-digestible plant components that are fermented in the gut to make compounds that feed the beneficial bacteria. I think of them as the fertilizers that help the good bacteria grow. Good prebiotic foods include legumes, most vegetables, and low-sugar fruits such as berries, apples, and pears.

Make sure you get enough fiber, which will help keep the body regular and will help remove cholesterol and other toxins from your body. **Aim for at least 30 grams of fiber per day.** Your good bacteria *love* fiber. Two other great prebiotics are plant compounds called fructooligosaccharides (FOS), which are compounds found in onions, garlic, leeks, rye, chicory, blueberries, and bananas; and inulins, which are found in chicory and artichokes.

Next, you need to add probiotics, which are live bacteria that you eat, either in food or as a supplement. The strains of bacteria in each product are chosen because they are known to be the beneficial bacteria in the human intestinal tract. Today, you can find many cultured or fermented foods at the supermarket. These words mean that live bacteria are grown as part of the food. You should add fermented foods like kimchi, sauerkraut, kombucha, yogurt, and kefir to your diet. I am not fond of dairy products (such as cheese and yogurt made from cow, goat, or sheep milk) because they contain the proteins casein and whey, which cause inflammation in the body for many people. Therefore, I suggest you try dairy-free alternatives such as coconut milk yogurt and kefir. If you really love dairy products, make sure you have tested yourself with an elimination/challenge experiment so that you know for sure if it is good for you.

You should **also add to your diet anything with live active cultures that include the following bacteria: lactobacillus species (such as** *L. reuteri, casei, rhamnosus,* **or** *acidophilus*) **and bifidobacterium species (such as** *B. infantis, lactis, longum, breve,* **or** *bifidum*). Most yogurt contains 1 to 3 billion live bacteria, in a four- to six-ounce single serving containing usually a blend of both lactobacilli and bifidobacteria. This is a good mix to have.

Tier 2: Using Herbal and Nutritional Supplements to Treat Your Dysbiosis

First, you need to **remove unfriendly bacteria, yeast, and parasites,** which is important if you scored 8 points or higher on the self-test. I recommend taking combination products made of the herbs mentioned below for a minimum of two to four weeks. (My favorite combination products can be found in the Supplement and Herb Guide in the appendix, page 329.) For mild symptoms, two weeks should be enough. For severe symptoms, I recommend four weeks. If your symptoms get better but don't completely resolve by the end of this time, I suggest you take these herbs for at least another two to four weeks, until your digestive symptoms go away completely. All herbs can be taken with meals or on an empty stomach— whatever your stomach likes best. Some herbs, such as oregano and thyme, can irritate the stomach lining if you already have heartburn.

The herbs I suggest are:

- Oregano oil capsules or tablets, 200 mg three times per day
- Thyme oil capsules or tablets, 100–200 mg three times per day
- Artemisinin capsules or tablets, 1–3 mg three times per day
- Berberine capsules or tablets, 200–400 mg three times per day
- Grapefruit seed extract capsules or tablets, 250–500 mg three times per day
- Garlic capsules or tablets, standardized to 5,000 mcg allicin potential three times per day

Keep in mind that these herbs will begin to kill off the bad bacteria and yeast that you have in your digestive tract. As they die off, you might get a headache, feel more gas and bloating, and/or feel really tired—symptoms that should pass after a few days. However, if you're really uncomfortable, drop the dosage of the herbs or take a day off completely. These symptoms are a sign that you have lots of bad bacteria or yeast and you might need to take it more slowly by using the herbs at a lower dose.

You also need to **restore the good bacteria with probiotics and prebiotics.** As I've mentioned, probiotics are the beneficial bacteria and prebiotics are the "fertilizer" to help them grow. Both are critical for repairing the intestinal lining. I recommend a combination formula with many strains of lactobacilli and bifidobacteria instead of single-strain products.

Here are the supplements I recommend:

- Lactobacillus (various species), 10–100 billion live organisms daily. You can take this as a capsule, tablet, or powder mixed in food or any beverage.
- Bifidobacterium (various species), 10–100 billion live organisms daily.
- *Saccharomyces boulardii*, 500 mg daily. This good yeast is especially useful for protecting your flora when you take antibiotics.

- Fructooligosaccharides (FOS), 500–5,000 mg one to three times per day
- Inulin, 500–5,000 mg one to three times per day. I recommend adding FOS and inulin *after* you have finished your dysbiosis herbs, not at the same time.
- Fiber: larch or acacia arabinogalactans, 500–5,000 mg each day.
- Modified citrus pectin, 3–5 grams two or three times per day.

Tier 3: Further Testing, Evaluation, and Treatment for Dysbiosis

If Tiers 1 and 2 have not completely resolved your symptoms, the next step is to get a functional stool analysis to see if you have a parasite or other imbalance that requires a clinician to supervise the treatment. There are two ways to find someone to help you. The first is to locate a functional medicine practitioner at www.functionalmedicine.org. They have a "find a practitioner" search section where you can put in your zip code and locate someone near you who has had the appropriate training. Most offer stool testing and know how to interpret the results. However, ask the practitioner's office specifically about this type of testing *before* making an appointment. The second is to visit the websites for the different stool testing companies and search for practitioners who use their services. The most frequently used stool testing is done by Genova Diagnostics, Metametrix Laboratories, Doctors Data Laboratory, and Enterolabs.

TREATMENT FOR IMPROVING DIGESTION

Results of Self-Testing

I need:

_____ Digestive support with pancreatic enzymes
_____ Digestive support with bile acids
_____ Digestive support with stomach acid

If you need help with your pancreatic enzymes, bile acids, or stomach acid, you should begin your treatment with Tier 1. It is possible that changing your diet to include foods that support your digestion will be all you need to cure your symptoms. I find that some of my patients really want to avoid supplements and only use food. If that's the case for you, follow Tier 1. However, if after one month of Tier 1, you haven't noticed

If you have heartburn or reflux, if you are taking antacids or proton pump inhibitors, or if you just feel like your stomach is irritated, it is a good idea to take a supplement to soothe your stomach at the same time you are treating your dysbiosis. You can take any of the following products alone, but I often suggest a combination product that includes some of the others on this list. You can find some of my specific suggestions in the Supplement and Herb Guide in the appendix. These include:

- Deglycyrrhizinated licorice (DGL): 500–1,000 mg three to four times a day. You can take chewable tablets, powder, or capsule versions; just do so on an empty stomach or twenty minutes before meals.
- Slippery elm: 2–4 grams three times per day. Slippery elm comes in capsules or as a powder. Take on an empty stomach or 20 minutes before a meal.
- Aloe: 50–100 mg two to three times a day. Look for aloe that has its laxative compounds removed so that only the soothing qualities remain; it should say so on the label. Aloe comes in many forms: capsules, powder, or liquid.

an improvement in your symptoms, it is time to move on to Tier 2 and try some supplements to help you.

Some of my patients are either impatient or not interested in trying the foods in Tier 1, and if this is you, you are welcome to start the supplements in Tier 2 right away. Please try to incorporate some food changes into your diet, too, as this lifestyle change will help you sustain your healing in the long run.

Tier 1: Foods to Support Enzymes, Bile, and Stomach Acid

Included in this list are **fermented and cultured foods,** such as kimchi, sauerkraut, and fresh pickles, because they contain enzymes that naturally help you digest your food and contain probiotics. All raw vegetables also contain digestive enzymes. Try eating sprouted veggies, which have dramatically increased amounts of enzymes, and cultured yogurt and kefir. As you already know, I am not fond of dairy, so stick to non-dairy alternatives for yogurt and kefir if possible. Green papaya contains the enzyme papain, and pineapple contains the enzyme bromelain; eat them at the end of the meal to aid your digestion.

You also need to **eat foods that will stimulate your liver to make and secrete more bile**, such as radishes (horse, red, and daikon varieties); dandelion, chicory, and other bitter greens; and artichokes. **Foods that support stomach acid are also important.** Although you cannot actually eat acid, you can stimulate your stomach to make more hydrochloric acid (HCL), which will keep the pH of your stomach close to 1.5. This acid will activate your digestive enzymes to work better. The strategy is to use a food much as you would a supplement: before meals to stimulate acid production. Do this by taking one tablespoon of apple cider vinegar or one umeboshi plum before each meal, especially large meals such as dinner.

There are also foods that aid other digestive symptoms. **Demulcents are soothing for irritated or inflamed internal tissues.** Examples include agar (used as a thickener for puddings), almond, barley, coconut oil, figs, flaxseed, oats, okra, parsley, plantain, pomegranate seeds, prunes, psyllium, pumpkin flesh, rice water, sage, and tapioca. Fenugreek seeds, marshmallow root, and slippery elm can often be found as a tea.

If you have gastroesophageal reflux disease (GERD), avoid alcohol, chocolate, citrus fruits and juices, tomatoes, peppermint, onions, garlic, high-fat meals, and carbonated drinks. Eat meals at least three hours before going to sleep. Do the elimination/challenge experiment and avoid foods that make your symptoms worse. Eat foods from the above lists to increase digestive enzymes and stomach acid to help you digest your food.

Tier 2: Supplements and Nutrients to Support Digestion

If your self-test revealed a need for digestive enzymes or if you have heartburn or reflux and are planning to taper off your antacids, try one of the following and see if you notice a change:

- Pancreatin (mixture of lipases, amylases, and proteases, standardized to lipase activity, animal derived), 800–24,000 USP units lipase activity, taken with meals. This formula is the most potent and usually my first choice unless you are a vegetarian or simply prefer the vegetarian enzymes.

- Vegetarian enzymes, usually aspergillus-derived, 800–24,000 USP units lipase activity, taken with meals. If you are allergic to mold, I suggest taking pancreatin instead.
- Bromelain (contains mainly proteases for digesting protein), 1,200–2,400 MCU, 250–500 mg taken with meals.
- Papain from papaya (contains mainly proteases for digesting protein), 50,000 USP units/mg, 100–200 mg taken with meals.

Include bile acids in your program if you scored positive on your self-test for bile acids or if you need more help with fat digestion even after taking the basic digestive enzyme.

- Bile salts (ox bile, which is actual bile from an animal; often you can find a digestive enzyme blend that includes ox bile), 500–1,000 mg with food.
- Taurine, 500–1,000 mg with food.
- Dandelion root, 2–4 grams three times per day with food, or 5 ml of 1:1 fluid extract three times a day with food.

If your self-assessment was positive for hypochlorhydria, you can now test yourself for low stomach acid. Before you start, make sure you are no longer on antacids, proton pump inhibitors, or H2 acid blockers and don't have heartburn, which is any kind of warmth or burning in your stomach or chest area. If you have been following the stomach treatment plan and your heartburn is now gone, you can do this treatment after 1 month of being heartburn-free and off antacids. However, if you have heartburn, *do not* do this test until your heartburn has been gone for at least one month. If you haven't done Step 1 or Step 2 and have heartburn, go back and do the stomach treatment before proceeding.

To test for hypochlorhydria, you will take betaine HCL tablets or capsules. Choose one that contains 250–350 mg of betaine and follow these instructions:

- Day 1: Take 1 tablet or capsule while you are eating a meal, not before.
- Day 2: Take 2 pills with each meal.
- Days 3–8: Each day you will take one more pill with each meal, until you reach a maximum of eight pills. However, if you notice a warmth or discomfort in your stomach, usually right after eating, then you have reached the maximum dose. This feeling might happen after taking two pills with each meal, five pills, or eight pills, or it might not happen at all.

When you notice anything uncomfortable, whether it is warmth or just not feeling right, the next time you eat reduce your dose by one pill. For example, if you found that five pills gave you some stomach discomfort, go back to four pills at the next meal. Keep taking that reduced dose until you feel the discomfort again, and then reduce your dose by one pill again. My patients who have gotten up to eight pills have come back down to four to five pills pretty quickly, but then stayed at that level for one to two months.

So what does this all mean? The higher the amount of betaine you needed before you feel any warmth, the more severe your hypochlorhydria or stomach acid deficiency really is. In that case, I suggest you stay at one to two pills (unless they cause discomfort in your stomach) for the next six months while you are healing your gut and getting your own juices flowing again. As an option to taking betaine pills, you can take these supplements to help stimulate your own acid production:

- Ginger, 500 mg–2 grams before meals
- Gentian, 1:5 tincture, 1–2 ml before meals
- Swedish bitters, 1–2 ml before meals

Tier 3: Further Testing, Evaluation, and Treatment for Digestion Problems

If the above treatment plans have not completely resolved your symptoms, the next step is to get a functional stool analysis to see if you have a parasite or other imbalance that requires a clinician to supervise the treatment. You can find someone to help you with this test in one of two ways. Find a functional medicine practitioner at www.functional medicine.org. They have a "find a practitioner" search area where you can put in your zip code and locate someone near you who has had the appropriate training. Most offer stool testing and know how to interpret the results. However, ask the office specifically if they do this type of testing before making an appointment. Or you can go to the websites for the different stool testing companies and search for practitioners who use their services. The most frequently used stool testing is by Genova Diagnostics, Metametrix Laboratories, Doctors Data Laboratory, and Enterolabs.

TREATMENT FOR LEAKY GUT SYNDROME
Your score on self-assessment 3: _____

0 or 1 point:	You don't have a leaky gut. But I do suggest that you follow Tier 1 so that you are eating in a way that supports your intestinal lining. You should also take a probiotic daily if you want to strengthen your immune system.
2 or more points:	You should complete Tier 1 and Tier 2 of the treatment plan for healing a leaky gut. It is best not to reintroduce problem foods (which you uncovered in Chapter 3, "Using Food as Medicine Workbook") for at least three months while healing the lining of the intestines. Some foods may need to be removed for six months or even a year to allow the immune system to recover before they are reintroduced.

Tier 1: Foods That Strengthen the Intestinal Lining

These are typically foods that improve the health of the cells that line your entire digestive tract, including your stomach and small and large intestines. The first is **ghee,** which is the same as clarified butter and is high in butyrate, a short-chain fatty acid that reduces inflammation and helps balance the immune cells in your gut. In the recipe section you will find instructions to make your own ghee from butter. You can eat ghee even if you have dairy allergies or sensitivities because the milk protein is removed. Use ghee in all your cooking anytime you would use butter, such as in hot breakfast cereals, frying eggs, gluten-free pasta, or rice. Another important food is **coconut oil** because it is loaded with medium-chain triglycerides, a source fuel for your cells. It also inhibits the growth of viruses and yeast. Because it is tolerant of high heat, coconut oil can be used to cook most foods. Add it to your hot cereal in the morning or use it to stir-fry meals for dinner.

You also want to **make sure your diet contains glutamine,** which is an amino acid that's critical for healing leaky gut syndrome because it is the most important food for the cells that line the intestines. Glutamine can be found in all animal protein, such as chicken, beef, and dairy, but also in beans, cabbage, beets, spinach, and parsley, so don't focus only on animal sources. Remember, the good bacteria in cultured foods are part of the barrier, so always include them when healing leaky gut.

Tier 2: Supplement and Nutrient Treatment for Healing a Leaky Gut

It takes time to heal the intestinal lining, so I recommend taking these supplements for at least three months, either in capsule form or as powders. There are many options in the Supplement and Herb Guide in the appendix. Make sure you follow your personalized nutrition plan and stay away from the foods you discovered were giving you symptoms. At the end of the three months, you can try reintroducing these foods to see if you can tolerate them; if not, remove them again and continue repairing your intestinal lining for another three months, then try again. That said, if you have an autoimmune disease, I recommend you stay off gluten even if you don't notice any symptoms when you eat it. (Note: If you also need treatment for dysbiosis, begin treatment for leaky gut at the same time as you are taking the herbs for dysbiosis.) The supplements you should take are:

- L-glutamine powder, 3,000 mg one to three times per day mixed with water
- Zinc, 15–30 mg per day

Probiotics and prebiotics are also crucial when it comes to healing a leaky gut. I have included this section in both the dysbiosis treatment and the leaky gut section because the beneficial bacteria (which are the probiotics) and the "fertilizer" to help them grow (which are the prebiotics) are critical for maintaining the barrier function of the intestinal lining. I recommend a combination formula with many strains of lactobacilli and bifidobacteria, instead of single-strain products. Here are the supplements I recommend:

- Lactobacillus (various species), 10–100 billion live organisms daily, taken in a capsule, tablet, or powder.
- Bifidobacterium (various species), 10–100 billion live organisms daily
- *Saccharomyces boulardii*, 500 mg daily. This good yeast is especially useful for protecting your flora when you take antibiotics.
- Fructooligosaccharides (FOS), 500–5,000 mg one to three times per day.
- Inulin, 500–5,000 mg one to three times per day.
- Fiber: larch or acacia arabinogalactans, 500–5,000 mg each day.
- Modified citrus pectin, 3–5 grams two to three times per day.

Tier 3: Further Testing, Evaluation, and Treatment for Leaky Gut Syndrome

If the above treatment plan has not completely resolved your symptoms, the next step is to get a functional stool analysis to see if you have a parasite or other imbalance that requires a clinician to supervise the treatment. You can also do an intestinal permeability test to confirm and determine the severity of your leaky gut, which is also called increased intestinal permeability. You can find someone to help you with this one of two ways. The first is to find a functional medicine practitioner at www.functionalmedicine.org. They have a "find a practitioner" search section where you can put in your zip code and locate someone near you who has had the appropriate training. Most offer stool testing and know how to interpret the results. However, ask the practitioner's office specifically about this type of testing before making an appointment. The second is to visit the websites for the different stool testing companies and search for practitioners who use their services. The most frequently used stool testing is done by Genova Diagnostics, Metametrix Laboratories, Doctors Data Laboratory, and Enterolabs.

Putting It All Together

While all four steps in this book are very important, fixing your gut is the most critical piece of healing your immune system and reversing your autoimmune disease. And as you may have noticed from reading through the workbook, it is also perhaps the most complicated to treat on your own. For that reason, I am going to show you the exact plan that Carol followed in order to illustrate how to put together all the pieces of the gut program for yourself.

Before we move on to Carol, I would like to give you some general advice for how to proceed. You should always begin with food. Work on the Tier 1 changes to your diet for all of the programs first. This means including food to balance your gut flora, support your digestion, and heal the intestinal lining to treat leaky gut, all at the same time. Choose one new food to include from each category, and when you are comfortable with this change, you can add more. Begin your gluten-free diet if you haven't done so already. After about two weeks, or when you are ready, you should move on to Tier 2 treatment for those programs where your score on any of the self-tests prescribed it.

In my view, if you have dysbiosis, you have leaky gut, and I always treat them both at the same time. After you finish treating the dysbiosis, which is usually about one month, the work to heal the intestinal lining continues for many more months, as I outlined in the Tier 2 program for leaky gut syndrome.

If digestive enzymes, stomach acid, or bile acids are also needed, you have the option of waiting until after the dysbiosis treatment is finished (about a month) and then adding what you need for digestive support. I suggest this because I like to change only one or two things at a time so that if you feel better, or worse, we know why. If you feel you can take supplements for dysbiosis, leaky gut, and digestion all at once, you certainly can start the digestive support at the very beginning, too. This is up to you, and it is what I did with Carol.

When Carol came to my office for our first visit, I diagnosed her with severe dysbiosis and leaky gut syndrome, based on my evaluation of her symptoms. She had so much gas and bloating after eating that I also gave her digestive support. Here is the program I put her on, using the brand names of the products I use in my office. Product details can be found in the Supplement and Herb Guide in the appendix.

I gave Carol a four-week program. First she started GI Cleansing Herbs. This is one of the formulas that I use at Blum Center for Health, and is a blend of berberine, black walnut, and artemisinin. The GI Cleansing Herbs are given as three capsules in the morning and three at night, with or without food. Most people prefer to take them with breakfast and dinner. Begin slowly when starting a new supplement to make sure that it doesn't cause any intestinal discomfort, such as diarrhea, nausea, or abdominal pain. I started Carol with one capsule twice a day on the first day, two capsules twice a day on the second day, and then the full dose of three capsules twice a day on the third day. On day four she started taking three oregano tablets twice daily, starting with one tablet twice a day and working up to the full dose over three days. She took the GI Cleansing Herbs and the oregano together for a total of four weeks.

As you follow this program, remember that these herbs will begin to kill off the bad bacteria and yeast that you have in your digestive tract. As they die off, you might get a headache, feel more gas and bloating, and/or feel really tired, symptoms that should pass after a few days. However, if you're really uncomfortable, drop the dosage of the herbs or take a day off completely. These symptoms are a sign that you have lots of bad bacteria or yeast and might need to take it more slowly by using the herbs at a lower dose.

At the same time that Carol took herbs to treat the dysbiosis, she took two Flora Support tablets at bedtime. Flora Support is a blend of lacto-bacilli, bifidobacteria, and *S. boulardii*. I always instruct people to take the Flora Support at bedtime while taking the dysbiosis herbs because you can't take these two supplements at the same time. The dysbiosis herbs will kill not just the harmful microbes we want to remove but also the probiotics that are in the Flora Support capsule. When you finish the herbs, you can take one Flora Support capsule with breakfast and one with dinner, daily for three months. After three months, you can drop the dose to one capsule a day.

Because Carol had severe gas and bloating immediately after eating, I gave her digestive support from the start. She took Complete Digestion Support, which is a combination of pancreatic enzymes, bile acids, and betaine. I told her to take one with each meal and to stay on these for at least three months.

There was no doubt in my mind that Carol had severe leaky gut syndrome. She had joint and muscle pain from many different foods, several different autoimmune diseases, and severe gut symptoms. We started treating her intestinal lining at the very beginning, using the simplest approach, which is with L-glutamine powder. Carol had 1 teaspoon of this very concentrated powder mixed with 4 ounces of water twice per day, on an empty stomach, or twenty minutes before a meal. Often this means when you wake up and when you go to sleep or before dinner. If you don't want to take a powder, you can take GI Repair Capsules or L-glutamine in capsule form. Then you need to take four capsules twice a day on an empty stomach or twenty minutes before a meal. Healing the lining takes time, and just like Carol, you will need to stay on these supplements for three months.

CHAPTER 10

Healing Your Gut Recipes

The recipes in this chapter are filled with the specific nutrients that support the beneficial bacteria living in your digestive tract and help heal your intestinal lining. I asked my culinary director, Marti Wolfson, to create recipes using cultured coconut milk to give your intestinal flora a boost because the cultures are filled with good bacteria and the coconut contains medium-chain triglycerides, which are great fuel for your intestinal cells and healing to the lining of your digestive tract. We also included foods such as chicken, turkey, and beans, which contain glutamine, an amino acid that helps maintain the health of the digestive system. Plus we added gut-healing ghee to as many recipes as possible, with the directions to make your own at the end of the chapter. Enjoy!

Recipes
Belly-licious Smoothie
Homemade Granola
Sprouted French Lentil Salad
Mung Bean Kitchari
Garlicky Greens in Coconut Oil
Orange, Fennel, and Golden Beet Salad
Turkey Burgers with Caramelized Onions
Chicken Stuffed with Red Peppers, Pine Nuts, and Spinach
Whipped Cauliflower
Blueberry Parfait with Cashew Cream
Ghee

Menu 1

Breakfast
Belly-licious Smoothie

Lunch
Mung Bean Kitchari
Garlicky Greens in Coconut Oil

Dinner
Turkey Burgers with Caramelized Onions
Orange, Fennel, and Golden Beet Salad

Menu 2

Breakfast
Homemade Granola

Lunch
Sprouted French Lentil Salad

Dinner
Chicken Stuffed with Red Peppers, Pine Nuts, and Spinach
Whipped Cauliflower

Dessert
Blueberry Parfait with Cashew Cream

Belly-licious Smoothie

Good bacteria are one of the key ingredients in a healthy gut. Yogurt and kefir are two probiotic foods that provide good bacteria to our digestive systems and are easy to incorporate into your daily diet. This satisfying smoothie is easy on the belly, while the citrus flavors transport the mind to a tropical island.

Makes 2 servings

1 cup mango, peeled and cut into chunks
1 banana
Juice of ½ orange
Juice of ½ lime
1 cup cultured coconut milk (or regular dairy kefir)
½ cup water
1 tbsp ground flaxseeds
1 serving protein powder (about 15 grams)

1. Combine all ingredients together in a blender and blend until smooth.

Homemade Granola

Most granolas are very high in refined sugar. Our recipe combines shredded coconut, honey, and spices to create a more wholesome sweetness and flavor. The coconut oil and the nuts provide good fats that fight inflammation. Brazil nuts are especially nutritious because they contain selenium, an essential mineral required for healthy thyroid function. Alter your ingredients according to your pantry or personal preference and enjoy.

Makes 16 servings (serving size ½ cup)

4 cups gluten-free rolled oats
1 cup shredded unsweetened coconut
½ cup Brazil nuts, coarsely chopped
½ cup almonds, coarsely chopped
½ cup walnuts, chopped
½ cup sunflower seeds

(*continued on next page*)

¼ cup coconut oil
⅓ cup honey
1 tsp vanilla extract
½ tsp cinnamon
½ tsp cardamom
2 tbsp maple syrup
⅓ cup dried currants or other fruit

1. Preheat oven to 325°F.
2. Place all the ingredients, except for the maple syrup and currants, in a roasting pan. Mix everything together with your hands until well combined. Bake for 15 minutes, then stir.
3. Bake for another 15 minutes, then drizzle maple syrup over the granola and stir.
4. Bake 10 minutes more or until golden brown. Remove from the oven. Stir in currants and serve.

Sprouted French Lentil Salad

Sprouting is a natural, no-heat way of preparing food that helps the stomach digest it better. When beans and lentils are sprouted, their enzymes are activated and made more available to the gut for easier digestion. The warm weather months are a nice time to eat sprouts because this is when our bodies crave more raw food. Every legume takes a different amount of time to sprout, with the larger ones such as chickpeas taking the longest.

Makes 4–6 servings

2 cups sprouted lentils (sprouting instructions below)
4 tbsp extra-virgin olive oil
Juice of 1 lemon
½ tsp salt
Pinch freshly ground pepper
1 tsp prepared mustard
1 tsp apple cider vinegar
1 heaping tbsp chopped parsley

1. To sprout lentils, rinse the lentils in a fine mesh strainer, picking out any small stones.

2. Drain lentils and then put them in a mason jar and cover with cheese-cloth and a rubber band.

3. Set the mason jar on its side in a cool dark place in the kitchen. Rinse lentils a couple of times per day to prevent any mold or bacteria from forming.

4. The lentils will take two to three days to sprout. The sprout should be at least ¼ inch long.

5. When they're ready to eat, whisk the remaining ingredients in a small bowl.

6. Pour over the lentils.

Mung Bean Kitchari

Kitchari is a classic dish in Ayurvedic medicine, the Indian science of life. Mung beans are one of the most digestible beans and when paired with rice become a complete protein. Classic Indian spices pop in flavor and nutrition when toasted in ghee, a clarified butter that is healing to the gut. This dish warms you inside and out. It's wonderful on a cold winter day or for periodic cleanses.

Makes 4–6 servings

½ cup mung beans, soaked overnight
1 cup basmati rice
3½ cups water
1 tbsp ghee
½ cup small-diced onion
1½ tsp ground cumin
½ tsp ground coriander
1½ tsp turmeric
Pinch cardamom
Pinch freshly ground pepper
½ tsp salt
Cilantro for garnish
Tamari or Bragg's Liquid Aminos for garnish

1. Put the beans, rice, and cold water in a pot, cover, and bring to a boil, then lower the temperature and simmer for 45 minutes.

(continued on next page)

2. Heat the ghee in a small pan over medium heat. Add the onions and cook until they soften, about 5 minutes.
3. Add the cumin, coriander, turmeric, cardamom, pepper, and salt to the onions and heat on low for another 5 minutes.
4. About 10 minutes before the mung beans and rice are finished cooking, add the onion-spice mixture to the lentils and rice and mix thoroughly.
5. Garnish with cilantro and tamari.

Garlicky Greens in Coconut Oil

Coconut oil, once wrongly deemed the bad fat on the block, has made a striking comeback because of all the health benefits it provides. It is made of medium-chain triglycerides, which are easily digested. Coconut oil is also antibacterial, antiviral, and an important saturated fat our bodies need in moderation. You have two choices when buying coconut oil: if you like the taste of coconut, choose virgin coconut oil because it tastes and smells like coconut. Choose the deodorized variety if you want the health benefits of coconut oil but don't care for the taste.

Makes 4–6 servings

1 tbsp coconut oil
3 cloves garlic, peeled and minced
5 cups Swiss chard or kale, ribs removed and leaves coarsely chopped
¼ tsp salt
¼ tsp freshly ground pepper

1. Heat the oil in a large sauté pan on medium-high heat.
2. Add the garlic and sauté until just softened.
3. Add the greens, stirring continuously, and sauté just until wilted.
4. Season with salt and pepper.

Orange, Fennel, and Golden Beet Salad

Nothing says spring like fennel and beets. This crunchy, colorful salad is a nice way to incorporate more raw vegetables as the weather warms up and our bodies crave less cooked food. This is a light dish that pairs well with fish and even balances out a heavier protein such as a burger.

Makes 4 servings

1 bulb fennel, shaved on a mandoline or thinly sliced
1 golden beet, cut into matchsticks
2 oranges, peeled, pith removed, and segmented
Zest of 1 orange
2 tsp chopped mint
1 tbsp brown rice vinegar
Juice of 1 lemon
2 tbsp olive oil
¼ tsp ground cumin
½ tsp salt

1. Combine the fennel, beets, and oranges in a medium bowl.
2. In a small bowl, whisk together the remaining ingredients and pour over the mixed vegetables.

Turkey Burgers with Caramelized Onions

Who says a burger can't have greens? Lean ground white meat turkey and spinach make this burger a healthy and hearty choice for you and the family. Spinach and turkey are rich in glutamine, the amino acid that is healing to the intestinal lining. Top this with caramelized onions for some added sweetness.

Makes 4 servings

1 lb lean ground turkey
1 medium onion, finely chopped
1 red bell pepper, seeded and chopped into small pieces
2 cups of spinach, chopped
3 cloves of garlic, minced

(continued on next page)

1 egg
1 tbsp gluten-free bread crumbs
1 tsp salt
1 tsp freshly ground pepper
Extra-virgin olive oil

1. Heat 1–2 tbsp oil in a large pan.
2. Add the onion and stir briefly until it is softened.
3. Add the red pepper and spinach and cook for 2 minutes.
4. Add garlic and stir for 2 minutes, then remove the mixture from the pan and allow to cool.
5. With a wooden spoon, mix together the turkey, egg, salt, pepper, bread crumbs, and spinach mixture. Form 4 patties.
6. In a nonstick pan, heat 1–2 tbsp oil on medium-high heat. Place the burgers in the pan and cook until slightly brown and cooked through, about 4–5 minutes per side. Slightly press the middle of each burger to make sure the center cooks.

Chicken Stuffed with Red Peppers, Pine Nuts, and Spinach

Spinach and parsley are high in glutamine, an amino acid that helps maintain the health of the intestinal lining. Here, chicken is pounded thin and wrapped around garlicky spinach, red peppers, parsley, currants, and pine nuts. The result is an elegant chicken dish that is satisfying to the eyes and stomach.

Makes 2–4 servings

Two 6-oz organic chicken breasts
1 tbsp dried oregano
Salt
Freshly ground pepper
4 tbsp extra-virgin olive oil
2 cloves garlic, minced
½ bunch spinach, chopped
Pinch red pepper flakes
2 small roasted red peppers, chopped
3 tbsp chopped parsley

2 tbsp currants
3 tbsp pine nuts, toasted
Any kind of butcher or kitchen string, presoaked in water

1. Preheat oven to 350 degrees.
2. Split each chicken breast in half and pound with a meat mallet between sheets of plastic wrap. Be careful not to make it too thin or the chicken will fall apart. Season on both sides with oregano, salt, and pepper.
3. Heat 2 tbsp olive oil on medium-high heat in a medium sauté pan. Add the garlic and cook for 30 seconds.
4. Add the spinach, a pinch of salt, a pinch of pepper, and the red pepper flakes to the garlic and sauté for a couple of minutes, or until the greens are wilted.
5. Remove from heat and add the roasted peppers, parsley, currants, and nuts.
6. Top each piece of chicken with one-quarter of the spinach mixture. Roll the chicken tightly around the filling and tie with the string.
7. In a medium pan heat the remaining 2 tbsp of olive oil on medium-high heat.
8. Add the chicken and brown on each side.
9. Place the pan in the oven and bake for 10 minutes or until the chicken is cooked through. Before serving cut the string. Then carefully slice each bundle into ½-inch pieces.

Whipped Cauliflower

Cauliflower is one of the few white foods that is nutritionally favorable, packed with vitamins, minerals, and phytochemicals. Here we puree it with ghee, a fat that is healing for the intestinal lining. A much healthier but equally tasty alternative to mashed potatoes, this side dish is simple enough for a weeknight and elegant enough for a special occasion. This is one of those great dishes that your kids will love, too.

Makes 6 servings

1 head cauliflower, broken into small florets
¼ cup minced parsley

(continued on next page)

2 tsp ghee or extra-virgin olive oil
Salt
Freshly ground pepper to taste

1. Bring a large pot of salted water to a boil.
2. Add cauliflower and cook until very tender, about 10 minutes.
3. Reserve ¼ cup of the cooking liquid and then drain the cauliflower well and transfer it to a food processor.
4. Add oil or ghee and reserved water, 1 tablespoon at a time, and puree until smooth.
5. Season with salt and pepper and garnish with parsley.

Blueberry Parfait with Cashew Cream

Agar is a healthful sea vegetable that has remarkable medicinal properties. In the kitchen, it acts as a gelatin, and it is typically used in puddings, parfaits, and tarts. This fiber- and mineral-rich vegetable from the sea soothes the digestive tract and reduces inflammation. You will find this parfait decadent while being light and creamy.

Makes 8 servings

4 cups apple juice
3 tbsp agar flakes (natural gelatin)
Pinch of salt
1 tbsp apple cider vinegar
2 cups frozen blueberries
1 cup plus 1 tbsp toasted cashews
1 tbsp maple syrup or agave syrup

1. In a large pot over medium-high heat, bring 3 cups of apple juice to a boil.
2. Immediately reduce to a simmer and stir in the agar flakes, salt, and vinegar. Continue to stir until the flakes have dissolved.
3. Remove from the heat, add the blueberries, and transfer to a 9-by-13-inch glass dish.
4. Refrigerate for about an hour or until it has firmly set.
5. Remove from the dish and blend with a handheld mixer or in a food processor until smooth.
6. Place 1 cup of cashews and the maple syrup in a food processor.

7. With the motor running, add the remaining 1 cup of apple juice slowly until you reach a smooth consistency.
8. Fill 8 dishes with a layer of the fruit mixture and add a layer of cashew cream.
9. Top with chopped cashews.

Ghee (Clarified Butter)
Reprinted with permission from Liz Lipski, PhD, CCN

Ghee is another name for clarified butter and is a traditional healing food in India. It is made by heating butter until it liquefies. The milk solids are removed, making it suitable for those who are dairy sensitive. You can also buy it already made in health food stores and Indian markets. Traditionally ghee has been used for ulcers, constipation, wound healing, and soothing the digestive tract.

1 pound unsalted organic butter

1. In a medium saucepan, heat butter on medium heat.
2. The butter will melt and then come to a boil. You will hear the butter snapping and crackling as it boils.
3. It will begin to foam at the top. Remove the foam with a spoon and discard.
4. After about 15–20 minutes you will hear the "voice" of the ghee change. It will get quieter. You'll see the oil become clear rather than cloudy.
5. Take it off the heat and strain it through cheesecloth or use a metal coffee filter and filter paper. You can wait 15 minutes or do this immediately. It's hot, so be careful.
6. Put into a ceramic, glass, or stone bowl and cover. This ghee will last for about a year unrefrigerated.

PART IV

Supporting Your Liver

Success is to be measured not so much by the position that one has reached in life as by the obstacles which he has overcome.

—Booker T. Washington

CHAPTER 11

Supporting Your Liver

It seems to me that we have been conducting a huge experiment on humans for the past sixty years. What do I mean? Since World War II, we have created and been exposed to thousands of chemicals and toxins with unknown health impacts and side effects. Some chemicals were removed from the market after it was discovered that they caused cancer. Examples include flame retardants that were once added to children's pajamas and the pesticide DDT, an insecticide for agricultural crops. But today we are discovering that some relatively new toxins may also play a role in the increasing prevalence of serious conditions such as cancer, diabetes, heart disease, and autoimmune diseases. What is important to understand is that the cumulative effect of all these toxins has created a big toxic load on your body without your knowing it.

My first goal in this chapter is to teach you about all the toxins that might cause or be associated with autoimmune diseases so that you can look around your environment and see which ones are lurking there. Removing your exposure to these compounds and reducing your toxic load is an important first step in your treatment. My second goal is to then help you clean the toxins out of your body.

A toxin is a substance that when ingested, inhaled, or coming into contact with your skin causes a reaction from the immune system because it is seen as foreign and dangerous. These toxic substances also cause direct damage to your cells and put a huge strain on your liver, the organ in charge of removing toxins from your body. Examples of toxins include:

- Dry-cleaning solvents
- Gasoline
- Auto fumes
- Tobacco smoke
- Resins
- Glue
- Paint

- Stain remover
- Heavy metals such as mercury, lead, arsenic, and cadmium
- Chemicals such as polychlorinated biphenyls (PCBs), of which dioxins are the most well known
- Pesticides such as organophosphates and organochlorides
- Toxic compounds found in plastics, such as BPA
- Some trace minerals, such as silica and iodine, that are good for us in very small amounts but make us sick when we are exposed to them in large quantities
- Drinking water that has become contaminated with high levels of prescription medications
- A group of compounds called xenobiotics, which include chemicals and compounds in the environment that act like estrogen in your body
- Toxins released by harmful bacteria, yeast, or parasites living in your gut

HOW YOUR LIVER HANDLES TOXINS

"Toxic load" is a term used to measure the total amount of all different kinds of toxins inside your cells and tissues. As the term implies, these toxins are difficult for your cells and liver to manage and for your body to process and remove so that you don't get sick. Your toxic load measures both how long and how high your exposure has been. The higher the load, the greater the chance that it is negatively affecting your health. In this section of the book, I want you to really get a sense of how high this toxic load is for you, which is why I mentioned a few of the different toxins you likely are exposed to. It's not that any one of them alone is causing your disease (although it might be; there isn't enough research to know); rather, the accumulation of all of them has stressed your detox system.

Your liver, your body's main detoxifying organ, does a heroic job every day trying to protect you from the bombardment of chemicals and toxins in the foods you eat, the air you breathe, and the water you drink. To imagine how your liver works, think of it like the strainer you use in the sink to drain cooked pasta. This strainer has lots of little holes, and when you pour the water and pasta into it, the water flows right through, leaving the pasta behind. Your liver is in charge of filtering all of your blood, which trickles through tiny vessels in the liver where the liver cells grab the toxins. Next, those cells transform the toxins so they are less dangerous and then either send them out of your body through your bile system or into your bloodstream to be filtered out through your kidneys. **If you are exposed to too many toxins for too long, they start clogging**

up your liver. To visualize this happening, let's go back to our strainer example. Imagine that the holes in the strainer are clogged. As a result, the bowl of the strainer fills up with water and pasta, which eventually overflow and spill out. In your body, this means that the liver is filling up with toxins that eventually overflow, spill out, and settle into all the tissues in your body.

Signs and symptoms of toxin-related illnesses include:

- Feeling tired all the time
- Not being able to think clearly (a.k.a. brain fog)
- Feeling puffy all over
- Headaches
- Muscle pain
- Tingling in your fingers or feet
- Unexplained weight gain

Healthy and beneficial nutrients found in food and supplements help your liver grab hold of the toxins you're exposed to and flush them out of your system. The higher your toxic load, the harder it is to process. As a result, the higher the load, the more nutrients (from foods such as vegetables, which we'll discuss in the next chapter) you need to consume.

Genetics play a role here, too, by influencing the functioning of the enzymes inside your liver cells and their ability to clear out toxins. If you are genetically handicapped, which means you were born with detox enzymes that don't work as effectively as they could, you need to be even more careful to reduce your toxic load and eat plenty of liver-supportive nutrients to stay healthy. I love to use the analogy of the canary in the coal mine. Miners used to bring a canary with them when they went to work down in the coal mines. The canary was much more sensitive to the presence of methane and carbon monoxide than they were, so when the canary died, the miners knew it was time to get out. The same goes for people with bad genetics in their detox system. I'm one of these people. I have had genetic tests done for my detox system, which revealed multiple handicaps in many of my pathways. I need to live cleaner than the person next to me because toxins will (and did) make me very sick. If you have an autoimmune disease, you might be a canary, too.

In the workbook chapter that follows, there is a self-assessment that will help you calculate your toxic load and another evaluation to see if you are experiencing toxin-related symptoms. This self-assessment will help you determine whether you are one of those people who might have bad genetics, and I will share information on genetic tests that are available, too.

YOUR ENVIRONMENTAL EXPOSURE: SOME EXAMPLES

Here are some interesting statistics to give you an idea of what you are up against in the world around you when it comes to toxins. There are numerous agencies involved in monitoring our exposures to chemicals and toxins from the environment, something that has become necessary because we are learning more and more about how these toxins are making us sick. In an effort to clean up our environment and reduce our exposures, the first step is to collect data. My hope is that when you see these lists, you will realize how big the problem is and that toxins are a problem for you, too.

The Centers for Disease Control and Prevention (CDC) conduct a large, ongoing survey to keep track of all the toxins that we are exposed to. Their *Fourth National Report on Human Exposure to Environmental Chemicals 2009* presents data for 212 chemicals that come from the thousands of people who participate in the National Health and Nutrition Examination Survey (NHANES).[1] They found widespread exposure to industrial chemicals, which means these chemicals were in the body of almost every American tested. Here are some examples:

- Polybrominated diphenyl ethers, fire retardants used in certain manufactured products
- Bisphenol A (BPA), found in plastics
- Polytetrafluoroethylene, which is used to create heat-resistant nonstick coatings in cookware. Choose anodized aluminum nonstick cookware for one safest alternative.
- Perchlorate, a chemical that is both naturally occurring and man-made and is used to manufacture fireworks, explosives, flares, and rocket propellant

(See the results for all 212 chemicals at www.cdc.gov/exposurereport.)

For at least three decades, scientists from the CDC's Environmental Health Laboratory have been using a technique known as biomonitoring to determine which environmental chemicals people have been exposed to. Biomonitoring measurements are the most health-relevant assessments of exposure because they measure how much of these chemicals actually get into our bodies. You can search their website for information at www.cdc.gov/biomonitoring/biomonitoring_summaries.html. Currently, more than three hundred environmental chemicals or their metabolites are measured in human samples.

Additional research by the Environmental Working Group (EWG) in 2005 found as many as 232 chemicals, including known carcinogens and neurotoxins, in the cord blood of ten newborns. Even though this study was small, it opened the door for many more studies now under way that look at the exposure to chemicals for both children and adults. In late 2006, the EWG in collaboration with *Commonweal* began a project called the Human Toxome Project with the goal of measuring the total amount of all types of toxins in humans. This project, which continues today, monitors more than five hundred different chemicals and toxins. (You can look up testing results and sort them by where you live or your age group at www.ewg.org/sites/humantoxome.)[2]

More and more attention has been given by the government, researchers, political action groups, and grassroots movements to uncover all the different toxins we are exposed to, to force companies to change and clean up the chemicals they use in their products, and to raise awareness about choosing better products. For example, for more than twenty years, the U.S. Environmental Protection Agency's Toxics Release Inventory (TRI) program has required industrial facilities to report the release, disposal, incineration, treatment, and recycling of 650 chemicals covered by the law.[3] While everyone agrees these companies need to report what they are releasing into the air, the debate still rages over what levels are considered too high and reportable.

MERCURY

Heavy metals have long been associated with autoimmune diseases, and mercury has the most data linking it to these conditions. Exposure varies among different people, but it is widespread because there are several ways you can come in contact with it. Mercury is found in dental amalgam (also called silver fillings), cosmetics, pesticides, and some vaccines. It's also a pollutant released into the air from many factories, especially those that burn coal. Then it settles in the soil and the bottom of the oceans, lakes, and rivers. There the small fish eat the algae, which contain mercury, and the big fish eat the small fish, so the mercury accumulates up the food chain, with the biggest fish, such as tuna and swordfish, having the highest levels. (Wild king salmon are the most immune to mercury because these fish are vegetarians, which is one reason this type of salmon is such a good source of protein and omega-3 fatty acids.)

The health impacts are highly dependent on which form of mercury you're exposed to. For example, dental amalgam is the major source of mercury vapor exposure. The most commonly used dental amalgam material contains approximately 50 percent liquid metallic mercury. Thus, when you get a silver amalgam filling, the preparation and placement of it in your mouth causes mercury vapor exposure for you, your dentist, and the technician. Usually your dentist and the technician are wearing a mask, but you aren't. Plus every time you chew, brush your teeth, or drink hot beverages, mercury vapor is released. Then you inhale it into your lungs and it enters your bloodstream. Studies have shown a direct correlation between the number of amalgam fillings and mercury concentration in the blood and urine.[4]

Occupational exposure to mercury occurs in gold mining and in the factory process for purifying and making chlorine. High levels of exposure may also occur with the use of skin lightening creams that contain mercury. In the body, inhaled inorganic mercury from breathing in mercury vapors can accumulate in and have toxic effects on the nervous system and kidneys. Mercury vapors cross over the blood-brain barrier very easily and can accumulate in the brain.

Methylmercury exposure is almost exclusively from seafood such as tuna and swordfish. Methylmercury is chemically different from inorganic mercury, and this difference changes how it acts in the body. Research has shown a direct correlation between the amount of fish consumed and methylmercury levels in the blood and hair. This type of mercury is toxic to the brain but doesn't cross over the blood-brain barrier as easily as the inorganic variety; instead, it accumulates in other tissues of the body. When you measure blood levels of mercury, if they are elevated, it is usually from methylmercury. All forms of mercury, once inside your cells, create free radicals, which are molecules that damage enzyme activity, cell membranes, and your DNA (the genetic code inside the cells).

Both forms of mercury (methylmercury and mercury vapor) pass easily through the placenta from a mother to her unborn child. Research has shown that methylmercury is absorbed into the placenta and stored in the fetal brain in concentrations that exceed maternal blood levels. The fact that it gets concentrated is even more dangerous, and some studies have linked prenatal mercury exposure to impaired cognitive function in children. High-level prenatal exposure may also result in developmental problems that include mental retardation, cerebellar ataxia, dysarthria, limb deformities, altered physical growth, sensory impairments, and cerebral palsy.

MERCURY

How does it feel to have very high levels of mercury in your body? Chronic low level exposure can cause:

- Tremors
- Gum disease
- Irritability
- Depression
- Short-term memory loss
- Fatigue
- Anorexia
- Sleep disturbance

High levels of methylmercury primarily affect the central nervous system, causing numbness and tingling; difficulty with balance, walking, and speaking; hearing impairment; and changes in vision. Acute, high-dose exposure to elemental mercury vapor may cause severe pneumonitis, which is inflammation in the lungs, according to the CDC's National Biomonitoring Program.

That said, many of my patients with high mercury levels do not have the classic signs of acute poisoning. Instead, I often see the typical fuzzy symptoms that bring you to the doctor. Unfortunately, your conventional doctor will do routine blood tests and declare you completely healthy despite the fact that you may be suffering from brain fog, muscle fatigue, overall fatigue, anxiety, depression, and difficulty concentrating and remembering things. You may also have difficulty exercising because you feel worse afterward, sometimes because of numbness and tingling in your hands, feet, or other parts of the body. These are the signs of low-level chronic exposure. If you do have any of these symptoms, and especially if you have some of the more severe symptoms of mercury poisoning, you need to follow my instructions in the workbook that follows and get tested.

ARSENIC

There are other heavy metals such as arsenic and lead that are not clearly associated with autoimmune diseases but which I want to mention. Because these other metals are metabolized in the body just like mercury, exposure to them makes it harder for you to remove any mercury from your body, which will increase your risk of autoimmune diseases. Arsenic can cause cancer in humans and contaminate drinking water. In 1975, passage of the U.S. Safe Drinking Water Act banned arsenic for use as a pesticide, and in 2003 it was banned for use in pressure-treated lumber, which was the main kind of wood used for outdoor decks and playground equipment. However, the U.S. Food and Drug Administration (FDA) has approved several organic arsenic compounds for use in small amounts as antimicrobials in animal and poultry feeds. Because the animals eat the arsenic and we eat the animals, our exposure to arsenic continues.

LEAD

Lead, which has a long history of human use, was finally banned in paint and gasoline in the 1970s, although it took until the 1990s for it to be completely removed from gasoline. Lead is a severe neurotoxin. It is absorbed easily from the gastrointestinal tract, especially in children. It also accumulates in the bone, where it can be stored for many years, only to be released into the blood after menopause, when bones increase their breaking-down/building-up cycles. I always review environmental exposures with my patients at our first consultation, and I am always shocked to find out that some people remember eating paint chips when they were children in older homes, or living in an old house during renovation and breathing in all the dust for months on end. Furthermore, drinking city water from the tap can cause lead exposure because the old pipes that bring the water to the tap from under the streets of the city are filled with lead. Just because the water is tested at a water treatment facility doesn't mean it isn't contaminated on the way to your kitchen. (I sometimes think that I should invest in a water filter company, because I tell everyone to get a reverse osmosis filter for their kitchen sink.) Cleaning up your exposures to all of these metals is important for your health, especially if you think that you have toxin-related illness, which we'll test you for in the next chapter.

Cosmetics (yes, cosmetics) are another issue. Many brand-name lipsticks contain lead. In fact, 61 percent of the thirty-three lipsticks tested by the Campaign for Safe Cosmetics in 2007 contained lead despite the fact that lead wasn't listed as an ingredient on any of them.[5] In 2009, the FDA released a study that found lead in all the lipstick samples they tested. That's surprising enough, but even worse was that the lead found ranged from 0.09 to 3.06 parts per million (ppm)—levels four times higher than those found in the Campaign for Safe Cosmetics study! The highest lead levels were in lipsticks made by three very well-known manufacturers: Procter & Gamble (Cover Girl brand), L'Oreal (L'Oreal, Body Shop, and Maybelline brands), and Revlon. An expanded FDA follow-up study in February 2012 found lead in hundreds of lipsticks at levels up to 7.19 ppm. Keep in mind that the latest scientific research indicates that there is no safe level of lead exposure. But there are safer cosmetics that are free of harmful chemicals and metals, and you can find them by visiting the EWG's website at www.ewg.org/skindeep.[6]

PLASTICS

Laboratory tests commissioned by the EWG have, for the first time, detected bisphenol A (BPA), a plastic component and estrogen-like compound, in the umbilical cord blood of American infants. An estrogen-like compound acts like the hormone estrogen inside your body, which is dangerous because it can have effects such as causing early puberty and difficult periods, and it may increase the risk of estrogen-related cancers such as those of the breast, ovaries, and uterus. Chemicals that act like hormones in the body are called endocrine disruptors and BPA is one of them. Where else can you be exposed to BPA? EWG testing found high levels of BPA on 40 percent of paper receipts that came from cash registers and ATMs sampled from major U.S. businesses and services.[7] Studies like this make it clear that our chemical exposure is sometimes where we least expect it.

Dioxins and polychlorinated biphenyls (PCBs) belong to a family of very toxic chemicals that were banned in the 1970s, but they still persist in the environment and our bodies. Dioxins are created during burning of forests or household trash, chlorine bleaching of wood pulp and paper, or manufacturing or processing of certain types of chemicals, such as pesticides. Until they were banned in 1979, PCBs were used in insulator fluids in heat exchangers and transformers, in hydraulic fluids, and as additives to paints, oils, and caulks.

Even though they are no longer manufactured, all of these chemicals remain in the environment, persisting in the soil and water. Animals are exposed to these chemicals first, and then we're exposed to them by eating high-fat animal foods such as milk products, eggs, meat, and some fish. These compounds build up in the body and are stored in fatty tissues and in fluids such as breast milk, and they can be passed on to fetuses and infants during pregnancy and lactation. In the CDC's *Fourth National Report on Human Exposure to Environmental Chemicals,* scientists measured twenty-six different dioxin- and PCB-related compounds in the blood serum of at least 1,800 participants twelve years and older. Also, PCBs have been found in all thirty-five people tested in the EWG/ *Commonweal* studies. The EPA has noted that these low-level exposures are unavoidable because the chemicals are widespread in the environment. As a consequence, exposures begin when you're in the womb, when chemicals cross the placenta, and newborn infants begin to ingest them from the very first days of life.

PESTICIDES, PRESCRIPTION MEDICATIONS, AND MORE

The most common pesticides are called organophosphates and organochlorines, which are used in agriculture to kill insects. Humans are exposed when they eat the plants that have been treated. According to the CDC, when people are exposed to small amounts of these pesticides over a long period of time, they may feel tired or weak, irritable, depressed, or forgetful. In the CDC's report, scientists found measurable levels of six different organophosphate metabolites in at least 1,903 participants ages six to fifty-nine.

Another form of toxin exposure is to prescription medications, and I'm not just talking about the drugs you take to treat an illness. I'm talking about drinking low-level mixtures of pharmaceuticals with every glass of water. It sounds unbelievable, but it's a reality. A wide range of pharmaceuticals, including antibiotics, sex hormones, and drugs used to treat epilepsy and depression, contaminate the drinking water supply used by at least 41 million Americans, according to a five-month study by the Associated Press National Investigation Team released in March 2008. Additional studies by the EWG have found that tap water across the United States is contaminated. To make matters worse, drinking-water treatment plants are not designed to remove these residues. In fact, the Associated Press National Investigation Team uncovered data showing these same chemicals in treated tap water and water supplies in twenty-four major metropolitan areas around the United States.[8]

The EWG's national drinking water database shows tap water testing results from forty thousand communities around the country. Since 2004, testing by water utilities has found 315 pollutants in the tap water that Americans drink, according to an EWG drinking water quality analysis of almost 20 million records obtained from state water officials. More than half of the chemicals detected, such as pharmaceuticals, are not subject to health or safety regulations and can legally be present in any amount. Not only has the EPA failed to set standards for pharmaceuticals, but they have also failed to require water treatment plants to test for these chemicals.

I know I am sharing a lot of frightening information, but I am not trying to scare you or make you feel hopeless. Yes, there is plenty of evidence that you are exposed to hundreds of chemicals and toxins foreign to your body, and yes, some of these have been linked to autoimmune disease. But there is a lot we can do to fix this problem, and that's my goal. What I am sharing with you is knowledge, and knowledge is power. **The first step is to understand the connection between toxin exposure and your health. The next is for me to help you identify where in your environment your exposures might be so that we can take steps to remove them.** We must find the tack and pull it out because there might be an association between your autoimmune disease and one or more of these toxins. Then we can help your liver get to work clearing out the toxic load that has accumulated in your body, which in turn will help your immune system come into balance again.

AUTOIMMUNE DISEASE AND TOXINS: HEAVY METALS AND XENOESTROGENS

Heavy Metals

Let's move on to what we know about the association between specific toxins and autoimmune diseases. First I will share with you the latest information about heavy metals, especially mercury. These metals have been used by humans for thousands of years and even though we know that they cause health problems, exposure to them continues and is even increasing in some parts of the world, especially in less developed countries.

There are a few theories about how mercury causes autoimmune diseases. The first is that it alters or damages the cells in your tissues, making them look foreign to your immune system, which then attacks the cell. The other is that mercury stimulates the army of cells in the immune system called lymphocytes and they grow abnormally, losing their tolerance and ability to tell the difference between self and not self. Then they either directly attack or make antibodies to attack your own tissue.

Among all heavy metals, mercury is the most important, and estimates are that environmental levels of mercury have grown threefold in the past century. As far back as 1986 there were reports of a connection between multiple sclerosis and chronic exposure to mercury from dental amalgam fillings. Researchers from Isfahan University of Medical Sciences in Iran studied a group of MS patients in Isfahan, a city with both industrial pollution with mercury and a high incidence of MS. They found a significant positive correlation between high mercury levels and MS.[9] A study out of the University of Milan reported the case of a patient with MS who had high levels of mercury, aluminum, and lead, and after he went through chelation (a toxin removal treatment that I'll explain more in the next chapter), his MS symptoms improved.[10] (I will share with you a similar story of my patient Steve in the next chapter.)

Many studies have shown that mercury exposure can cause autoimmune diseases in rats. In these studies, the mice were given mercury and then the researchers watched the mice develop autoimmune diseases such as MS and lupus.[11, 12] Of course, you can't do similar studies in humans, so most of the studies are based on self-reports (which is when people are asked about their past mercury exposure) or they compare the characteristics of people with autoimmune diseases to those who don't have them (called case-control studies). A study from the National Institute of Environmental Health Sciences in North Carolina found a strong link between lupus and self-reported mercury exposure and also a connection between lupus and working in a dental office.[13] Other research has found a connection between higher levels of mercury (diagnosed by looking at the mercury level in hair, which is a way to measure chronic high exposure) with a positive ANA, which is the first sign of an autoimmune process that can lead to lupus.[14] In yet another study, scleroderma patients had a higher concentration of mercury in their urine compared to patients without scleroderma antibodies.[15]

But the evidence is strongest for the association between mercury and autoimmune thyroid disease. Studies show that people with higher mercury exposures have an increased risk of getting an autoimmune thyroid disease. And if you have an autoimmune thyroid disease, there's an increased likelihood that you also have high levels of mercury in your body.

There is evidence that mercury accumulates in the thyroid gland and is one cause of autoimmune thyroid diseases. There are two types of autoimmune thyroid diseases: Graves' disease, where antibodies are stimulating the thyroid gland to be overactive, and Hashimoto's thyroiditis, where there are anti-thyroid antibodies blocking the thyroid gland's ability to make hormones, making it underactive. Keep in mind that you can have these antibodies for two to seven years before your thyroid becomes damaged enough to show signs of thyroid hormone imbalances. The autoimmune process starts first, and unless your doctor tests you for antibodies, you might never know that you have it until one day you notice that you are extremely tired, have gained weight, are losing your hair, have no sex drive, are constipated, and/or feel cold all the time. If you develop hyperthyroidism from the Graves' disease antibodies, you can experience heart palpitations, weight loss, and insomnia, and your eyes can begin to look like they are popping out, a condition called exophthalmos. Once you develop these symptoms, your thyroid hormones are out of balance, caused by years of damage from the undetected antibodies from the autoimmune disease. (In my office, I check everyone for antibodies at the first visit, because I want to catch this problem early and fix it before your thyroid hormones are affected.)

What have we learned from the research about mercury and autoimmune thyroid diseases? Researchers in the Department of Preventive Medicine at Stony Brook University looked at blood levels of mercury and anti-thyroid antibodies in women over the age of twenty who were not using birth control pills, not pregnant, and not lactating and found that those with the higher mercury levels had a much greater risk for having higher thyroglobulin antibodies.[16] This information has important implications for everyone with Hashimoto's thyroiditis and for people with other autoimmune diseases who also have elevated thyroglobulin antibody levels. Elevated thyroglobulin antibody levels are very common in patients with rheumatoid arthritis, lupus, pernicious anemia, fibromyalgia, chronic hives, and type 1 diabetes and suggests that these other diseases are associated with mercury as well. Therefore, the association found between mercury and these antibodies could indicate a broader relationship between mercury and other immune-related disorders.

Vaccinations

Before leaving our discussion about mercury, it is important to mention the use of heavy metals in vaccinations. Mercury is added as a preservative and aluminum is added to some vaccines to enhance the immune-stimulating effect so that these shots work better. (Something added to increase the immune response to a vaccine is called an adjuvant.) In other words, aluminum is being used to irritate the immune system so that it will react to the mumps, measles, or other virus in the vaccine in a bigger way to make more antibodies. While this process must have made sense to the people who were just concerned about making a successful vaccine (success meaning that the people receiving the vaccine would become immune to the disease), they ignored the dangers of what they were putting into the mix.

The most-studied links between vaccines and autoimmune conditions involve Guillain-Barré syndrome (an autoimmune disease of the nerves and muscles) after the 1976 swine influenza vaccine; immune thrombocytopenic purpura, which is when your platelets are destroyed by antibodies after the measles, mumps, and rubella vaccine; and myoperi-carditis, an inflammation in and around the heart after smallpox vaccination. There have also been reports of an increased risk of developing rheumatoid arthritis, MS, or thrombocytopenia (low platelets) in adults receiving the hepatitis B vaccine. The question remains whether the illness was caused by the infectious agent in the vaccine, the mercury in the preservative, or the adjuvant (aluminum). There are also almost twenty-five cases in the literature linking lupus and vaccines, specifically those for typhoid-paratyphoid A and B, scarlet fever, and hepatitis B. In fact, a new phrase has been coined, "autoimmune/inflammatory syndrome induced by adjuvants" (ASIA), because so many people are developing immune issues after vaccinations.[17]

Mercury, when put in vaccines as a preservative, is called thimerosal. Because many studies in mice have shown that exposure to low levels of mercury induces autoimmune reactions, it seems obvious that giving it to people, especially babies and children, could be a dangerous idea. In fact, one of the most active areas of research right now is looking at the association of mercury in vaccines with the development of autism in children. While, to date, studies have not proven the cause, the debate still rages and has many parents concerned. And while vaccinations have proven to be remarkably efficient in preventing infectious diseases, questions have been raised about the possibility that the mercury or aluminum might be triggering autoimmune diseases in people who have a genetic susceptibility. (However, no controlled trial has yet confirmed that this triggering of an autoimmune disease could happen.) While most of the recent focus has been on mercury, almost every vaccine has aluminum used as an adjuvant because it is such a potent stimulator of the immune system. While you can't avoid aluminum, they are now making mercury-free immunizations, and I suggest you look for these. If you have an autoimmune disease, speak to your doctor before getting any immunizations. If you are on any immune-suppressing medications, you should know that vaccines don't work very well, and so the benefit might not be worth the risk of exposure to the aluminum or mercury in the vaccine.

Let me be clear: I am not against vaccines. As a public health measure, they are necessary to keep us safe from dangerous infectious diseases that killed many children and adults in the early part of the twentieth century. I am just pointing out that studies are increasingly showing evidence that these adjuvants (and aluminum is still being used in most vaccines) might be causing severe immune stress with unknown consequences. There has to be a better, safer way to immunize both children and adults to reduce infectious diseases in the general population.

Xenoestrogens

For the last fifty years, there has been much evidence that environmental chemicals, such as pesticides and industrial chemicals, can cause hormone-like effects. When these chemicals mimic the effects of estrogen in the body, they are called xenoestrogens, and they are all around us in food, soil, air, water, and household products. Some of these toxins are stored in your body fat, so when you go on a diet, they are released, and you can feel sluggish. But they also cause symptoms like estrogen does—women, for example, have fuller and more tender breasts, heavier and more painful periods, bloating, and water retention. If you are a man, you might notice more breast tissue or a low sex drive. Xenoestrogens are one important type of xenobiotic, which is an environmental substance of synthetic, natural, or biologic origin that can mimic the effects of estrogen in the body. You need to know about these because they play a role in the development of autoimmune diseases.

Xenoestrogens are found in plastics, detergents, surfactants, pesticides, and industrial chemicals. They're also found in conventional dairy and meat you eat because those animals are treated with hormones to grow faster and make more milk, which is why I suggest you buy organic dairy, eggs, beef, chicken, turkey, and pork. These environmental estrogens have spread all over the globe. Amazingly, high levels of dichlorodiphenyltrichloroethane (DDT), a pesticide, have even been found in the Arctic, far from any people or factories. A group of researchers from the University of Milan conducted a review of all the studies looking at the role of environmental estrogens and autoimmunity. Over and over, they found a positive association between exposure to different agricultural chemical pesticides and rheumatoid arthritis, lupus, and a positive anti-nuclear antibody (ANA) laboratory test. They also reported that exposure to PCBs has been linked to rheumatoid arthritis and dioxins linked to a positive ANA. Humans have always been exposed to phytoestrogens and mycoestrogens (plants and fungi that have mild estrogenic activity), but our exposure to this new class of environmental chemicals increased dramatically in the twentieth century.[18]

The first sign that something was amiss came years ago when aviation crop dusters handling DDT were found to have low sperm counts and factory workers working closely with pesticides were found to have low libido, low sperm counts, and impotence. Then came the headlines that feminized male fish were found near sewage treatment plants. The fact that estrogen-like substances were polluting the environment couldn't be denied anymore. Next came the discovery that chemicals in plastics, among them BPA, which I mentioned earlier, were being metabolized in our bodies into estrogen-like compounds. These xenoestrogens have also been called estrogen mimics because they bind to estrogen receptors and increase estrogen activity in the body.

My point is that there are many, many problematic chemicals out there, and every chemical you are exposed to adds to your toxic load. **Having a high toxic load makes it harder for your liver to handle mercury, pesticides, and environmental estrogens, toxins that we know will affect your immune system.**

Autoimmune diseases are much more prevalent in women; 75 percent of autoimmune diseases affect women, while 25 percent affect men. This statistic makes it seem like estrogen is involved in some way. We know that estrogen affects the immune system, because all immune cells have estrogen receptors and these hormones also encourage your immune cells to begin to make too many antibodies. The role of estrogens in autoimmune diseases has been well studied in women with lupus. Researchers from the National University Health System, Singapore, did a thorough review study looking at the role of estrogens in autoimmunity. They report evidence that oral contraceptives and the use of postmenopausal hormone replacement therapy (HRT) increased the risk of lupus and that the incidence of lupus rises after puberty and drops after menopause, when estrogen levels are lower.[19] These findings make sense because estrogen causes a shift toward Th2 (lymphocytes that make antibodies) and women with lupus are already Th2 dominant; thus the extra estrogen makes the disease worse. The severity of symptoms in patients with lupus often gets worse as estrogen levels climb, such as during the menstrual cycle and during pregnancy.

But what about xenoestrogens and lupus? Reports from the Research Laboratory on Immuno-Rheumatology in Milan, Italy, reveal that several pesticides (chlordane, HCB, PCP, and chlorpyrifos) have been associated with an increased prevalence of a positive ANA and that farming and agricultural pesticide use has been associated with lupus. A weak association has also been reported for organochlorine pesticide exposure

KAREN

When I think about pesticides, I'm reminded of a forty-eight-year-old patient of mine named Karen. She had numbness and tingling in her fingers, was exhausted, and had signs of high estrogen, with tender breasts, PMS, and heavy periods. The many doctors she went to see before me found only a positive ANA. The most interesting thing I discovered from her story was that she had been in Europe for five years before she got sick and lived in a valley next to vineyards. Every day the crop-dusting planes would fly overhead and drop clouds of pesticides on her house. Honestly, uncovering her pesticide exposure was one of the easiest pieces of detective work I ever had to do! So we went to work on her detox system, as I will show you how to do in the next chapter. At the time I'm writing this, my work with Karen has only just begun, but I am confident that she will make a full recovery. I share this story with you to prove that pesticide exposures are not a thing of the past—they are still happening on a large scale. Do you remember seeing trucks going through your neighborhood when you were young, spraying a big white cloud of pesticides behind them? I have many patients who tell me they remember running and dancing in the clouds behind the trucks. At the time it seemed fun, but in retrospect they realize that this was a really bad idea and might have started the accumulation of toxins that are now making them sick.

and rheumatoid arthritis. The Women's Health Initiative Observational Study looked at seventy-six postmenopausal women ages fifty to seventy-nine and found that personal use of insecticides was associated with an increased risk of rheumatoid arthritis and lupus. This risk was also associated with long-term and frequent insecticide application among women with a farm history.[20] While these are only a few studies and they need to be replicated in other populations to confirm results, they do suggest a connection between environmental pesticide exposure and the development of autoimmune rheumatic diseases such as lupus and RA.

Why am I telling you this story about estrogens in the detox chapter? Because environmental estrogens coming into your body and behaving like revved-up, supercharged, harsh estrogen is a big problem. We are beginning to understand that there are different kinds of estrogens in the body and they each have different effects on your cells and health. **Some estrogens are gentle, but some are what we call toxic, because they are more likely to cause cancer or cause autoimmune diseases, and your liver has a vital role in determining which kind you will have.** The idea that toxic estrogen metabolites made in the liver could be responsible for triggering lupus has been supported by many human clinical observation studies and experimental animal studies.

Let's talk about how the liver metabolizes estrogens. You make estrogen in your body, and you take it intentionally if you are on birth control pills or hormone replacement. You also know now that you are filled with xenoestrogens from the environment. All of this estrogen doesn't just sit around; it is constantly moving, and your liver is supposed to detoxify it by changing its structure so that it can be less active and excreted through your bile. The first step in estrogen detoxification happens in what is called the cytochrome P450 system in the liver; afterward it can be made into either good, soft, gentle estrogen or bad, harsh, more toxic estrogen. This process is very important to understand because when you have symptoms of too much estrogen, it is usually too much of the toxic estrogens.

Researchers at Boston University School of Medicine have looked at the metabolism of estrogens in women with lupus and found that they are making more of the harsh estrogens, possibly triggering their disease or making it worse.[21]

How does it feel to have too many toxic estrogens in your body? You might have noticed you have more PMS symptoms, such as breast tenderness or fullness, anxiety or other mood changes, water retention, and insomnia, and you might also have noticed that your period is heavier, longer, or irregular. These are all symptoms of what we call estrogen dominance—too much estrogen activity. Estrogen and progesterone help balance each other, and so estrogen dominance symptoms are worse when progesterone is low, which can be caused by chronic stress. Therefore, in addition to supporting your estrogen detox pathways by optimizing your liver function, as we are doing in this chapter and the workbook that follows, you need to support your body's production of progesterone by following the treatment discussed in Chapter 6, "Understanding the Stress Connection Workbook."

Why do some people make toxic estrogens in their liver and some people don't? One reason is genetic. Some people have genes that predispose them to make more of the bad estrogens and not enough of the good. But genetics do not determine a guaranteed outcome. Toxins can be a bad influence on the enzymes made by these genes, but food can make a big difference, with healthy fats and plant compounds influencing them in a good way. **So the first step is to clean up your environment and remove all of the xenoestrogens and other toxins around you. The next step is to help your liver do a better job removing toxic estrogens from your body.** The following chapter, "Supporting Your Liver Workbook," will help you do just that.

IMPROVING DETOXIFICATION, REMOVING METALS, AND REVERSING DISEASE

I have described the relationship between autoimmune diseases, mercury, and environmental xenoestrogens, how they make you sick, and the importance of detoxifying estrogens in your liver. Now it is time to explain how to help your body remove all harmful compounds, including mercury and xenoestrogens. Toxins are stored in every cell in your body, and you need to get them out.

The first way to remove toxins from your body is to optimize your liver function. Our goal is to help all of your cells process and remove toxins better. Think of your detox system as a little engine that is inside every cell, with the biggest engine in the liver. Just like the engine in your car, these motors need gas to keep them running. If you overwork your car by driving too far without enough gas in it, the engine will stall. If you overwork your liver by burdening it with too many toxins without giving it enough nutrients to run, it stalls, too, and the toxins begin to accumulate in your body and tissues because the engine isn't running. When I talk about optimizing your liver function so that it is able to process and remove toxins better, I am referring to giving your detox engine the fuel it needs to do its job better. So part one of our program is to get the engine going, which may be all you need to feel better. Boosting the estrogen detoxification pathways is an easy add-on to this part of the program.

The second way is to focus on mercury and what we know about removing it from the body safely. For some people, just doing the liver support mentioned above will be enough. But if you have high mercury levels (you will need to have the test done to know), you might have to go to the next step, which is treatment that specifically helps your body remove mercury. Here I will explain glutathione, metallothionein, and chelation. There are circumstances where it makes sense to use particular chelation compounds to grab the metals and pull them out. For this part of our discussion I will share my experience, discuss the circumstances under which I recommend specific chelation compounds, and review the research on using chelation to treat heavy metal overload.

Improving Detoxification: The Place to Start

Your liver is filled with enzymes that are grouped into different detox systems. There are three different detox pathways in the liver, called Phase 1, Phase 2, and Phase 3. You can think of them like steps in a recipe. You start with an ingredient (the toxin), add some antioxidants or other B vitamins, and process them together in some way (the enzyme). Just like cooking, the enzyme changes the structure of the ingredients, so the toxin is transformed into something that is less toxic. After the first step, you add some new ingredients, maybe some amino acids from protein, process again (another enzyme), and presto—you have a completely new compound that is harmless and ready to be excreted from the body. This last step, removing the new end product, is the last phase and requires the toxin in its new form to be sent out into the bile and then your stool, or into the blood and then your kidneys into your urine.

All of the enzymes involved in these different steps in the detox system in your liver have to be working really well so that there is a constantly fast-flowing river carrying the blood into the liver, where the toxins are removed, transformed, and released into the bile and your stool. Remember the strainer I mentioned earlier? What happens if the river can't flow through here because the strainer is all clogged? The toxins overflow from the liver and you get sick because the toxins start to pool in your tissues. When the liver (strainer) is clogged with toxins, it is hard for the filter to work well, and it slows down.

The good news? All of these enzymes in your liver can be made to work better, and we can clear the toxins out and open up the filter so the strainer isn't clogged anymore. Boosting your liver enzymes, including those I talked about earlier that help you remove toxic estrogens, will get things moving. All of these enzymes have nutritional needs that are outlined in the workbook chapter that follows. **When you give the liver enzymes what they need, you turn on the engine, and the toxins sitting in the cells all over your body start to move into your liver to be transformed into a less harmful compound and then excreted.** Your estrogens go into the liver and are transformed into the less harmful type, too. If you want to reduce your toxic burden, making your liver enzymes work better is the place to start.

Removing Metals: Glutathione

Now I want to focus on specific strategies that have been used to get the river flowing and move the metals out of the body. Let's start our discussion on removing metals with a focus on mercury, because as you already know, it is associated with autoimmune disease and there is a lot of it in our environment. First I want to explain how your body protects itself from exposure to metals.

The term "heavy metal" encompasses a number of essential and nonessential metals. Among the latter, cadmium, mercury, and lead are toxic even in trace amounts. Although zinc and copper, which are essential heavy metals, are integral parts of your tissues and enzymes, an excess of these metals is also toxic. So you can see how important it is for your body to be able to hold on to the metals it needs and get rid of those it doesn't. For this purpose, your body has developed elaborate systems to import, sequester, store, transport, and expel all of these different metals. The most important players in this metal balancing act are glutathione and the metallothioneins. Both of these systems need to be working really well so that you don't accumulate too many metals, especially mercury.

Glutathione is the most important antioxidant. It's in every cell in your body, but it's found in highest concentrations in the liver. **Not only does glutathione clean up heavy metals such as mercury, cadmium, and arsenic, but it also aids in protecting the body from pesticides, solvents, and plastic residues such as BPA.** It has a natural role in mopping up the everyday end products of your body's metabolism, called free radicals, which are activated oxygen molecules that were generated inside your cells as a result of energy production and which can damage your cells. Glutathione's ongoing and important job is to disarm these oxygen molecules. With so much work to do, glutathione is always getting used up and constantly has to be made by the body. If you have environmental exposures to heavy metals, solvents, and pesticides, the glutathione levels in your body can get depleted. This depletion begins a process that can lead to damage to your tissues.

As you already know, one theory of how you get an autoimmune disease is that your tissue gets damaged and then your immune system attacks it. The first and most important way that mercury is removed from your body is by glutathione, especially in your liver, where it is secreted into bile and then into your stool. **The bottom line: if you don't have enough glutathione, you can have trouble removing mercury, which can build up, harm your cells, and cause autoimmune diseases.** Studies have shown that increasing glutathione levels will increase the excretion of mercury in the bile.

How do you become low in glutathione? Here is where it gets interesting. Glutathione is made by an important enzyme called glutathione-S-transferase (GST), and some people have a handicapped version thanks to their genes. If you're one of them, your glutathione levels get depleted very easily, making it harder to remove heavy metals and toxins from your body. Remember my story about the canary in the coal mine? People with low-functioning GST because of genetics are canaries. I know that I am one of them because the genetic testing that looks at your detox pathways showed that my GST genes are the worst possible. Because of my genetic handicap, I got sick from mercury at one point in my life, while my husband did not, even though our exposure was probably very similar.

But your genetics are not your destiny. Think of them like a roadblock, not a dead end; there is plenty we can do to help the handicapped enzymes work better. We can get past the roadblock by first removing as many toxins as possible from your body and environment and then using strategies and supplements to increase the amounts of glutathione in your body. We will tackle this obstacle in the workbook chapter that follows.

Another way you can get low in glutathione is if your diet lacks the raw materials required for making it. Glutathione is made from three amino acids: cysteine, glutamic acid, and glycine. Of the three, cysteine is the most important because it contains sulfur, which is the component that grabs on to and binds the mercury. Food sources of cysteine include poultry, yogurt, egg yolks, red peppers, garlic, onions, broccoli, Brussels sprouts, oats, and wheat germ.

The other important molecule you need to keep your glutathione levels high is alpha lipoic acid, a fat-soluble molecule that crosses into all your cells, including those in your brain. When glutathione does its job mopping up the free radicals, it gets oxidized itself and can no longer mop up anything else. Alpha lipoic acid, the second most potent antioxidant, cleans up the glutathione and makes it ready to go back to work. Sources of alpha lipoic acid include dark green leafy vegetables (including spinach, collard greens, and broccoli), animal foods (such as beef), and organ meats (such as calf's liver). These molecules are often used to support the process of detoxifying mercury and help repair your cells when you have been sick with a toxin-related illness. In Chapter 12, "Supporting Your Liver Workbook," you will take the self-assessment to see if you have a high toxic load and/or toxin-related illness; then I will give you instructions on how to use these important supplements.

Glutathione protects you from mercury in three ways. First, it binds to the mercury so that it can't cause direct damage to your tissues (which it will do if it is left alone to float freely in your blood and inside your cells). Second, the glutathione links up with the mercury, creating a glutathione-mercury complex, which is then excreted through the kidneys or into the bile. Reports reveal that increasing the levels of glutathione in the body will increase the levels of these glutathione-mercury complexes in the bile and that glutathione can increase excretion of mercury from brain cells and the kidneys. So people with low glutathione levels can't effectively get rid of the mercury they are exposed to or the mercury that has accumulated in their tissues. The third way that glutathione helps you is that it protects the inside of every cell in your body by mopping up all of the harmful free radicals released by mercury when it is running amok inside your cells. Mercury can get into every cell in your body, and once inside it can damage the mitochondria, which are the little energy-producing furnaces inside every living cell. Glutathione is the key protector against this type of mitochondria damage.

Removing Metals: Metallothioneins

In addition to glutathione, your body has an important metal management system called metallothioneins (MTs). These are a family of sulfur-rich, mercury-binding proteins that also live inside each cell and actively bind heavy metals. MTs are in charge of regulating zinc and copper levels inside the cells, but they also bind tightly to cadmium and mercury and are found in highest concentrations in the liver, the kidneys, and the cells lining your intestines.

In the case of mercury, MTs grab on to it, preventing it from wreaking havoc inside the cell. Like glutathione, metallothioneins also act as anti-oxidants separately from their metal-binding activity, to protect the cell from damage. Researchers in the Department of Environmental Health Sciences at the University of Michigan found that MTs also have different genetic variations in the population, which means that some people have really good metallothionein activity.[22] This discovery may also partly explain why some people are better at excreting metals than others.

How can you get your body to make more metallothioneins? It turns out that when you are exposed to heavy metals of any kind, including increasing your intake of zinc, your cells start to make more of it. Zinc is the best stimulator of activity, either from supplements or from the diet, but studies have also shown that cadmium, copper, and mercury can do it as well.

Removing Metals: Chlorella, Cilantro, and Fiber

Heavy-metal chelating agents are compounds that, when ingested, grab on to metals and pull them out of the body. These chelators can be food, supplements, or prescription medication. They vary in strength and ability to remove metals from your cells and tissues, and I believe that when used wisely they can be an important part of a general preventive health or treatment program. Because there is so much exposure to heavy metals from our environment, especially lead and mercury, it is important to be eating and living in a way that is protective, and so in this section I mention some gentle and simple options to enhance your body's ability to excrete metals.

Chlorella

Because chlorella is sold in vitamin stores and advertised as a heavy-metal chelator, I wanted to briefly mention it here. Chlorella is a unicel-lular green algae that has been eaten as a nutritional food in Japan since 1964 because it contains high levels of powerful nutritional components such as proteins, vitamins, minerals, and dietary fiber. There are numerous studies showing positive health benefits from adding it to your diet.

Animal studies have also found it useful in removing toxins such as dioxins, cadmium, and lead. Researchers at the National Institute for Minamata Disease in Minamata, Japan, who looked at using chlorella in the treatment of mercury toxicity in mice found that chlorella intake can increase the elimination of methylmercury in the urine and stool. They also found that giving chlorella to pregnant mice at the same time that they were exposed to mercury reduced how much mercury crossed the placenta to the fetus and how much accumulated in the blood and brain of the mother.[23] Other mouse studies revealed similar findings, showing less accumulation of mercury in the tissues of mice fed chlorella at the time of their exposure to mercury.

This research makes a good argument for the possibility that chlorella might be useful in reducing humans' mercury levels. However, I haven't seen any studies proving this theory. Because chlorella is generally very safe, I often recommend it to my patients who are eating lots of fish, in order to prevent mercury from getting stored in their tissues. I will tell you more about how to choose chlorella supplements in the treatment plan section of the next chapter.

Cilantro

What about cilantro (coriander)? I was unable to find any studies in the literature that prove that cilantro is a chelator of metals, though there is evidence that cilantro is a great antioxidant and boosts glutathione levels, which might be the mechanism behind its support for treating heavy metal toxicity.[24] Because I love food as medicine, I recommend eating lots of cilantro, and I put a handful in my green shake every morning. You should, too.

Fiber

This chapter would not be complete without mentioning the role of dietary fiber in removing toxins from the body. There are two kinds of fiber. Insoluble fiber is the kind that does not dissolve or get digested; it helps with constipation by providing bulky stools that get pushed along more easily by your intestines. The other is soluble fiber, which dissolves easily in water or in the liquid environment of your stomach and intestines. There this fiber is able to bind to various compounds and keep them in the stool for elimination. Soluble fiber's ability to bind to cholesterol and keep it from getting reabsorbed by the intestines is one way this nutrient helps lower cholesterol. The same thing happens for estrogens and toxins—they are pulled out of the body by fiber. Soluble fiber is found in oats, lentils, apples, oranges, pears, strawberries, nuts, flaxseeds, beans, dried peas, blueberries, psyllium, cucumbers, celery, and carrots. Insoluble fiber is found in all whole grains, nuts, barley, zucchini, celery, broccoli, cabbage, onions, tomatoes, carrots, cucumbers, green beans, dark leafy vegetables, all fruit (fresh and dried), and root vegetable skins.

Most Americans get only about 15 grams of fiber per day in their diet, but you should aim for more like 30. Don't worry about what kind of fiber you are getting. Instead, focus on eating a healthful diet rich in fruits, vegetables, whole grains, legumes, nuts, and seeds, which will provide a variety of soluble and insoluble fibers and all of their health benefits. Just note that as you increase the fiber in your diet, you may experience more intestinal gas. Increasing fiber gradually will allow your body to adapt, and because some fibers absorb water, you should also drink more water as you increase fiber.

Removing Metals: Chelation

I am going to tell you about chelation, because understanding how to test and treat yourself for mercury toxicity is an important final step in reversing autoimmune diseases. While I don't know if you have an overload of mercury in your body, because of the relationship between mercury and autoimmune diseases you need to think about it and perhaps get tested, especially if you have been eating lots of fish or have lots of dental amalgam fillings. Many people are very confused about what chelation is and whether they should do it or not. I am not going to go through a complete review of chelation programs, because that is outside the scope of this book. But here's a brief overview.

Chelating agents are compounds that bind on to toxins and pull them out of the body. There are a whole bunch of them, but the common ones used in functional medicine are dimercaptosuccinic acid (DMSA), which is a pill you swallow; 2,3-dimercapto-1-propanesulfonic acid (DMPS, also called unithiol), which is done through an IV; and EDTA, which is good for lead and can be done either by IV or by rectal suppository. Chelation agents are used as treatment to remove heavy metals from people who have been tested and found to have high levels.

You can't tell how much of a heavy metal such as mercury is stored inside the tissues of your body by doing a blood test from a routine laboratory. A blood test will only tell you if you have been exposed to mercury in the past few weeks, and it also will only be looking at the serum portion of your blood (the liquid part without any cells), which is not where most of the mercury is stored. Instead, one option for testing is to do a red blood cell test for mercury (and other metals), which will be more accurate because the metals get absorbed into the red blood cells floating in your blood. However, since red blood cells live for only three to four months, this test tells you only how much exposure you've had to metals during this period, not how high your body burden might be.

Body burden is the total amount of any toxin that is stored in your body's cells and tissues. The most widely accepted test for body burden, and the one I use in my office, is called a provoked urine test. You take a chelating agent (I use DMSA), and over the next eight hours the DMSA pulls metals out of your tissues and into your urine. You collect all your urine during this time and then send a sample of it to the lab to see how much mercury, lead, arsenic, cadmium, aluminum, nickel, and other toxic metals have been grabbed by the chelation agent. The higher the levels, the more likely it is that a lot is stored in your body and is making you sick. I will tell you more about how to get this test in the workbook chapter that follows.

The chelation program that I use most often in my office is DMSA because it has a long history of safe use in treating metal toxicity and it can be given by mouth instead of intravenously. It also doesn't cause a redistribution of metals from one organ to another. I use it for all metals, including mercury. In 2000, the journal *Alternative Medicine Review* published a review of the use of DMSA in chelating mercury and found when compared to treatment with other chelating agents, DMSA resulted in the greatest urinary excretion of mercury and was the most effective at removing mercury from the blood, liver, brain, spleen, lungs, large intestine, skeletal muscle, and bone. Another study indicated that mercury excretion was greatest in the first eight to twenty-four hours after taking DMSA orally. Animal studies show that following intravenous administration of methylmercury, DMSA removed two-thirds of the brain mercury deposits.[25]

Because chelating agents are imperfect and don't always get into every cell or grab every metal, newer approaches are now being studied where you take multiple agents at the same time. Examples of these agents are DMSA with EDTA, N-acetylcysteine with DMSA, or alpha lipoic acid with DMSA, and using antioxidants such as vitamins C and E, beta-carotene, or melatonin at the same time to reduce the damaging effects of the metals on the cells and tissues and to enhance the excretion of the metals. These other antioxidants can also be used on their own to reduce the toxic effects of metals in your body.

You should never do these treatments with DMSA, DMPS, or EDTA on your own, because they have side effects if you are not careful. You need to be very respectful of moving metals around your body. Always do them with a doctor. The biggest side effects involve pulling out other good minerals, such as copper, manganese, molybdenum, and zinc, when you pull out the heavy metals. These side effects are why you need to replenish these minerals on the days when you aren't doing the chelation. The other big concern is that the metals might not find their way out of your body properly and instead recirculate and settle in other tissues. To prevent this, your detox system has to be tuned up and your bowels should be moving at least once each day so that the metals make their way out of the body. In my experience, a detox system that is not functioning optimally is the most common reason why some people get headaches when they do chelation. If they do get headaches, I always stop the treatment and go back to doing more basic liver detox support and optimizing gut health. The possibility of side effects is why I am very cautious and do chelation only after several months of preparation and why you should never do this treatment on your own.

Does removing metals from the body by chelation cause an improvement in symptoms or reversal of disease? There are some case studies where chelation resulted in improvement. One study showed a reversal in MS symptoms when the mercury was removed, and another showed a complete resolution in RA in a woman with high levels of aluminum and lead after chelation removed the metals in her body.[26] There aren't many studies looking at chelation of mercury and its effect on autoimmune diseases, but to me this approach makes logical and scientific sense based on all the research and information I have shared with you in this chapter.

I have seen mercury chelation positively affect autoimmune diseases in my own practice. But chelation isn't the only way to remove mercury from your body. In this chapter, you learned that toxins are all around you and that you need to clean up your environment to reduce your toxic load. You also learned that supporting your liver enzymes is critical to remove stored environmental chemicals and metals and also to prevent them from accumulating in your body and making you sick in the future. Just working to support your liver can remove metals from your body, and that is the best place to begin.

CHAPTER 12

Supporting Your Liver Workbook

In 2007, Steve, a married father of two, came to see me complaining of a strange feeling. He was experiencing a combination of numbness and tingling in his left foot, and it had been bothering him for about seven months. The sensation was there all the time and got worse during his weekly runs on the treadmill. When these symptoms initially started, Steve, thirty-eight, had gone to the emergency room, where the neurologists examined him and didn't find anything unusual, but they suggested an MRI as the next step. So Steve was referred to a neurologist, who sent him for the MRI. When they reviewed the results, his doctor said there was a pattern that looked like multiple sclerosis. By this he meant that there were spots on the brain or spinal cord where the nerves had lost their myelin sheath, a characteristic of this autoimmune disease. However, you are not diagnosed with MS if you have only one episode of symptoms with one abnormal MRI. The diagnosis is made only after you have new symptoms for a second time, with new spots on your MRI. Since this was Steve's first episode and because doctors couldn't tell if the spots on the MRI were new or old, Steve wasn't formally diagnosed with MS. Instead, he was told that he probably had this potentially debilitating autoimmune condition and was basically sent home to wait and see if he experienced these symptoms again, which would then confirm his diagnosis.

The potential of having MS was very alarming to Steve, a fit, healthy man with a physically active job as a construction worker. Understandably, he was anxious and distressed at the possibility of developing this disease because it would ruin his career, not to mention his health. He came to see me for two reasons. The first was that the numbness and tingling had not gone away and he was worried about those symptoms getting worse. The second was that he had heard about functional medicine and wanted to know if I could help him not only get better but also avoid developing a full-blown autoimmune disease.

At our initial appointment I noticed that Steve was very disciplined and willing to do whatever it would take to get better and stay healthy. I was impressed by his calm and easygoing nature, even though he was deeply concerned about his diagnosis. After giving him a thorough physical exam, carefully reviewing his medical paperwork, and listening to his story, the only issues I could find were more fatigue than usual and the numbness and tingling in his foot, especially after working out. Otherwise, he was in excellent health, physically fit and lean.

By now you've probably already guessed that the first thing I did was put Steve on a gluten-free diet. I also had him change the kinds of fats he was eating, from fried foods and beef to white meat chicken and turkey and vegetables stir-fried in olive oil. I also took him off dairy. Next, I took a look at the stress in his life and how he was handling it. But after talking to him for a while and doing the assessments that you did in Chapter 6, "Understanding the Stress Connection Workbook," I saw that he was managing his stress well. It was clear to me that stress was not a big contributing factor to his illness—something that is actually pretty unusual because most people have lots of stress and don't handle it well.

From there, I decided to focus on the third step described in *The Immune System Recovery Plan*, healing his gut, and the fourth step, supporting his liver. To do so, I ordered a stool test to look for infections and a heavy metal test to look for mercury in his body. As part of his autoimmune evaluation and because he was excessively tired, I also ordered tests that looked at his thyroid and testosterone levels, screened for other autoimmune diseases, tested for celiac disease, looked for chronic infections, and checked many of his vitamin levels. When I asked Steve about his diet, it turned out that he had been eating tuna sushi at least once a week for over five years and regularly ate swordfish. Both of these fish are high in mercury, so I was concerned that this heavy metal was stored in his tissues and in turn damaging his immune system and nerve cells. This is why I also had Steve's mercury levels evaluated.

As I explained in the last chapter, there are several types of tests you can do for heavy metals. One is a blood test through a regular laboratory. However, this will tell you only if you are being exposed to that metal right now. This is because these metals last in your bloodstream for only a short time before they are excreted by your liver and kidneys or before they leave the blood and settle into your tissues. Because your red blood cells live for three to four months, a red blood cell test will tell you if you've been exposed to high levels of metals during that time period.

While it is helpful to see if you have high levels of metals in your blood using these tests, they tell you only one part of the story. The real question is whether you have metals inside the tissues in your body. This is where they cause damage and promote autoimmune disease. So for Steve, as I do for many of my patients, I used another test that looks deep inside your tissues. You have to find a doctor, naturopath, nurse practitioner, or osteopath to give it to you, but it basically involves taking DMSA pills. This substance goes into your tissues, grabs on to any mercury and other metals that are there, pulls them out, and carries them to your kidneys, where they pass into your urine, which is then tested.

Steve returned one month later for his next visit to go over his test results. When he walked into my office, he was bursting with excitement because his numbness and tingling had improved. Yes, he was still having the tingling in his foot when he ran on the treadmill or did any exercise, but it wasn't as severe. To me, this was a great start and showed me that gluten was definitely part of the problem. But results of his tests also revealed a few other things. His thyroid was a bit sluggish, which explained why he was feeling tired. Also, he had yeast, called candida, in his digestive tract; this damages the intestinal lining and releases toxic compounds that cause fatigue and brain fog. It can also provoke digestive symptoms such as constipation, gas, and bloating after eating, and it can spark an immune reaction that creates inflammation at distant sites, especially the brain.

As you know from Chapter 8, "Healing Your Gut," a healthy digestive tract is important for people with autoimmune diseases, especially those with MS, so my next step was to focus on his gut. Because of this, I put Steve on a low-sugar diet (yeast loves sugar, so removing it helps starve the yeast) and gave him both a prescription for nystatin and the herb oregano to kill the yeast in his digestive tract. His vitamin D level was 24 ng/ml. At the time, this was considered in the normal range of 20–80 ng/ml. (Recently the normal range was changed to 30–80, so in fact his levels would be considered low by today's standards.) Though many traditional doctors would have dismissed this, vitamin D deficiency has been associated with MS, so I wanted to get Steve's levels up over 50 ng/ml. This is why I had him take 5,000 IU per day of vitamin D. (I discussed vitamin D levels in Chapter 2, "Using Food as Medicine," and will again in the MS section in Chapter 14, "Infections and Specific Autoimmune Conditions.") For his thyroid, I had Steve take a thyroid formula that contains vitamin A, zinc, selenium, and iodine.

One of Steve's test results that concerned me was a urine test that showed a mercury level of 15 mcg/gram of creatinine. The normal level for this test is below 3, so this was a problem. My suspicion was that mercury was playing a role in Steve's symptoms and maybe even the damage seen on his MRI. There are a few ways to get rid of the mercury in your body. One is the chelation process, which I don't recommend you do on your own. But you can start removing toxins, including heavy metals, by supporting your liver with a detox program at home. Doing this is the first part of your heavy metal treatment program, and for some people it is the only treatment they will need. For others, supporting the liver isn't enough by itself and they will ultimately need some form of additional treatment such as chelation. With my patients, I always spend three months preparing their bodies for chelation, because you don't want to pull mercury or other metals out of the tissues unless the liver is working well enough to properly excrete them. The digestive tract also needs to be in top shape for the excretion process, so fixing the gut by removing any bad bacteria, yeast, or parasites also comes first.

To start Steve's mercury treatment and to get his detox system up and ready, he took liver support herbs and vitamins for three months. We also added lots of dark leafy greens such as kale, chard, collards, and spinach and cruciferous vegetables such as broccoli, cauliflower, cabbage, Brussels sprouts, and bok choy to his diet to help support his detox system.

Steve was supposed to follow up with me in three months, but he got busy and pushed his follow-up off for six months. Even though he hadn't come back sooner, Steve told me that he had followed the treatment plan religiously during the entire time. Results of his repeat lab tests were evidence of this. His thyroid had improved slightly, and his vitamin D level had gone up to 65 ng/ml. Still, he was concerned because his numbness and tingling hadn't changed since our previous visit. As I mentioned before, the constant numbness and tingling were gone, but came back when he was running outside or on the treadmill. To me this was a sign that the mercury might still be a problem for him, because this heavy metal is known to cause these kinds of neurological symptoms. While he had treated his high mercury levels by taking supplements to support his liver for six months, Steve was still having symptoms. I felt that we should be more aggressive in our approach to get all of the mercury out of his body, and so I moved to a chelation treatment program that involved taking DMSA for three days, and then not taking it for eleven days. During the eleven days off, he took other supplements to rebalance the minerals that are pulled out with the mercury during the three days of chelation. This went on for three months. Then he stopped taking the chelation pills for one month and retook the heavy metal test to check his mercury levels.

By the time he came back to see me I had good news for him: his mercury levels were down to 5.9 from 15 mcg/gram of creatinine. But the minute I saw him, I could tell that I wasn't the only one who was excited. He could hardly contain himself. Before he even walked into my office, Steve announced that his numbness and tingling were completely gone. We were both convinced that removing the mercury from his body was what had finally cured him. I am also certain that the mercury was harming his thyroid gland because his thyroid had begun working much better (we had repeated that test, too) and his energy was back to normal.

Steve wanted to continue a program that would remove the last of the mercury from his body (he wanted to get his level down to 3 or less). But this time, instead of chelation, I gave him a supplement that I use for people who have only mild elevations in their metal levels, called MetalloClear. This herbal formula, from a company called Metagenics, is taken for one month to boost metallothionein and enhance the body's excretion of metals for two to three months afterward. It isn't as strong as doing chelation, so I often use it as the second step in someone who starts out with very high levels of any metal, whether mercury, lead, arsenic, cadmium, or aluminum.

One year later, we retested Steve's mercury level. At 3.0, it was now normal. By that point Steve and I had been working together for two years. His symptoms were all gone, and he went back to his neurologist, who did another MRI. We were all relieved to see that it was excellent, with no change. This was three years ago, and all repeat MRIs since then continue to be unchanged *and* Steve remains symptom free. He never got a formal diagnosis of MS, and I believe he never will. But I also believe he would have ended up with MS if we hadn't put him on a gluten-free diet, cleaned up and healed his gut, and removed the mercury. Now he just returns to my office every year for what I call "a good look under the hood" to make sure his systems are all functioning optimally.

Self-Assessment

Self-Assessment: How Do You Know if You Need a Detox Program?

Most of the time, the reason to do a detox program is not because you are getting ready for chelation but because you have symptoms caused by too many toxins in your system. Most people who come into my office, whether they have an autoimmune disease or not, have a body burdened with toxins from everyday exposure to things such as pesticides, plastics, and heavy metals. After carefully taking a patient's history of environmental and toxin exposure and then listening to all his or her symptoms, I can diagnose toxin overload disease. I have created a questionnaire that will help you diagnose yourself and determine if *you* need a detox program, just as I would if you were in my office. Depending on your results, you can treat yourself with food alone or with supplements.

The purpose of the assessment for toxic load is for you to find out how much exposure you have had to toxins over your lifetime. If you score high in this section, then your detoxification system has been, and might still be, carrying a large toxic load. Depending on your genetics and how well you have been taking care of yourself (eating a healthy diet, exercising, sleeping, managing stress, etc.), you might be handling this load okay. But if you are like most people, the toxins are probably spilling out of your liver and irritating all the other tissues in your body—brain, joints, muscles, fat cells, and immune cells. In fact, every cell of your body can be affected.

How will we know if your toxic load is making you sick? That's where our second assessment comes in. I will help you find out if the symptoms you are having right now are related to toxin overload. The results here will help us decide what kind of detox support you need. Perhaps using food for detox support will be all you need, but it is also possible you will benefit from targeted supplements to boost your liver detox system.

Assessment for Toxic Load

In your work or home environment, have you ever been exposed to:

	Occasionally = 1	Frequently = 2
Chemicals or chemical smells at work		
Electromagnetic radiation (for example, you live or work near wires, high-voltage machinery, or a cell tower)		
Mercury from fish (swordfish, tuna, king mackerel) or dental amalgam fillings		
Mold (moldy smell or actual mold you can see)		
Lead (from old pipes or old paint from before 1970)		
Asbestos (from exposure to construction debris from a pre-1950 building)		
Pesticides (from your lawn, a golf course, a farm, or another outdoor location)		
Insecticides (for example, from inside your house if you frequently use an exterminator)		
Solvents (from paint, furniture, and household cleaners)		
Paint (especially oil-based paint, either on the outside of your house or if you are an artist)		
Dry-cleaning chemicals		
Drinking alcohol in the past ten years		
Smoking cigarettes or being exposed to secondhand smoke in the past ten years		

(continued on next page)

	Occasionally = 1	Frequently = 2
Recreational drugs in the past ten years		
Fast-food chicken, beef, and fish, or eating nonorganic dairy products		
Total		

YOUR SCORE

Less than 6: low toxic load Congratulations, you have been living a very clean life!

6–15: moderate toxic load You have been exposed to a fair amount of toxins. Your score on the next assessment for symptoms of toxicity will determine if you need a Tier 2 detox program or if food is all the support you need.

16–30: high toxic load You have a very high toxic load and should do the Tier 2 detox program.

Assessment for Symptoms of Toxicity

Now we will take a look at symptoms you are having. Rate each of the following symptoms based upon the past thirty days. Use the following scoring to do so:

0—You never or almost never have the symptom.
1—You occasionally have it but the effect is not severe.
2—You occasionally have it and the effect is severe.
3—You frequently have it and the effect is not severe.
4—You frequently have it and the effect is severe.

	Never (score = 0)	Occasional, not severe (score = 1)	Occasional, severe (score = 2)	Frequently, not severe (score = 3)	Frequently, severe (score = 4)
Headaches					
Dizziness					
Insomnia					

Bags or dark circles under eyes					
Itchy ears					
Ringing in ears or tinnitus					
Sinus problems					
Sneezing attacks					
Canker sores					
Chronic coughing					
Swollen or discolored tongue					
Chronic acne					
Excessive sweating					
Hot flashes					
Hives or rashes					
Hair loss					
Irregular or skipped heartbeats					
Asthma or bronchitis					
Chronic constipation					
Chronic nausea					
Bloated feeling after eating					
Pain or aches in your joints					
Arthritis					
Pain or aches in your muscles					
Feeling weak, tired, or sluggish					

(*continued on next page*)

	Never (score = 0)	Occasional, not severe (score = 1)	Occasional, severe (score = 2)	Frequently, not severe (score = 3)	Frequently, severe (score = 4)
Water retention					
Weight gain					
Craving certain foods					
Restlessness or irritability					
Poor memory					
Poor concentration					
Mood swings					
Anxiety					
Depression					
Get sick often					

TOTAL: _____

Scoring:

Low: <35
Moderate: 35–69
High: 70–99
Severe symptoms of toxicity: >99

Putting It Together: Toxic Load Plus Symptoms

Use the table below to determine your treatment plan. First, find your score from the assessment for symptoms of toxicity in the left column. Then follow that row to the right, until you find your score from the *assessment for toxic load*. Read the treatment program for the box that matches the two scores.

		Assessment for Toxic Load		
		Low toxic load (< 6)	**Moderate toxic load (6–15)**	**Severe toxic load (16–30)**
Assessment for symptoms of toxicity	Low symptoms of toxicity (< 35)	Congratulations! You are living clean and your liver is keeping up with your toxin exposure. Follow Tier 1 for ongoing prevention and maintenance.	Your liver has done a good job keeping up with your toxin exposure. Follow Tier 1 for ongoing prevention and maintenance.	Because you have high levels of exposure to toxins, you should do both Tier 1 and Tier 2. Even though you aren't having symptoms right now, you are at high risk of getting them.
	Moderate symptoms of toxicity (35–69)	You are having symptoms of toxicity even though we haven't identified your exposure. You have the option of completing only Tier 1, but if you have an autoimmune disease, I suggest including Tier 2 as well.	You should do both Tier 1 and Tier 2 because you have exposure to toxins and it is affecting your health.	You should do both Tier 1 and Tier 2 because you have exposure to toxins and it is affecting your health.
	High symptoms of toxicity (70–99)	Even though you seem to have a low toxic load, your body is sick from too many toxins. You might have a genetic handicap in your detox pathways. You need Tier 1 and Tier 2.	You should do both Tier 1 and Tier 2 because you have exposure to toxins and it is affecting your health.	You have a high toxic load, and the toxins are making you sick. You need Tier 1, Tier 2, and Tier 3 treatment.

(continued on next page)

		Assessment for Toxic Load		
		Low toxic load (< 6)	Moderate toxic load (6–15)	Severe toxic load (16–30)
Severe symptoms of toxicity (> 99)		Even though you seem to have a low toxic load, your body is very sick from too many toxins. You might have a genetic handicap in your detox pathways. You need Tier 1, Tier 2, and Tier 3 treatment.	Your toxic load, even though moderate, is making you very sick. You need Tier 1, Tier 2, and Tier 3 treatment.	You have a high toxic load, and the toxins are making you very sick. You need Tier 1, Tier 2, and Tier 3 treatment.

Supporting Your Liver Treatment Program

If you've been following the program in this book in order, you have already taken the most important steps in cleaning up your body and supporting your liver. In Part I, "Using Food as Medicine," you learned how to eat an anti-inflammatory diet and cleaned up what you eat by eliminating processed sugar and white flour products as well as trans fats and saturated animal fats. You're also eating more antioxidant-rich, colorful foods and healthy fats and have started the process of identifying foods causing inflammation for you, such as gluten, dairy, soy, and corn.

In Part II, "Understanding the Stress Connection," you began the process of healing your stress system, sleeping better, and eating more mindfully. You learned to eat enough protein (not just meat but vegetarian sources, too) during the day and not to skip meals.

In Part III, "Healing Your Gut," you took very important steps to remove toxins in your digestive tract and bring balance to the bacteria that live there, adding foods rich in natural digestive enzymes and probiotics that heal your intestinal lining. This not only strengthened the part of your immune system that lives below your intestinal lining but helped your liver by reducing all those bacterial and yeast toxins that your liver had to deal with every day. You may not have realized it, but you already started your detox program with these three steps.

So what's left? Two things. First, we still need to figure out if there are any more foods that you might be sensitive to that might be causing inflammation and that your liver might view as toxic. Second, we need to give your liver some detox support with food and possibly supplements.

Tier 1: Using Food as Medicine

Step 1: Complete Detox Elimination Diet

Whenever I first mention a complete elimination diet to my patients, I can see a glint of panic in their eyes. Don't worry! This book has helped you start slowly, and you've already removed many foods on this list.

The purpose of doing a complete detox elimination diet for three weeks is twofold. First, we need to find out if you have any food sensitivities besides gluten, dairy, soy, or corn that we haven't tested for yet. (We tested for these four in Chapter 3, "Using Food as Medicine Workbook.") If you skipped that chapter, now is your opportunity to go all out and do all the foods at once. It is critical that we create a personalized food plan for you, and that means identifying and removing any foods you are sensitive to, which will reduce inflammation and lower the stress on your immune system.

The second reason we need to do a complete detox elimination diet as part of the liver support program is that your liver is the organ that processes all the food you eat. After food is digested, nutrients and possibly toxins are absorbed into your bloodstream, and all the blood vessels from your entire digestive tract (which includes your stomach and small and large intestine) go straight to the liver first. The liver then processes everything, looking for toxins and packaging the fat and sugar into cholesterol. This is a lot of work for your liver every day, so a complete detox elimination program gives it a break from having to deal with heavy animal foods, sugar, alcohol, and processed foods, and at the same time gives it a boost with specific nutrients it needs to work better. Therefore, even if you already tested yourself for sensitivities to gluten, dairy, soy, and corn in Chapter 3, no matter the results of that experiment, you will remove these foods again for this complete detox elimination program. My goal in this chapter is to take you the last few yards to the finish line. You are almost there!

Here is the summary for the three-week complete detox elimination diet. As we did in Part I, we will reintroduce foods one at a time when the three weeks are over. We will be eliminating:

- Gluten, dairy, soy, and corn
- Processed sugar and bad fats
- Eggs, shellfish, beef, pork, sausages, and deli meat
- Peanuts
- Oranges
- Coffee, caffeine, alcohol, and chocolate (sorry!)

Food Category	Food to Include	Food to Remove
Vegetables	All vegetables, steamed or sautéed in olive oil or coconut oil	Whole corn, corn syrup, cornstarch (check ingredients on food labels)
Bread, starch, cereal	Whole-grain gluten-free bread, pasta, crackers, and wraps; brown or wild rice, quinoa, whole buckwheat, whole millet, brown rice	White flour, wheat, spelt, barley, kamut, rye flour, white potatoes, white rice
Legumes	Lentils, chickpeas, all beans	All soy products, including tempeh, tofu, edamame, soy sauce, tamari, and soy listed as an ingredient on food labels
Dairy	Dairy substitutes: almond, rice, coconut, and hemp milks, coconut milk yogurt and kefir	All cow, sheep, and goat milk, yogurt, kefir, cheese, and butter; casein and whey as ingredients on food labels
Protein	Turkey, chicken, lamb, wild game (free-range and organic if possible); fish from low-mercury list at www.edf.org	Eggs, shellfish, deli meat, sausage, pork, beef

Nuts and seeds	Almonds, walnuts, Brazil nuts, all nuts and seeds except peanuts	Peanuts
Fruit	Best choices are low-sugar fruit such as berries, apples, pears, peaches, and plums	No oranges; steer away from high-sugar fruit such as pineapple and melon
Animal fats	Fish, fish oil supplements, grass-fed beef, ghee (clarified butter)	Cheese, milk fat, beef raised on corn, shortening
Vegetable fats	All cold-pressed oils: olive, canola, flax, safflower, sesame, almond, sunflower, walnut, pumpkin; avocado, coconut oil, coconut milk, palm oil; nuts, seeds, leafy greens	Margarine, salad dressings, mayonnaise, or other products made with trans fats (look on labels for partially hydrogenated oils)
Sweeteners	Raw unprocessed agave syrup, stevia, brown rice syrup, blackstrap molasses, concentrated fruit juice sweetener	All artificial sweeteners, including aspartame, sucralose (Splenda) and saccharin; high-fructose corn syrup, white and brown sugar, honey, evaporated cane juice, maple syrup
Drinks	Filtered water, decaffeinated herbal teas, seltzer, mineral water; limit caffeinated coffee or tea to one cup each day	Soda, fruit juices, other drinks sweetened with high-fructose corn syrup; limit caffeine and alcohol
Condiments	Organic ketchup, mustard, vinegar, all spices	Anything with high-fructose corn syrup, corn syrup, or added cane sugar, such as ketchup, barbecue sauce, hot sauce, teriyaki sauce

(continued on next page)

Food Category	Food to Include	Food to Remove
Desserts	Coconut milk yogurt or ice cream, fruit (fresh or dried), unsweetened chocolate, low-sugar dessert recipes in this book	Frozen yogurt or ice cream, sorbet, cookies, cakes, candy
Snacks	Gluten-free whole-grain crackers with hummus, almond butter, or guacamole; coconut yogurt; nuts (except peanuts); fruit such as apples, pears, peaches, plums, and all berries	Pretzels, potato chips, corn chips, tortilla chips, popcorn, white-flour crackers, white-flour and white-sugar cookies, cakes, muffins

Tips for Getting Started

Preventing and treating toxin-related illness involves a combination of identifying what you're being exposed to and removing it, then helping the liver to cope by giving it nutrients to support metabolic detoxification. What is metabolic detoxification? Think of it as boosting the liver's metabolism. By increasing the metabolism of the detoxification process, it is easier to clear out toxins. But before we do this, you need to do some detective work to find out if your environment is making you sick. Then you need to take steps to clean it up and reduce your exposure.

- Use the most natural cleaning supplies and household products that you can find.
- Use a HEPA air filter.
- Don't spray pesticides around or in your home.
- Look for cosmetics and skin care products that don't contain synthetic fragrances, parabens, and phthalates.
- Go organic when it comes to fruits and vegetables (see www.ewg.org for a list of the "Dirty Dozen," the produce that tends to contain the most pesticide residues) and dairy products.
- Opt for free-range, organic meats and eggs.
- Drink clean water. It varies depending on where you live, but in general it's a good idea to filter your tap water.
- Plastic bottles and containers with the numbers 3, 6, and 7 on them

(usually on the bottom) are believed to leach plastic into any foods or drinks they hold, so avoid using them.

- Microwave food in microwaveable glass containers, not plastic.
- If you have a cavity, talk to your dentist about not using dental amalgam (silver) fillings. Find a holistic dentist if you have to.
- Visit the following websites: www.everydayexposures.com, the Environmental Working Group (www.ewg.org), and the Environmental Defense Fund (www.edf.org).

Getting Ready for the Detox Elimination Diet

Be sure to drink at least six to eight 8-oz glasses of water daily during the detox program. This helps the body flush out toxins. The first few days, you may feel some fatigue, achiness, headache, or fogginess depending on how toxin-filled your body is. If this becomes too much, you might not be eating enough, so make sure you are eating protein throughout the day. Keep in mind that for people whose bodies are carrying a lot of toxins, the fog doesn't clear until the second week. Although light exercise such as walking, gentle yoga, or a short relaxed jog helps the body clear toxins while you are doing the program, avoid vigorous exercise. Be sure to get plenty of sleep, at least eight hours a night, to give your body the rest it needs while it is doing this extra metabolic work. If you are a coffee drinker, I recommend tapering off coffee *before* you begin the program to avoid caffeine-withdrawal headaches. If you've been living on sugar, you may also want to taper your sugar consumption down for a few days before starting this program, which requires you to eliminate it completely. Sugar, like caffeine, is a very addictive substance, so quitting cold turkey rather than slowly tapering can give you a bad headache or other detox reaction.

I suggest you take time to prepare your pantry before starting the program. Make sure you have all the food you will need to make your shakes, and bring snacks to work if you are not home during the day. It will be very hard to stick to the food restrictions or to find something to eat when you're hungry unless you plan ahead. I also recommend that you make our Green Detox Soup (see recipe on page 282) and freeze it in small batches so you have it on hand to drink during the program. You can have as much broth as you like, and it is nourishing, liver supportive, and filling. When eating produce or poultry, try to go organic if possible, especially during this program, as you will be eating lots of these foods and the pesticides in nonorganic produce will add an extra burden to your liver.

Remember, even if you don't take the detox supplements in Tier 2, this elimination diet plus foods that support your liver (coming up next) will be enough for you to feel the powerful effects of a detox program. This means you might experience some of the side effects mentioned above, but it also means you will feel great!

After the three weeks on the elimination program, do the following:

- Reintroduce one food at a time. Eat that food at least twice each day for two days, noticing how you feel. On day three, don't eat the food, but continue to observe how you feel. If you have no reaction to the food, you are ready to move on to challenge the next food on day four.
- If you *do* have a reaction, such as headache, rash, brain fog, fatigue, digestive reaction, or other symptom you are familiar with, write it down in the following table so you don't forget later. Once you know a particular food isn't good for you, remove it again. The food reaction should go away within a day or two, but for some people it can take longer.
- Once that reaction goes away, then it is time to try reintroducing the next food.
- A reminder about gluten, something we already discussed in Chapter 3, "Using Food as Medicine Workbook": finding out if you are having a noticeable reaction to gluten is important. If you don't have a reaction and don't have an autoimmune disease, you can add it back into your diet. However, even if you don't react, make sure to remove it again if you have an autoimmune disease.
- Be patient—it will take you another three weeks or so to reintroduce all the foods you have eliminated.
- Record your reactions in a table like the one below. You can also download a similar one from www.immuneprogram.com.

Symptom	Gluten	Dairy	Soy	Corn	Eggs	Peanuts	Oranges	Beef	Other
Bloating									
Headache									
Joint pain									
Hot flashes									
Your symptom									
Your symptom									

Congratulations! You should now know whether any of the foods from the table above create an immune reaction in your body by causing either familiar or new symptoms when you eat them again. If you found that you were sensitive to more than one, that is okay and very common. All these symptoms are caused by inflammation that affects different parts of the body. How long should you avoid these foods? My recommendation is to remove these foods from your diet for at least six months. Once you finish healing your gut (which you should have already started in the previous step, Part III, "Healing Your Gut"), you can try reintroducing all the foods again, one at a time, just as you did after the three-week elimination program, following the instructions above.

Remember, if you have had a positive test for celiac disease (including anti-gliadin and anti-deamidated gliadin antibodies), your diet should stay gluten free for life. If you have an autoimmune disease but don't have celiac disease, you should remain 100 percent gluten free until your autoimmune disease is gone, which means you no longer have symptoms and your lab tests are normal. Once that happens, you can live 95 percent gluten free, which means that you should live 100 percent gluten free in your daily work and home life. Then, if you go out to eat or travel, you can go off the wagon, but limit this to once or twice a month. Just remember to get right back on it again when you come home.

Step 2: Eating for Better Detoxification and Liver Support

We live in a world filled with toxins such as pesticides and hormones in our food, solvents and mold in our homes, and heavy metals in the fish we eat and in the water we drink, among others. Since your liver is the body's main detoxifying organ, your body's ability to remove these toxins depends on it! The liver's detoxification process happens in several phases, and different foods, vitamins, and herbal supplements play an influential role in each one.

During Phase I of detoxification, enzymes in your body (known collectively and more formally as the cytochrome P450 system) use oxygen and vitamins, especially antioxidants, to modify any toxic compounds, drugs, or steroid hormones in your system. After altering them, the enzymes send the toxins, drugs, or steroid hormones to the next phase of detoxification. But before they get to Phase II, they are called "intermediary metabolites." This is where antioxidants are very important, because these activated molecules have lots of free radicals, and unless they move along into Phase II, they build up and damage the tissue in your liver. In

Phase II, amino acids and other compounds are added to toxins, making them easier for the body to eliminate (either when you urinate or in your feces). These are called conjugation reactions, and the most important nutrients for this step come from vitamin B_{12}, folate, and amino acids.

Foods to Improve Detoxification

Your liver loves fruits and vegetables. They provide much-needed antioxidants, B vitamins, and minerals. Their ability to help improve Phase I and Phase II detoxification partially explains why vegetables and fruits protect against many cancers.

The following are especially potent: cruciferous vegetables such as broccoli, Brussels sprouts, cauliflower, watercress, and cabbage. This is also where kale, Swiss chard, and collard greens shine. They are potent detox boosters and, like the rest of the cruciferous vegetables, are especially important for the estrogen metabolism pathway. Others include garlic, onions, grapes, berries, soy, green and black teas, and herbs and spices such as rosemary, basil, turmeric, cumin, poppy seeds, black pepper, and cilantro (also called coriander).

Many people ask me about doing a three- or seven-day detox program where they live on liquid green drinks. I love the idea of green drinks and welcome you to use them to supplement a detoxification program. However, they come up short when used alone, for a few reasons. First, they aren't always organic, so I worry that you will be consuming a big, toxic load of pesticides while thinking you are doing something good for your body. Second, while these drinks supply your liver with plenty of antioxidants for the Phase I Detox pathways, they leave you short on amino acids, which are the building blocks of protein. If you aren't eating some form of protein during your juice cleanse, especially if you have a high toxic load, your liver will start processing the toxins better, but it will get stuck halfway through the process without a supply of amino acids. How will you feel? Crummy! This is why many people who try juice cleanses get overwhelming headaches, exhaustion, muscle aches, or brain fog on the second or third day: the liver got overwhelmed without all the nutrients it needed to do its work.

For this reason, we add the following food requirements for any medically sound detox program: vegetarian protein (lentils, beans, nuts, seeds), animal protein (organic free-range chicken and turkey), and protein powders (rice, hemp, pumpkin seed, and vegetarian blends). Soy and whey are not allowed on the elimination diet.

Tier 2: Supplements for Liver Support on a Medical Detoxification Program

While we love the idea of getting all the nourishment you need through food and green drinks, this isn't realistic for most people, especially if they have a high toxic load. After doing the self-assessments in the beginning of this chapter, did you learn that you are one of those people? If you need Tier 2 treatment, then you need a medical detoxification program. I call this a medical program because we are using the supplements like a prescription, treating you for liver fatigue, a term I use often in my practice.

Here are my suggestions for putting together a liver support detox program. The dosages I am suggesting are *daily dosages.* This means you might need to take a particular capsule or tablet more than once each day to reach the necessary amounts.

For everyday support, **you need a B-complex vitamin.** Each day you should take 25–50 mg each of vitamins B_1, B_2, and B_3; at least 100 mg of vitamin B_5; at least 50 mg of vitamin B_6 (as pyridoxal-5'-phosphate); at least 1,000 mcg of vitamin B_{12} (as methylcobalamin); at least 800 mcg of folate (as l-5-methyltetrahydrofolate); and 400 mcg to 1 mg of biotin.

You also need **an antioxidant.** Put together a program that will give you each day 1,000–2,000 mg of vitamin C; 200–400 mg of vitamin E (mixed tocopherols); 1,000–5,000 IU vitamin A (as retinyl palmitate); 3,000–8,000 IU of mixed carotenoids (including beta-carotene); 200–600 mg of alpha lipoic acid; and 250–500 mg of EGCG.

A supplement that contains minerals is also important. Look for a multivitamin/multimineral supplement that contains 15–30 mg zinc, 200 mcg selenium, 250 mcg manganese, and 500 mcg copper.

Additionally, you need a **liver and heavy metal support formula.** Each day you need 100–400 mg milk thistle, 400–600 mg N-acetylcysteine (NAC), and 300–600 mg alpha lipoic acid.

You should also take **supplements that target estrogen metabolism pathways.** These include 100–150 mg indole-3-carbinol twice a day or 100–150 mg diindolylmethane (DIM) twice a day.

Amino acids are another important part of everyday support. I recommend that you **eat protein with every meal**; this can be animal protein (organic free-range chicken or turkey, grass-fed beef, or fish) or vegetarian sources such as legumes, nuts, seeds. The guidelines for daily protein intake are 1 gram of protein per kilogram (2.2 pounds) of body weight. So if you weigh 132 pounds, you are 60 kilograms and should eat 60 grams of protein each day. You can see how much protein is in your meal by reading the label on the package to see how many grams of protein you are getting per serving. To figure out how much protein you are getting in a piece of chicken or fish, use the general rule that 1 ounce of meat or fish has 7 grams of protein. I usually recommend splitting up your protein during the day into 4 meals: breakfast, lunch, afternoon snack, and dinner.

In addition to eating enough protein in your diet, you also need to be digesting it well so it breaks down into the building blocks, which are the amino acids. This is the only way your body can actually absorb and use the protein you eat. You must have good digestive power, and if you aren't sure about your digestion, go back to the self-assessment in Chapter 9, "Healing Your Gut Workbook" to find out, and treat if necessary.

If you are having reflux, gas, and bloating right after you eat, and a feeling of fullness in your stomach that hasn't gone away two hours after you finished your meal, you might need some extra digestive support. I suggest an enzyme formula with each meal to guarantee that you get the amino acids you need. Again, see Chapter 9 for more specifics.

If you want to take an amino acid supplement, **use a blend of amino acids** together, instead of taking one at a time. This can be done as capsules or as a protein powder that you can drink as a smoothie or breakfast shake. Glycine is the most important of all the amino acids for Phase II detox support; supplement with 1,500 mg/day as part of an amino blend. If you are interested in drinking a detox shake, look for products that are in a rice, pea, or vegetable protein base. I have some specific suggestions for you below.

Detox Program to Go with the Detox Elimination Diet

For a three-week intensive liver support program as part of your three-week detox elimination diet, add a detox breakfast shake each morning to your everyday supplements. You can make a breakfast smoothie by mixing any fruit (except oranges, since it is restricted on the elimination diet), water, ice (optional), and two scoops of one of the following metabolic detoxification protein powders:

- Metagenics: Ultraclear plus line of detox shakes
- Designs for Health: Paleocleanse
- Xymogen: Opticleanse
- Thorne: Mediclear
- Blum Center for Health: Liver Support Powder

You can also add your detox powder to the Blueberry Spinach Smoothie recipe in the next chapter, page 282. (You can get more info on where to find these products in the appendix.)

With the detox shake, you must take extra antioxidants, B vitamins, and herbs to balance the different enzymes in your liver detox pathways. I use the following products:

- Metagenics: Advaclear, 2 capsules/day
- Designs for Health: Detox Support Packets, 1 packet/day
- Xymogen: Liver Protect, 2 capsules/day
- Blum Center for Health: Daily Detox Support, 2 capsules/day, and Detox Booster, 2 tablets/day

You can get more information in the appendix on where to find them. These supplements are also good to take for detox support even if you don't drink the detox shakes.

Tier 3: Functional Medicine Options from a Health Professional

It can be very difficult to do a detox program on your own if you have a very high toxic load and you are very sick with what might be an environment-related illness. (We talked about this at the beginning of our toxin discussion in the previous chapter). If you know that you want to do a metabolic detoxification program but feel overwhelmed by the prospect of doing it on your own, you can get help from an integrative medicine practitioner. Also, if you are concerned that you might have high levels of mercury, lead, or other environmental toxins that you want to measure, an integrative medicine practitioner, especially one who focuses on functional medicine, can do these tests for you.

Health professionals who are trained in working with detox elimination diets and metabolic support for your liver are physicians, naturopaths, chiropractors, osteopaths, nurse practitioners, physician assistants, and nutritionists who have a background in functional medicine. Find one at www.functionalmedicine.org. A new certification program is currently being established, and soon there will be a list of certified practitioners. You can also go to one of the functional medicine laboratory websites, such as Genova Diagnostics (www.gdx.net) or Metametrix labs (www.metametrix.com), and find a practitioner who is regularly using their services. That is a great way to locate someone who is actively practicing functional medicine.

If you want to do heavy metal testing, find a functional medicine practitioner or naturopath who uses Doctors Data for the overnight urine collection test for heavy metals.

CHAPTER 13

Supporting Your Liver Recipes

The recipes in this chapter were created to supply many of the nutrients that your liver needs to do its best job. This is very easy when you eat a whole-foods diet, which means that every food looks like it did when it was grown or picked and is filled with protein, fiber, antioxidants, minerals, and vitamins. On the other hand, if your diet consists of processed foods (many of which come out of a box or bag), snacks filled with sugar and white flour, and pesticide and hormone-filled produce and meat, you are not eating in a way that supports your body's natural detox system. In fact, you are taking in even more toxins that add an extra burden to your liver. Whenever possible, choose organic dairy, fruits, vegetables, and animal products, following the guidelines in the previous chapter.

Recipes
Green Detox Soup
Blueberry Spinach Smoothie
North African Red Lentil Soup
Sautéed White Beans and Garlicky Greens
Chickpea Salad
Kale Salad with Tahini Dressing
Harvest Wild Rice
Maple Teriyaki Salmon
Black Bean Burgers
Asian Slaw

Menu 1

Breakfast
Green Detox Soup

Lunch
Chickpea Salad
Kale Salad with Tahini Dressing

Dinner
Maple Teriyaki Salmon
Sautéed White Beans and Garlicky Greens

Menu 2

Breakfast
Blueberry Spinach Smoothie

Lunch
North African Red Lentil Soup
Harvest Wild Rice

Dinner
Black Bean Burgers
Asian Slaw

Green Detox Soup

This soup is one of the best gifts you can give your liver to help it with its critical role in cleansing and filtering the blood. Sulfur-containing foods, such as onions and garlic, will keep your glutathione levels and antioxidant power high. Cruciferous vegetables are great for all of your detox pathways, especially estrogen. Enjoy this soup for breakfast, as a snack or any time of day. You can make a big batch and freeze it in small containers, so it will be on hand during your detox program whenever you get hungry.

Makes 4–6 servings

1 tbsp extra-virgin olive oil or coconut oil
1 small onion, diced
1 tsp minced ginger
2 cloves garlic, minced
1 celery stalk, chopped
3 cups chopped broccoli, florets and stems
½ head fennel, chopped
1 tsp salt
3 cups water
⅛ tsp freshly ground pepper

1. Heat the oil in a medium pot on medium-high heat.
2. Add the onion and ginger and cook until the onion is translucent.
3. Add the garlic, celery, broccoli, fennel, and a generous pinch of salt and continue to cook another 2 minutes.
4. Add the water, remaining salt, and pepper.
5. Bring to a boil, then cover, reduce the heat, and simmer for 20 minutes.
6. Place the soup in a blender and blend until smooth and creamy. Adjust salt.

Blueberry Spinach Smoothie

When most people think of smoothies, they think of all-fruit drinks. But smoothies are also a great vehicle to pack in vegetables and add the antioxidants, vitamins, and minerals that your liver needs to eliminate harmful substances. If you are not used to having greens in your smoothie, don't worry—you won't even know they are there. Try adding a handful of cilantro for an extra antioxidant punch for your heavy-metal detox system.

Makes 2 servings

1 cup almond, coconut, or rice milk
¾ cup frozen blueberries
1 banana
1 medjool date, pitted
1 tbsp ground flaxseeds
1 scoop protein powder (about 15 g)
1–2 handfuls of spinach or kale
1 handful cilantro (optional)

1. Blend all ingredients until they reach the desired consistency.
2. Add a little water if a thinner consistency is desired.

North African Red Lentil Soup

This soup has been made often in our teaching kitchen at Blum Center for Health for its yum factor, easy preparation, and many health benefits. Lentils are a rich source of fiber, which aids in healthy elimination and binds toxins in the gut so you excrete them better. The generous amount of cumin adds digestive and anti-inflammatory support, and garlic and onions provide the sulfur we love for heavy-metal detox support. Make a big batch of this and store in small containers in the freezer to enjoy all year long. During the winter, I eat this for lunch at least once a week. It is wonderful either alone or served over some cooked quinoa or other gluten-free grain.

Makes 8 servings

2 tbsp olive oil
1 medium yellow onion, chopped
1 large carrot, diced
2 tsp ground cumin
3 cloves garlic
1½ tsp salt
2 cups red lentils   (continued on next page)

8 cups water or stock
Freshly ground pepper
Lime wedges, for garnish
Chopped parsley, for garnish

1. In a large pot, heat the olive oil over medium-high heat.
2. Add the onion, carrot, cumin, garlic, and 1 teaspoon salt. Cook, stirring, for about 5 minutes, or until the onion is soft.
3. Add the lentils, water or stock, and the remaining salt to the onion mixture.
4. Bring to a boil, then turn the heat all the way down to the lowest possible setting.
5. Partially cover and simmer gently for about 30 minutes, or until the lentils are completely soft.
6. For a thicker soup, allow the lentils to cook until they are nearly dissolved.
7. Grind in a generous amount of pepper and stir to blend.
8. Serve hot, with a lime wedge on the side. Garnish with parsley.

Sautéed White Beans and Garlicky Greens

When beans and greens come together, it's a detox match made in heaven. The fiber from the beans and the antioxidants and B vitamins in the greens make this a detoxifying meal unto itself. Use any dark green leafy vegetable you prefer, such as collard greens, bok choy leaves, spinach, or kale, because they all supply indole-3-carbinol, the nutrient that helps you detoxify your estrogens.

Makes 4–6 servings

3 tbsp ghee or olive oil
3 cloves garlic, chopped
5 cups chard, leaves only, coarsely chopped
½ tsp salt
Pinch red pepper flakes
½ cup dried white cannellini beans, soaked overnight and cooked, or one 14-oz can
Freshly ground pepper
Extra-virgin olive oil, for drizzling
Squeeze of lemon juice, for drizzling

1 roasted red pepper, thinly sliced
Toasted pine nuts, for garnish

1. Heat 2 tbsp ghee or olive oil over medium-high heat in the widest skillet you have.
2. Add the garlic and sauté for 30 seconds.
3. Add the chard, ¼ tsp salt, and red pepper flakes. Sauté the greens until they just start to wilt.
4. Add the white beans, remaining salt, and a pinch of pepper.
5. Stir to combine and cook until the beans are heated through. Drizzle olive oil and a dash of lemon.
6. Plate the beans and greens and garnish with a few slices of roasted red pepper and some toasted pine nuts.

Chickpea Salad

Beans are rich in fiber, which helps eliminate toxins through the digestive tract. When cooked with the sea vegetable kombu, the chickpeas are richer in essential minerals for good thyroid function. Here chickpeas get an abundance of flavor from fresh herbs and a vitamin C punch from lemon and red peppers. We've added rosemary for its flavor, and also because it helps support the detoxification of estrogens in the liver. Serve this along with the Kale Salad with Tahini Dressing for a high-protein meal.

Makes 6 servings

2 cups cooked chickpeas
¼ cup chopped red onion
¼ cup carrot, diced small
¼ cup red bell pepper, diced small (if you are avoiding nightshade vegetables, substitute cucumbers or radishes)
1 tbsp fresh lemon juice
2 tbsp apple cider vinegar
4 tbsp extra-virgin olive oil
2 small sprigs rosemary, minced
2 tbsp minced parsley
Salt
Freshly ground pepper

(continued on next page)

1. Combine all ingredients in a serving dish.
2. Serve right away or chill for a few hours to allow the flavors to come together.

Kale Salad with Tahini Dressing

This salad was created for my appearance on the Dr. Oz show when I was featured as one of his top four "disease detectives." Kale is one of the most nutrient-dense vegetables, filled with vitamins A, K, D, and E and fiber, which are all important in the liver pathways. Not only will your liver be working better, but so will your thyroid from all the zinc, iodine, and selenium in the kelp and seeds. Zinc is a wonderful support for the immune system and helps stimulate the excretion of heavy metals. This salad can be made in advance and refrigerated overnight. The kale will break down and become softer from the lemon juice the longer it marinates.

Makes 2–4 servings

1 bunch kale, either curly or Tuscan, finely chopped with ribs removed
¼ cup thinly sliced radishes
½ to 1 tbsp kelp flakes
1 small red or yellow bell pepper, diced
¼ cup finely chopped cilantro
2 tbsp tahini
Juice of 1 lemon
1 tsp agave syrup or honey
½ tsp salt
2 tbsp water
2 tbsp olive oil
¼ cup toasted walnuts or brazil nuts, finely chopped

1. Combine the kale, radishes, kelp, pepper, and cilantro in a large bowl.
2. Mix the tahini, lemon, agave, salt, water, and olive oil until blended.
3. Pour the tahini dressing over the kale mixture and mix very well.
4. Let it sit for at least an hour.
5. Add the walnuts.

Harvest Wild Rice

Rich in protein, folate, magnesium, and vitamin A, wild rice makes a hearty and comforting side dish in the fall and winter seasons. We've added lots of veggies for an extra antioxidant punch.

Makes 6 servings

1½ cups wild rice
Salt
2¾ cups water
2 tbsp extra-virgin olive oil
1 small onion, finely chopped
2 garlic cloves, minced
2 cups mushrooms, preferably cremini, stemmed and quartered
½ cup finely chopped celery
Squeeze of fresh lemon juice
¼ cup finely chopped parsley
¼ cup toasted chopped pistachios or walnuts
¼ cup dried cranberries
Freshly ground pepper

1. Bring rice, ¼ tsp salt, and water to a boil in a saucepan.
2. Cover, reduce heat to a simmer, and cook until all the water is absorbed, about 30 minutes.
3. Heat oil in a large pan over medium heat. Add the onion and a pinch of salt and cook, stirring occasionally, until soft, about 8 minutes.
4. Add the garlic and cook another 2 minutes, stirring often.
5. Add mushrooms, celery, and lemon juice, cover, and cook for 5 minutes.
6. Uncover and cook for another 5 minutes, stirring, letting the excess juices evaporate and the mushrooms and celery finish cooking.
7. Let the mushroom mixture cool slightly and then mix with the rice in a serving bowl.
8. Gently fold in the parsley, nuts, and cranberries. Add salt and pepper to taste.

Maple Teriyaki Salmon

Salmon is one of the richest sources of omega-3 essential fatty acids. A 4-oz serving also delivers vitamin B_{12}, niacin, and selenium. Look for wild or organically farmed salmon to ensure you're getting the cleanest fish free of contaminants. Unless it's organic, farmed fish often has high levels of PCBs, dioxins, and food dye.

Makes 4 servings

1 lb wild salmon, cut into 4 fillets
2 cloves garlic, minced
2 tsp minced fresh ginger
1 tbsp maple syrup
2 tbsp mirin
1½ tbsp balsamic vinegar
Juice of ½ lemon
Pinch of sea salt
1 tbsp thinly sliced scallion

1. Wash and dry the salmon fillets.
2. Mix the garlic, ginger, maple syrup, mirin, vinegar, lemon juice, and salt well and pour ¾ of this marinade into a freezer bag, saving the remainder in a small bowl in the refrigerator.
3. Add the salmon to the marinade in the bag and place in the refrigerator for 1–4 hours.
4. Preheat the oven to broil.
5. Bring the salmon to room temperature.
6. Place the salmon on a broiling pan and set the pan 4 inches from the top of the oven. Broil for 5 minutes.
7. Brush the salmon with the marinade frequently as the salmon continues to cook for another 10 minutes or just until the salmon flakes. Cooking time will vary depending on the thickness of the salmon.
8. Garnish with scallions.

Black Bean Burgers

This black bean burger may lack meat, but it doesn't skimp on being hearty. It is important to get adequate protein at every meal, which is why this burger is great at lunchtime or for a casual dinner with your family. You can also freeze these uncooked or cooked, then defrost when you are ready to eat them.

Makes 4 servings

1½ tsp ground flaxseeds
2½ cups cooked black beans
½ jalapeño pepper, seeded and chopped
1 clove garlic, chopped
1 tsp ground cumin
¾ tsp salt
1 tbsp tomato paste
2 tbsp gluten-free bread crumbs
1–2 tbsp gluten-free flour
¼ cup carrot, diced small
1 avocado, for topping (optional)
2 tbsp olive oil

1. In a small bowl mix together the ground flaxseed with 1½ tbsp water. Let sit for 5 minutes. This will act like an egg binder.
2. Place the beans, jalapeño, and garlic in a food processor and pulse to combine. Add cumin and salt and pulse mixture until it resembles a chunky black bean dip.
3. Transfer the beans to a large bowl and stir in the tomato paste, bread crumbs, flour, carrot, and flax mixture. Stir well until everything is combined.
4. Heat the oil in a skillet on medium-high heat.
5. Form the black bean mixture into 4 patties and fry for about 4 minutes per side, until golden and crusty.
6. Top with avocado slices, if using.

Asian Slaw

Slaws are great for summer side dishes or tossing into your favorite taco. Cabbage is most commonly used in slaws, which provides an easy way to pack in essential nutrients to support liver detoxification, including anti-oxidant vitamins C and E, vitamin A, B vitamins, and indole-3-carbinol, a compound that reduces the levels of toxic estrogens in your body.

Makes 4 servings

4 cups shredded red cabbage
1 carrot, cut into matchsticks
1 red bell pepper, thinly sliced
½ cup red onion, thinly sliced
2 tbsp light sesame oil
2 tbsp toasted sesame oil
2 tsp lime juice
2 tsp brown rice vinegar
1½ tsp salt
2 tsp grated ginger
2 tbsp toasted sesame seeds
¼ cup chopped cilantro

1. In a large bowl combine the cabbage, carrot, pepper, and onion.
2. In a small bowl whisk together the oils, lime juice, vinegar, salt, and ginger.
3. Pour over the cabbage mixture and toss. Taste and adjust salt.
4. Refrigerate 10–20 minutes to let the salad marinate.
5. Toss with sesame seeds and cilantro and serve.

PART V

Additional Considerations

The best way out is always through.

—Robert Frost

CHAPTER 14

Infections and Specific Autoimmune Conditions

As you have seen, all autoimmune diseases have a lot in common. We have detailed the association between gluten and many autoimmune diseases, how stress can trigger or exacerbate these diseases, the importance of your gut bacteria in maintaining balanced immune function, and how dysbiosis and leaky gut syndrome are associated with all autoimmune diseases. We have also described how many environmental toxins, such as mercury, can trigger autoimmune diseases and how reducing your exposure, enhancing your detox system, and boosting glutathione can heal your liver, your body's natural detoxifying system, and cure your symptoms.

But there are some unique features and treatment strategies for the different autoimmune diseases, so I have included this chapter to highlight additional considerations for MS, RA, lupus, autoimmune thyroid disease (Graves' disease and Hashimoto's thyroiditis), celiac disease, and Sjögren's syndrome. I have chosen to highlight these six because these are the conditions I see most frequently in my office.

While the focus when treating autoimmune diseases is to fix the functioning of the foundational systems—food, stress, gut health, and toxins—there are some special considerations and treatments that are specific to each disease. I will talk about them here and also add a brief review about what each disease is, possible symptoms, the conventional approach, and the functional medicine approach.

But before we begin our review, I want to tell you about another possible trigger for autoimmune disease that I haven't fully discussed yet: infections. There is a lot of research examining the role infections, especially viruses, might play in triggering autoimmune diseases in general, and before we go into detail about each health condition, I will provide a little background information.

THE ROLE OF INFECTIONS IN SPECIFIC DISEASES

In Chapter 8, "Healing Your Gut," we talked about the relationship between the bacteria in your intestinal lining and your immune system. As we discussed, sometimes there can be an overgrowth of harmful bacteria, yeast, or parasites in your gut. These can cause subclinical infections. This means that they don't produce the typical symptoms of an infection, such as fever, fatigue, muscle aches, localized redness, pain, and swelling. Instead these infections are under the radar, causing chronic irritation to your immune system. In this chapter, I will focus on the viruses and other infections that do not come from your gut but which can live in your body and contribute to autoimmune conditions.

Let's start with what we know about infections and autoimmune disease. Over the years there has been an array of studies trying to prove that a particular microbe (meaning a bacteria, virus, parasite, spirochete, or yeast) causes a particular autoimmune disease. Unfortunately, not a single study has been able to prove that a microbe caused an autoimmune disease. In order to do that, you would need to find that infection in every person with the disease, which hasn't happened. So why do we still think microbes are involved? Because research on animals and results of epidemiological studies (research that looks at the numbers of people with the disease and how many of them have the infections) have shown a clear association between some viruses and bacteria and many autoimmune diseases. An association is an increased risk of getting a disease if you have the virus or infection. Though an association does not prove cause, it does tell us that the infection is probably one of the triggering events.

HOW INFECTIONS TRIGGER AUTOIMMUNE DISEASES

There are many theories about how infections can cause, trigger, or be involved in autoimmune diseases. The first is that the immune system makes a mistake: after it creates antibodies against the microbe, these antibodies also attack your own tissues. The tissue being attacked determines which autoimmune disease you have. For example, if this happens to the myelin in your brain, then you get MS; if it's your thyroid, then you get Hashimoto's thyroiditis or Graves' disease. This is called *molecular mimicry*, something we have talked about throughout this book, because both gluten and chronic dysbiosis in the gut are believed to cause autoimmune disease this way. The antibodies made against the gluten protein and against microbes in your gut are also reacting against your tissues.

Another possibility for infections as a trigger for autoimmune disease is that the microbe infects the cells directly, living inside them and causing direct cell and tissue damage. There are two things that can happen as a result, both of them bad. The first is that your immune system reacts to the virus living inside the tissue and your body gets damaged in the crossfire. This is called a bystander effect. The second is that the infection inside your cell causes the cell to develop a different "name tag" on the outside of its cell surface. As a result, the immune system begins to see your own tissue as foreign. If the infection becomes a chronic situation, the immune system will continue attacking your cells because the infection is still inside. An infection can persist anywhere, including but not limited to your joints, brain, and thyroid. It is even possible for an infection to live inside your immune cells themselves, which can cause your immune cells to lose their tolerance for your own tissue.

The final way that infections can exacerbate autoimmune conditions is when your tissues are already damaged from an autoimmune disease and then a virus is drawn to the inflammation and takes up residence in this tissue as a secondary problem. In studies that find viruses at the site of autoimmune damage, it is unclear whether the damage came first or if it was caused by the virus.

Why do some people recover from an infection, whereas other people don't? **There is some evidence that in certain people bad genetics or damage from an environmental toxin or exposure has made their immune systems unable to get rid of a chronic infection.** As a result, the infection triggers autoimmunity either right when the person first gets sick or because the infection persists. As we start to talk about the different autoimmune diseases and their associations with viruses and bacteria, keep in mind that this is an area of active investigation in the scientific literature.

IS YOUR IMMUNE SYSTEM HANDICAPPED?

Emerging research on the association of chronic infections and autoimmune disease suggests that a handicapped immune system might be part of the problem.[1] This means you will have trouble getting rid of infections, which in turn makes it easier for the virus to take advantage of you. How does your immune system become handicapped? Genes appear to be part of the problem, but the environment plays a role, too. Genetics are not destiny; they are simply a blueprint for what could happen. Your environment dictates how this blueprint will be read and transcribed. In this book, you have learned how **the food and nutrients you eat, the stress you experience, environmental toxins, and having a gut full of harmful microbes all affect your immune system at the deepest cellular level.** So even if you have bad genetics, you can overcome them by positively influencing the function of your immune system so that it can better clear out viruses and infections and lower your risk of autoimmune diseases. This is why the four steps in this book are the ultimate answer if you have chronic infections: you need a healthy immune system to fight these infections so that they won't stay persistently active in your body, possibly contributing to your autoimmune disease.

How do you know if you have a handicapped immune system, with genes that make you more susceptible to getting an autoimmune disease? One clue is if you have family members—parents, grandparents, aunts, uncles, or siblings—with an autoimmune disease. This makes it more likely that you could have one, too. In other words, a family history makes the genetic connection more likely. There aren't many genetic tests for specific autoimmune diseases, but research has slowly been identifying parts of the genes, called HLA regions, that are involved. I believe that someday, as these genes get sorted out, we will have useful tests that can help you know if you have a gene for a specific autoimmune disease. For now, family history is best, and HLA testing for a few diseases is available. (One of these is celiac disease; I will discuss this below.)

There are a limited number of genetic tests that are available that allow you to see if you have any handicaps in the way your immune cells function. Some of these I do in my office, although not very often, because they are very costly and not covered by insurance. The test I use is called the ImmunoGenomics Profile from Genova Diagnostics (www .gdx.net). Keep in mind that if you have an autoimmune disease, chances are you have a genetic predisposition, and you don't need the test to tell you that. But the ImmunoGenomics profile can help me know if you have handicaps in your immune system that are making it hard for you to clear chronic infections from your body.

Now that you know the basics about the possible role of infections as triggers for autoimmune diseases, you are ready to review the six specific autoimmune diseases: MS, RA, lupus, autoimmune thyroid disease (Graves' disease and Hashimoto's thyroiditis), celiac disease, and Sjögren's syndrome.

MULTIPLE SCLEROSIS (MS)

As you learned from reading about Steve in Chapter 12, "Supporting Your Liver Workbook," MS is a serious chronic neurological disorder in which the myelin sheathing around the nerve cells is destroyed—a condition called demyelination. This causes the nerves to malfunction and spurs inflammation that damages the central nervous system, which includes the brain and spinal cord. There are four types of MS, and which one you have depends on your symptoms. Relapsing-remitting MS is where you have symptoms and then they go away completely until the next relapse or attack. The other three are called progressive and in all of them your symptoms never seem to go away. They are primary progressive (you have never had a remission), secondary progressive (you had remissions at the beginning but not anymore), and progressive relapsing (you had progressive disease from the beginning, but you occasionally experience remissions).

Common symptoms of MS:

- Eye pain
- Numbness, tingling, or a pins-and-needles sensation anywhere in the body that doesn't go away after two weeks
- Swelling of the limbs or trunk
- Intense itching sensation, especially in the neck area

Tests to ask your doctor or other health care professional for:

- There are no antibody tests for MS. Instead, it's diagnosed when lesions are seen on an MRI. It's important to note that the diagnosis is made only after having neurological symptoms twice or a second episode that shows a new lesion in the brain or spinal cord. One episode that resolves and never comes back is not considered MS.

The clinical course of MS is variable, but 85 percent of patients begin with the relapsing-remitting type. It is believed that something triggers the immune cells to attack the myelin that surrounds the nerve fibers. The results are flares, ongoing inflammation and destruction in the central nervous system. The question has always been what starts this process. Is there one trigger or cause? Or are there many triggers happening at once? Are the immune cells making a mistake and attacking healthy myelin? Or is something damaging or changing the myelin so that it looks foreign and then it gets attacked? Infectious disease has emerged as the number one suspect when looking for MS triggers.

The Role of Infections as Triggers for MS

Chlamydia pneumoniae

Many studies looking at the statistics and patterns of disease occurrence have suggested that MS is acquired, not genetic, although as with all autoimmune diseases, a genetic predisposition is likely. When researchers look at the cerebrospinal fluid (CSF) of MS patients, they always find elevated amounts of immunoglobulins, molecules made by your immune cells. In fact, 95 percent of MS patients have high concentrations in their CSF, which suggest that the brain is actively trying to fight an infection.[2] Further research has shown that these immunoglobulins are directed against *Chlamydia pneumoniae*, a bacterium that is distributed worldwide and lives inside your cells. It is known to infect humans and for continuing to cause problems long after you think you are better. Some people never know they have this infection because they have no symptoms; others have a respiratory illness such as bronchitis, an upper respiratory infection, or pneumonia. *Chlamydia pneumoniae* can cause a persistent brain infection, and in the past fifteen years there has been emerging evidence of a strong association between chlamydia and MS.

Antibodies to *Chlamydia pneumoniae* are consistently found in the CSF of MS patients, leading researchers to believe that this bacterium might be causing chronic infection in the brains of these patients. Researchers from the Department of Neurology at Vanderbilt University School of Medicine have shown that these antibodies are also being made inside the central nervous system, suggesting the infection is there, too. In fact, these authors report that *C. pneumoniae* antibodies are found in the blood of only 50 percent of MS patients (remember, your blood travels outside your brain), and since the levels are higher when measured inside the brain, the infection is most likely localized in the brain.[3]

Chlamydia pneumoniae was implicated as a cause of MS after the bacterium was isolated from the CSF of a patient with rapidly worsening MS who improved after being treated with antibiotics. Since then, there have been many studies looking for this bacterium in the tissue cultures from MS patients. Several centers have continued to report that they find the bacteria in the tissues, although others have not been able to replicate these results. At this time, even though the presence of *Chlamydia pneumoniae* is clearly more likely in MS patients, the findings are insufficient to establish firmly that it causes MS. However, because *C. pneumoniae* is easily treated with antibiotics, it seems reasonable to treat all MS patients with minocycline. Although I generally avoid giving antibiotics because they can harm the good bacteria in the gut, for patients with MS I will prescribe minocycline, and make sure to give probiotics as well to protect the gut.

Epstein-Barr Virus (EBV)

EBV is the most well-studied chronic viral infection associated with autoimmune diseases. EBV is the virus that causes infectious mononucleosis (mono). Positive antibody tests for EBV are found in up to 95 percent of the general population but almost 100 percent of MS patients, raising possibilities that EBV may be associated with MS. Epidemiological studies have shown that people who have had infectious mononucleosis are twice as likely to later develop MS, and that higher levels of EBV antibodies have been consistently found in patients with multiple sclerosis compared with control individuals. Research also has found that in some studies of MS patients, EBV itself is present in areas of the brain with myelin damage.[4]

Even though many studies have shown this association, this does not prove that EBV causes MS. And this is where all the debate still rages, because research has not uncovered whether the virus came first and actually *caused* the autoimmune condition or if it is just taking advantage of the poorly functioning immune system to persist in the body as a secondary problem.

While the connections between MS and EBV and between MS and *Chlamydia pneumoniae* seem real, the question still remains whether the autoimmune disease was caused by the infections, and if it was, whether the primary problem is the infection itself or a failure in the immune system to adequately get rid of the infection. Because we are all walking around with hundreds of viruses inside of us, and most of us live in balance with them, I would suggest that the issue is a weak or dysfunctional immune system. So following the four steps described in this book to fix your immune foundation is the first step you can take to combat the disease.

Other Possible Triggers for MS

Vitamin D

There has been a strong association found between MS and low vitamin D levels and also an association between MS and people living in locations with low UVB radiation, which helps the body make vitamin D. It turns out that inside your body vitamin D is converted to 1,25 vitamin D, a hormone that stimulates antibacterial and antiviral properties in the body. In the brain, 1,25-dihydroxyvitamin D increases the amounts of a compound called cathelicidin, which helps keep the brain sterile. It is therefore likely that the vitamin D deficiency is allowing chronic infections to persist in the central nervous system, something that is especially important in MS. One study found that women who took supplemental vitamin D had a 40 percent lower risk of getting MS.[5]

Your Program: Additional Testing and Treatment

If you have MS, in addition to focusing on the four foundational steps in this book, I also suggest the following treatment guidelines:

- There is enough research on *Chlamydia pneumoniae* to support using the antibiotic minocycline. You will have to get a prescription from your neurologist. Ask for 100 mg capsules and take one twice a day for three weeks. You can give your neurologist the references at the end of this chapter if he or she is skeptical.
- Always get tested for the yeast candida with IGG and IGM in the blood and as part of a stool analysis as well. If any of these tests are positive, treat with diflucan for three weeks (100 mg twice a day).
- I learned these treatments from David Perlmutter, M.D., a brilliant neurologist who has helped develop the functional medicine approach to MS.

When it comes to the brain, it's best to follow a slightly different approach to using food as medicine. We recommend that MS patients focus on maintaining a ketogenic diet. Ketones are simple fat molecules that are used as fuel, and it turns out the brain and your mitochondria really like them. The focus of the paleo diet, where you eat no grains and focus on healthy fats (from avocados, coconut oil, and grass-fed organic animals), vegetables, berries, some nuts and seeds, and whole, unpasteurized, organic dairy products from grass-fed animals has some good support in the literature. This kind of diet increases ketones in the brain, which is anti-inflammatory and helps the myelin repair itself. I would recommend you follow this type of diet and refer you to *Primal Body, Primal Mind: Beyond the Paleo Diet for Total Health and a Longer Life* by Nora T. Gedgaudas if you want to learn more.

The gut is very important as a foundational problem for people with MS, so you need to do Tier 2 of the dysbiosis and leaky gut programs in Chapter 9, "Healing Your Gut Workbook," even if you don't have gut symptoms. Additional considerations for supplements are those that focus on nerve repair. These include glutathione with NAC, which we discussed in Chapter 12. Dr. Perlmutter created a great line of products for Xymogen that I use for this: NRF2 for boosting glutathione, and Brain Sustain for additional nerve and membrane support. NRF2 has broccoli seed extract, which provides sulforaphane, turmeric, black pepper extract, green tea, and pterostilbenes. Brain Sustain has DHA, coenzyme Q_{10}, N-acetylcysteine, alpha lipoic acid, phosphatidylserine, and acetyl-L-carnitine. Good fats are also important, so I suggest 1 tablespoon of an oil that provides medium-chain triglycerides (such as coconut oil) twice per day and at least 500 mg a day of DHA.

SYSTEMIC LUPUS ERYTHEMATOSUS (SLE OR LUPUS)

Systemic lupus erythematosus, more commonly known as lupus, is a chronic inflammatory autoimmune disease that is widespread throughout the body. It is a multisystem disorder that affects not only the central nervous system, like MS, but also several organs. Lupus mostly attacks the skin, joints, kidneys, and nervous system, but it can damage any other organ as well. The disease is nine times more common in women than in men. African Americans have a three times higher risk than Caucasians. There is a strong genetic predisposition: identical twins have the disease together 25 percent of the time, but fraternal twins have the disease together only 2 percent of the time. On the flip side, there must also be a strong environmental influence, to explain why 75 percent of the time only one of a pair of identical twins gets lupus and the other one doesn't. So while genetics play an important role and lays the foundation for risk, there is clearly an environmental trigger.

Throughout this book I have shared with you the multiple environmental triggers that are associated with lupus; here I will summarize them all in one place. Studies have shown an association with:

- High estrogen levels
- Exposure to silica dust, pesticides, aromatic amines (as in hair dyes), and hydrazines
- Exposure to mercury
- High-fat/low-antioxidant diet
- Ultraviolet radiation
- Cigarette smoking
- High infection rate with viruses and bacteria
- Molecular mimicry after infections as a possible trigger (the association with EBV is most significant; some other studies show an association with *Chlamydia trachomatis* and with pneumococcus)

All lupus patients have IgG antibodies directed against themselves, and researchers have discovered more than fifty different types. The laboratory testing looks for the most common ones to make a diagnosis. Those specific to lupus are:

- Anti-Sm
- Anti-ribosomal P
- Anti-double-stranded DNA

Found in lupus and other rheumatologic autoimmune diseases:

- ANA (anti-nuclear antibody)
- Anti-phospholipid
- Rheumatoid factor
- Anti-single-stranded DNA
- Anti-La (SS-B)
- Anti-nuclear ribonucleoprotein (anti-nRNP)

The antibodies in lupus are not focused on a specific organ, so the inflammation and damage occur throughout the entire body. Research has shown that you can have these autoantibodies for years before you show any clinical signs or symptoms of lupus. This is why it is good to get these tests if you aren't feeling well but your doctor can't find anything specific. Why? Because if you catch these antibodies before you have symptoms of the disease, you can more easily stop the disease in its tracks by following the steps in this book.

What does it feel like to have lupus? Symptoms include:

- Fatigue
- Muscle pain and weakness
- Fever when the disease is active

- Symptoms specific to the organ involved, such as joint pain, muscle pain, and difficulty breathing
- Butterfly rash over the cheeks and nose that appears after sun exposure
- Hair loss (but not baldness)
- Oral or nasal ulcers that are not painful
- Cold- or emotion-induced color changes of the fingers or feet

Tests to ask your doctor or other health care professional for:

- Antinuclear antibodies (ANA)
- Anti-phospholipid antibodies
- Antibodies to double-stranded DNA
- Anti-Smith (Sm) antibodies

The ANA test is the first screening test for lupus. As I explained, a positive test doesn't mean you have lupus unless one of the three other tests is positive as well.

Just like with all other autoimmune diseases, you need to go through the four steps in the treatment program of this book, which will help your immune system function better. **For lupus patients, I focus on two additional pieces: EBV activity, to see if it is chronically active or reactivated, and hormones, especially estrogen and DHEA.**

Epstein-Barr Virus and Lupus

Systemic lupus erythematosus has been associated with EBV infection for decades; however, researchers have never been able to determine the exact mechanism for this link. Most human adults are infected by EBV and carry the virus for life without clinical symptoms. However, for unknown reasons EBV induces infectious mononucleosis in some individuals, during which cross-reactive antibodies specific for both virus and the self have been detected. Interestingly, the same antibodies are also frequently found in lupus patients, another example of molecular mimicry. This cross reactivity of anti-EBV antibodies with self proteins is a compelling hypothesis to explain how the autoimmune process begins in lupus. Researchers at the Oklahoma Medical Research Foundation found that anti-EBNA-1 antibodies, found in people with EBV, react with self-proteins common in lupus (such as anti-Ro and anti-Sm). Many studies have shown that EBV antibodies and viremia (viruses detected in the blood) are more frequent in lupus patients than in healthy individuals, and this has further supported the possibility that EBV triggers autoimmunity.[6]

How does this happen? Researchers at the University of Queensland found that the immune systems of lupus patients are less capable of controlling EBV viremia and were unable to target and kill the EBV-infected cells. Their theory of how EBV works to cause lupus is that the persistent infection causes an accumulation of EBV-infected B cells inside the tissues of the body, and that these sick B cells lose their tolerance and make antibodies targeted against the self.[7]

This is another possible mechanism for how EBV causes lupus, but it also shows that a fundamental problem in the immune system came first, which allowed the EBV to persist in the body. I think this argument is the most compelling explanation. In my office, I have been measuring and looking for EBV activity in all of my autoimmune patients, and over and over I find that the virus is there, sometimes dormant, sometimes active. I recently had a new lupus patient, Maggie, who was thirty-eight years old when she came to see me. She told me that she had developed lupus six months after a terrible case of mono when she was in high school. Chances are that she has a genetic susceptibility. It's also possible something like low vitamin D, for example, was the reason her immune system wasn't able to fight the EBV. But I have no doubt that for her, the EBV infection was the trigger that set her autoimmune disease in motion. When I tested her antibody levels, she had signs that the EBV was active in her body. Because there is no antiviral treatment for EBV that is hiding inside your cells, the answer for Maggie is to fix all the foundations and help the immune system to work better.

What to do? As I told you in the last chapter, we need to help your body do a better job by healing your gut, improving your diet, replenishing nutrients you might need (such as vitamin D), removing toxins, and balancing your hormones. This will help your body fight EBV better.

Lupus and Hormones: Estrogen, Progesterone, DHEA, and Testosterone

What about your hormones? Because there have been many studies linking exacerbations or flares in disease activity with increased estrogen levels, it is important to make sure your estrogen and progesterone are in good balance. Women with lupus should never take hormone replacement therapy after menopause and should not go on birth control pills.

Your Program: Additional Testing and Treatment

Testing

For EBV activity, I run the full panel of four different blood tests: EBV EA IgG, EBV VCA IgG, EBV EBNA IgG, and EBV VCA IgM.

- The EA will tell you if you have chronic active viral infection.
- The IgM test will tell you whether you have a reactivated or new infection.
- The EBNA and VCA will be positive if you ever had an infection, and most doctors will tell you this means you had an infection in the past. But the EBNA also tells you that the EBV is actively replicating inside your B cells, and the higher the number, the more activity is still going on. So even though most doctors ignore and dismiss the results of this test, if the EBNA is > 8, I believe that means you have an ongoing problem with the virus that is perhaps continuing to trigger production of autoantibodies.

Hormone-related testing that I do for lupus patients:

- Estrogen metabolism testing from Genova Diagnostics Laboratory (I explained this in Chapter 12, "Supporting Your Liver Workbook.")
- Adrenal saliva testing to check cortisol (cortisol will affect your progesterone levels). You can get this test from a number of functional medicine labs, including Genova Diagnostics and Metametrix.
- Blood tests for progesterone, DHEA-S, and testosterone from your routine laboratory. Your doctor can order this.

Treatment

The treatment focus should be optimizing estrogen metabolism in the liver. Some of this I explained in Chapter 11, but I will summarize it here again for you.

- Clean up your diet and your environment from all xenoestrogens (see page 241) and pesticides.
- Support your liver enzymes and eat dark leafy greens and cruciferous vegetables every day (see page 276).
- Increase your consumption of non-GM organic soy, ground flaxseeds, and fish oil. Increase fiber in your foods. All these will help you detox estrogen better.

- As far as supplements, I suggest indole-3-carbinol or DIM, broccoli extracts, and sulforaphane, because all of these help detox estrogens.
- Also, make sure you heal your gut, because bad bacteria can increase the recirculation of toxic estrogens.
- You also need to focus on supporting your adrenal hormones. Have your doctor measure DHEA-S in the blood, and take supplements of DHEA to get your levels over 100 mcg/dl. I told you about the study where the researchers gave lupus patients very high doses of DHEA (200 mg), which helped them lower their prednisone dosages. The usual dose I recommend is 25 mg, but you should have your DHEA-S level checked to make sure this is the right dose for you. Make sure you are practicing your self-care and helping your adrenal glands stay healthy. Go back to Part II, "Understanding the Stress Connection." Get an adrenal saliva test to find out if you have adrenal fatigue.

CELIAC DISEASE

As I described in Chapter 2, "Using Food as Medicine," celiac disease is caused by an allergy to gluten and is marked by destruction of the microscopic, finger-like protrusions called villi that line the small intestine. It may take many years of gluten exposure before the villi are damaged and a laboratory confirms that you have celiac disease, but in the meantime gluten in your diet can cause other digestive and autoimmune issues. Celiac disease has become the most well-known autoimmune disease because so many people have developed sensitivities to gluten.

Symptoms:

- Gluten can cause autoimmune disease in other organs in addition to the gut, so there is a wide range of symptoms, from numbness and tingling in the extremities to fatigue from low thyroid function
- Arthritis
- Generalized brain fog
- Generalized fatigue
- Digestive issues such as diarrhea, gas, and bloating after eating

Your Program: Additional Testing and Treatment

Tests to ask your doctor or other health care professional for:

- There is a lot of confusion about how to diagnose celiac disease. Gastroenterologists will give you this diagnosis only after a small bowel biopsy showing damage to your villi. This is very restrictive since you might have silent celiac disease for decades before this test is positive.

- Instead, ask your doctor for anti-gliadin antibodies (AGA) and anti-deamidated gliadin antibodies (ADGA). The ADGA test is the newest and most sensitive for picking up gluten allergies, and both the AGA and the ADGA can be positive for many years before there is any damage to your small intestine. If either of these is positive, it's a sign that an autoimmune attack is taking place somewhere in your body. In that case, you should assume you have very early celiac disease that hasn't affected your intestines yet but is doing plenty of damage in your body, perhaps showing up as Hashimoto's thyroiditis, Graves' disease, MS, or another autoimmune disease.
- Just to add to the confusion, even if all the above tests are negative, you might *still* be sensitive to gluten. That's because these tests were designed to pick up celiac disease only, and gluten can cause other autoimmune diseases as well. Therefore, it is good to do the tests above, but if they are negative, you should still remove gluten from your diet, based on research showing a connection between gluten and many other autoimmune diseases.
- There is a genetic test you can ask for to see if you have an increased risk of developing celiac disease. Ask your doctor to test your HLA DQ2 and HLA DQ8. When you get the results from the lab, the report will explain your risk of developing celiac disease based on the results. If the rest of your tests for celiac disease are normal, this test can be useful information, because if you are genetically susceptible, you must stay on the gluten-free diet as best as you can for the rest of your life.

If you were diagnosed as having celiac disease, just going on a gluten-free diet won't be enough to allow your whole body to recover from the damage it has suffered. If you had a positive anti-gliadin antibody test or a positive anti-deamidated gliadin antibody test, you have *potential* celiac disease and should follow these guidelines even if your gastroenterologist is saying you don't need to because there is no sign of damage to your intestines. (I explained the research behind this in Chapter 2, "Using Food as Medicine.") People with celiac disease often have trouble absorbing nutrients.

If you get a positive result on any of the tests I mentioned, you need to do the following things, in addition to going on a gluten-free diet:

- First, restore your vitamins by taking a daily multivitamin/multimineral supplement. Also take a sublingual (under the tongue) B_{12} supplement.

- Heal your gut lining and healthy bacteria following the program in Chapter 9, "Healing Your Gut Workbook," for leaky gut syndrome. Because the gluten was causing stress in your gut, probably your bacteria are out of balance and you have leaky gut syndrome, too. It isn't enough to just stop eating gluten; you must help your intestinal lining and therefore your immune system get healthy again. Take a probiotic every day—at least 25–30 billion live organisms of mixed strains of *Lactobacillus acidophilus.*
- You are at an increased risk of other autoimmune diseases, so have your doctor check your thyroid for antibodies and screen you for lupus, RA, and Sjögren's. If these tests are positive, going off gluten will help them too. There is a genetic risk, so make sure to test your children, as young as possible.

RHEUMATOID ARTHRITIS (RA)

If you have arthritis, it's often difficult to tell the difference between RA and common osteoarthritis, which can occur with aging or after injury. Rheumatoid arthritis occurs when your immune cells attack your joints, causing tissue damage, inflammation and pain. It is a very specific form of arthritis, and sometimes the only way to know which kind of arthritis you have is to do the blood test below.

Symptoms of RA include:

- Muscle pain
- Fatigue
- Low-grade fever
- Weight loss
- Depression
- Morning stiffness that lasts at least one hour for at least six weeks
- Swelling of three or more joints for at least six weeks
- Swelling of wrist or fingers for at least six weeks
- Symmetric joint swelling
- Nodules or bumps under the skin and over an affected joint

Tests to ask your doctor or other health care professional for:

- Hand X-ray
- Blood tests for ANA, rheumatoid factor (RF), and anti-citrullinated peptide/protein antibodies (anti-CCP)
- Blood tests for inflammation: ESR (erythrocyte sedimentation rate) and high-sensitivity C-reactive protein (sometimes called Cardio CRP)

It is good to get all the above blood tests because they will help you know if you have rheumatoid arthritis. It is possible to have a positive ANA yet have all the other tests come back negative. If this happens, then you don't have RA. And you can have RA because you have a positive RF or anti-CCP but a normal ANA. The ESR and the Cardio CRP are indicators of how much inflammation might be happening at the moment, helping to monitor flares in the disease.

Rheumatoid Arthritis and Leaky Gut Syndrome

Of all the autoimmune diseases, RA has the strongest association with dysbiosis, leaky gut syndrome, and immune-complex disease. This means that research has worked out the mechanism for how an overgrowth of bad bacteria in the gut can cause leaking of foreign proteins into the bloodstream, which causes the release of significant amounts of antibodies by immune cells. When the antibodies attach to the foreign proteins, they form immune complexes, which deposit in the joints, causing inflammation and destruction. This is the model most widely accepted for the development of RA. Because lupus, Sjögren's, and all of the rheumatologic autoimmune diseases (which have a positive ANA in common) can have joint involvement, this process is important for all of them.

There is another category of arthritis called reactive arthritis, and it's the same as RA, but there are no positive blood tests. All the symptoms might be the same, but none of the tests for autoimmune rheumatoid arthritis are positive. The important thing to remember here is that your arthritis is caused by the same process, so the treatment is the same as if you had RA. You are having an inflammatory reaction in your body, and most likely this inflammation is coming from a bacterial infection in your gut or urinary tract. For you, cleaning up your gut, as we did in Chapter 9, "Healing Your Gut Workbook," is the place to start. Reactive arthritis includes people diagnosed with psoriatic arthritis and spondylarthritis. Genetics play a role in RA, but not as strongly as for lupus. When looking at pairs of identical twins in which one twin has the disease, only 15 percent of the time the second twin had the disease, too. This means that something in the environment, probably microbial, caused the disease for at least 85 percent of RA patients.

Infections and RA: *Proteus mirabilis* and EBV

Proteus mirabilis *and RA*

Since the mid-1980s, many studies have emphasized the role of *Proteus mirabilis* microbes in RA. These bacteria cause recurrent urinary tract infections (often with undetected involvement of the kidneys) with the production of large amounts of cross-reactive antibodies, which could bind and attack the targeted antigens within the synovial tissues, causing destruction in joint structures and the eventual development of RA. Infections with *Proteus mirabilis* can go undetected and without symptoms such as severe pain and burning with urination. This process is a classic example of molecular mimicry or cross-reactivity between bacterial and self antigens, which means that the immune response to *Proteus mirabilis* is also active against tissues in the joints of people with RA.

Several independent groups have found that antibodies to *P. mirabilis* were significantly elevated in patients with RA compared to those with other diseases or corresponding healthy subjects recruited from fifteen different countries throughout the world.[8] These immunological, molecular, and microbiological findings support the notion that there is a crucial role for *P. mirabilis* microorganisms in the initiation and perpetuation of RA. Does this mean that this infection can cause RA? Maybe. Does this mean the infection is the cause in everyone who has RA? Definitely not, but I would suggest that there is probably another infection, coming from the gut perhaps, that *is* causing RA by molecular mimicry, as well as immune-complex disease.

EBV and RA

As with all autoimmune diseases, RA is presumed to have a genetic basis triggered by interaction with the environment. And as with lupus, research has found that antibodies in RA patients cross-react for both EBV and joint tissue, suggesting that molecular mimicry might play a role in this disease as well. Some studies have detected EBV in the joints of patients with RA. Researchers in the Faculté de Médécine in Marseille, France, found that the T cells in RA patients don't do a good job of fighting EBV. As a result, RA patients have a higher viral load than people who are healthy. This suggests that persistent EBV could trigger RA. The antibodies could be directly attacking the joints or causing immune complexes to deposit there.[9] (Remember, immune complexes are when the antibody binds onto the foreigner and they become stuck together in very large molecules that settle into tissues and joints and cause local inflammation and damage.) So if people with RA don't do a good job clearing out their EBV infection and have persistently higher loads of virus and antibodies in their blood, they might experience ongoing elevated amounts of immune complexes, causing chronic joint inflammation. This is the theory that researchers have been discussing for many years.

A recent study by researchers at Brigham and Women's Hospital followed women with positive EBV over time and found they did not have an increased risk of RA, suggesting no association between EBV and RA.[10] This is one of the first prospective studies to really answer the question whether having EBV puts you at a higher risk for RA, and this study suggests that the answer is no.

Your Program: Additional Testing and Treatment

Here are my suggestions:

- Do a complete elimination and challenge diet, including removing the nightshade vegetables (tomatoes, potatoes, eggplant, and peppers). Food is a big trigger for you, and you need to figure out which foods you are sensitive to and remove them.
- Do Tier 2 of the dysbiosis and leaky gut treatment program, even if you don't have symptoms.
- Remove all the foods you are sensitive to from your diet for at least six months while you focus on healing your gut.
- Take 450–500 mg/day of the omega-6 oil gamma linoleic acid (GLA). Studies have shown this will help your inflammation.
- Take anti-inflammatory herbs such as curcumin and boswellia to reduce pain and inflammation in the joints, which will help them heal. You can use curcumin alone or in a combination product. (See my product guide, page 329.)
- If you have no improvement after three months, get a stool analysis. Dysbiosis in the gut is strongly associated with RA, and you must make sure your gut flora are very healthy. You can get a stool analysis from a functional medicine practitioner, with listings at www.functional medicine.org.

SJÖGREN'S SYNDROME

Sjögren's syndrome, which can occur on its own or in conjunction with RA, lupus, or other systemic autoimmune disease, is an attack on the mucus-secreting glands, causing a reduction in excretions. Lymphocyte cells infiltrate these glands and prevent them from working properly. Therefore, the first symptoms can often be dry eyes and mouth because of the immune damage to the salivary glands, which are in the mouth, and lacrimal glands, those that secrete tears. The biggest challenge in the conventional medical world is making an accurate diagnosis for Sjögren's syndrome because many of its clinical features, such as arthritis, fatigue, and muscle pain, can be seen in other diseases. Also, the Sjögren's antibodies can be present in people with lupus, RA, systemic sclerosis, mixed connective tissue disease, and antiphospholipid syndrome. The fact that so many different diseases have similar and overlapping symptoms and lab results is further evidence that these are all variations of the same underlying process. Just as with lupus, 90 percent of people with Sjögren's are female.

Symptoms:

- Dry mouth and dry eyes
- Dryness in the vagina, skin, lungs, sinuses, and digestive tract
- Fatigue
- Joint pain
- Muscle pain
- Cognitive dysfunction

Tests to ask your doctor or other health care professional for:

- ANA, anti-SSA, and anti-SSB antibodies

Sjögren's and DHEA

Research has shown that treating Sjögren's patients with DHEA can result in symptom improvement.[11] DHEA is a pre-hormone made by the adrenal glands that, for women, helps the body make the androgen testosterone. Since DHEA is made in the adrenal glands, this is a reminder that if you have Sjögren's, you need to focus on making sure your adrenal glands are healthy, as we discussed in Chapter 5, "Understanding the Stress Connection." But it turns out that your estrogens and your androgens need to be in good balance to keep your immune system in balance, too. Estrogen pushes one way (toward Th2 dominance), and DHEA and testosterone push the other way (toward Th2 dominance). Therefore, if your DHEA and testosterone get low, you will become more estrogen dominant, which is not good for your immune system. This is why for my Sjögren's patients I pay extra attention to supporting DHEA and testosterone and making sure they are in good balance.

Sjögren's and EBV

Research has also shown a strong association between Sjögren's syndrome and EBV, which is why Sjögren's patients are at a higher risk for a type of lymphoma caused by EBV. There is some evidence that viruses are involved in triggering the disease, especially EBV, because it infects the throat and nose cells, which are right next to your salivary and lacrimal glands. Researchers at University Hospital Jean Minjoz in Besançon, France, reported that EBV DNA has been found in the saliva and/or salivary glands of Sjögren's patients more frequently than in those of people in control groups.[12] However, other researchers have not found this to be true. But there is agreement that, just as in RA and lupus, antibodies against EBV are higher in patients with Sjögren's compared to healthy people. While there have been some descriptions of patients who developed Sjögren's after acute EBV infection, there is no consistent evidence that having EBV increases your risk of getting Sjögren's.

Your Program: Additional Testing and Treatment

In addition to the four foundational steps in this book, people with Sjögren's need to focus on hormone balance and supporting androgens. And just as I explained for lupus, I recommend that they measure and follow EBV levels.

- Measure DHEA-S and take a supplement to boost your levels over 100 mcg/dl. If your doctor doesn't want to follow your levels, show him or her this book.
- Measure testosterone, too. Taking DHEA will boost testosterone levels in women, as will 1–2 tablespoons of ground flaxseed per day. I always recommend taking both; the flaxseed contains an aromatase inhibitor and will prevent all the testosterone from being turned into estrogen, which happens when you are stressed.
- Follow the instructions for detoxing estrogens in the section on lupus, page 301.

- If you have joint involvement, follow instructions in the section on RA (page 308) and focus on treating your leaky gut.
- Make sure you have your EBV antibody levels done, including all four tests (see page 305) to check for chronic or reactivated disease.

AUTOIMMUNE THYROID DISEASE: HASHIMOTO'S THYROIDITIS AND GRAVES' DISEASE

I put these two conditions together in one section because they have a lot in common. As you remember, Hashimoto's thyroiditis is a condition in which your body makes antithyroid antibodies, which slowly destroy the thyroid gland, eventually causing hypothyroidism. In Graves' disease, your immune system makes stimulating antibodies, which cause the gland to produce too much thyroid hormone, resulting in hyperthyroidism. You can have both of these antibodies for a long time before you develop signs of hypo- or hyperthyroidism. Picking up these antibodies early is a golden opportunity to fix the autoimmune problem and save the thyroid from damage. I screen for all of these antibodies in all of my patients, even if they have normal thyroid hormones, and most commonly I find anti-thyroid antibodies. So **get tested for the antibodies, especially if you have another autoimmune disease, and even if your thyroid function appears normal on the surface.**

Viruses and Autoimmune Thyroid Diseases

Viruses have been long implicated in causing subacute thyroiditis. This is an inflammation of the thyroid gland that happens right after a viral illness, such as an upper respiratory infection, influenza, or mono, and causes neck pain or a severe sore throat. Some people are sick for a few weeks or even months and then get better. When they are sick with subacute thyroiditis, they can have symptoms of too much thyroid hormone (rapid heart rate, weight loss, insomnia) or too little thyroid hormone (feeling tired and sluggish, weight gain, hair loss, feeling cold all the time). There is good evidence that this condition is caused by an infection, but the question remains whether this infection of the thyroid gland can go on to cause Hashimoto's thyroiditis or Graves' disease. While this seems possible and there have been some reports of this happening, it is not common. So if there is an infectious cause for subacute thyroiditis, it only continues on and causes autoimmune thyroid disease in a minority of cases.

But separate from subacute thyroiditis, there is plenty of evidence that infectious agents may trigger autoimmune thyroid diseases. For example, studies have shown seasonality and geographic variation in the incidence of Graves' disease. And other studies have found evidence in the blood for a recent bacterial or viral infection in 36 percent of newly diagnosed Graves' disease patients versus only 10 percent of people in the control group. Microbes that have been implicated in this process include coxsackie B virus, retroviruses, hepatitis C virus, *Yersinia enterocolitica*, and *Helicobacter pylori*. Direct evidence of the presence of viruses or their components in the thyroid tissue itself has been found for retroviruses in Graves' disease, and for HTLV-1, enterovirus, rubella, mumps, herpes simplex virus, Epstein-Barr virus, and parvovirus in Hashimoto's thyroiditis.[13]

Do these viruses or bacteria cause the disease? More and more we are beginning to think that these infections might take hold and persist in damaged tissue where there is inflammation and immune activity, so it is possible these viruses are just innocent bystanders. Further research will have to sort this out. But again, this is another example of how viruses seem to be present in areas of tissue damage and inflammation, either possibly as the cause or collecting there after the fact.

GRAVES' DISEASE

Graves' disease happens when your body makes antibodies that stimulate your thyroid gland, causing it to secrete high levels of the hormone thyroxine (also known as T4). This condition is called hyperthyroidism. Conventional treatment involves medication aimed at destroying the thyroid gland, so it stops making the hormones that have gone out of control. If you have severe symptoms, such as dangerous heart palpitations or severe weight loss and insomnia, this may be an urgent medical situation and this treatment might be a wise course of action. But I have had many patients who did not have these extreme symptoms, and so we had time to work on treating the autoimmune issue and quiet down the antibodies. They were therefore able to avoid thyroid-damaging medication.

Symptoms include:

- Weight loss
- Rapid pulse
- Protruding eyes
- Insomnia

- Feeling too warm
- Restlessness
- Diarrhea
- Irritability
- Heart palpitations

Tests to ask your doctor or other health care professional for:

- TSH
- Free T4
- Free T3
- Thyroid-stimulating immunoglobulins (TSI)
- TSH receptor antibody

Here is the pattern of test results you would expect if you have Graves' disease:

- TSH is low, typically < 0.5 mIu/L, often lower or undetectable
- Free T4 elevated, usually over 2.5 ng/dl
- Free T3 might be normal but is usually over 4.0 pg/ml
- Either the TSI or the TSH receptor antibody will be positive; if they are both normal, than you don't have Graves' disease

The above pattern is what the numbers would look like in a typical, classic case of Graves' disease. However, sometimes only one of the numbers looks out of range, like a high free T4 with a normal TSH, which is a sign that you might have caught the problem early and that this is the perfect time to go through the steps in this book and reverse the problem before the disease starts.

Hashimoto's Thyroiditis

Also called chronic autoimmune thyroiditis, this is the most common autoimmune disease. Here, the immune cells invade the thyroid. Usually this autoimmune condition is diagnosed only after you become hypothyroid, which is when the thyroid is not making enough hormone. Once you become hypothyroid, the conventional treatment is to give you hormone replacement. This approach treats only the hypothyroid problem, not the autoimmune problem. Wouldn't it be better to find out you have Hashimoto's thyroiditis even before your thyroid gland is damaged, causing you to need a prescription for thyroid hormone replacement? If you catch it early and follow the steps in this book, you can stop the autoimmune attack on your thyroid even before you become hypothyroid.

Remember, when it comes to the thyroid gland, there are two potential problems: the autoimmune disease and the functioning of the gland. You can have Hashimoto's with normal thyroid function, and you can have Hashimoto's with hypothyroidism. The symptoms can be the same either way, and therefore blood tests are crucial to make the proper diagnosis.

Symptoms:

- Enlarged thyroid (called a goiter)
- A sore throat in some people with an actively inflamed thyroid
- Fatigue
- Hair loss
- Weight gain

Tests to ask your doctor or other health care professional for:

- TSH
- Free T4
- Free T3
- Anti-thyroglobulin and anti-thyroid peroxidase antibodies

Hashimoto's Thyroiditis with Normal Thyroid Function

- One of your antibody levels will be elevated, either thyroid peroxidase antibodies or anti-thyroglobulin antibodies. If both are normal, you don't have Hashimoto's.
- TSH, free T4, and free T3: if these levels are normal, it is the perfect time to follow the steps in this book because you have caught the problem early while it is reversible, preventing damage to your thyroid gland. Here are my suggested normal values for the hormones for screening purposes:
  - TSH: <3.0 mIu/L
  - Free T4: > 1.0 ng/dl
  - Free T3: > 2.6 pg/ml

Hashimoto's Thyroiditis with Borderline Hypothyroid

- One of your antibody levels will be elevated, either thyroid peroxidase antibodies or anti-thyroglobulin antibodies
  - TSH: Between 3 and 4.5 mIu/L
  - Free T4: < 1.0 ng/dl
  - Free T3: < 2.6 pg/ml

If your TSH is less than 4.5, you wouldn't be diagnosed as hypothyroid, but you might be on your way and feeling the effects of a sluggish thyroid gland. Give yourself three months to complete the steps in this book, especially the additional treatment below, and you can probably avoid ever needing to take a prescription thyroid hormone replacement.

Hashimoto's Thyroiditis with Hypothyroidism

If your TSH is over 4.5, you might want to consider taking a prescription thyroid hormone replacement. It is outside the scope of this book to review the different options for medication, but my rule of thumb is that I avoid glandular products such as Armour Thyroid and Naturethroid for my Hashimoto's patients. I have seen anti-thyroid antibodies go up after treating some people with these glandular prescriptions, and therefore I prefer to use a T4/T3 non-glandular hormone from my compounding pharmacy, or the prescriptions Levoxyl/Cytomel from the regular pharmacy. Because prescribing the right hormone replacement is very personalized and specific, if your TSH is over 4.5, I suggest discussing with your doctor whether it is a good idea to take a prescription thyroid hormone replacement, and what would be the best option for you.

Your Program: Additional Treatment

There are three major things to focus on if you have either Graves' disease or Hashimoto's thyroiditis:

- You must remove gluten from your diet because autoimmune thyroid disease is associated with celiac disease, even if you have no signs in your blood or intestines that you have celiac disease.
- You need to take 200–400 mcg of selenium every day, because selenium is needed for the thyroid cells to be healthy and make hormones, as I talked about in Chapter 3, "Using Food as Medicine Workbook."
- You must focus on reducing your mercury exposure. Because of the thyroid gland's location, it is especially susceptible to toxins coming from the mouth, and this is one very important way that it is different from the rest of the autoimmune diseases. There are studies showing an association between dental amalgam (silver) fillings (especially for those people who have a mercury allergy, meaning they make antibodies to the mercury), mercury exposure, and autoimmune thyroid disease.

If you have an autoimmune thyroid disease, when you go through the four foundational steps in this book, make sure you focus on determining if you have exposure to mercury. Do you have multiple cavities with silver fillings? If yes, then make a plan with your dentist to remove all of your amalgam fillings. Go to the website for the International Academy of Oral Medicine and Toxicology at www.iaomt.org to find the instructions for safe removal. Do you eat fish every week that are on the high-mercury list, such as tuna, swordfish, and Chilean sea bass? If so, switch to low-mercury fish and focus on taking selenium and N-acetylcysteine to boost the glutathione and antioxidant levels inside your thyroid cells. These levels get low from mercury exposure and then your thyroid cells get damaged from the inside. Follow the Tier 2 program in Chapter 12, "Supporting Your Liver Workbook," and follow the three-month program to begin getting your metals out. Lastly, consider getting tested by an integrative practitioner.

Conclusion

Right now you are turning the final pages of this book. Yet you are at the start of an exciting, life-changing journey. Whether you have completed one part of *The Immune System Recovery Plan* or all four (or are somewhere in between), you are on your way to reversing your autoimmune disease and, ultimately, to a richer, fuller life. I know that living with your autoimmune disease has not been easy. I suspect that it has been a roller-coaster ride of emotions filled with a lot of frustration, confusion, and "why me?" moments. And I know this because I've been there.

I, too, was diagnosed with one of these conditions and I, too, was told by my doctor that my life as I knew it had changed. I was inspired and motivated to find the path to full recovery rather than accept that there was nothing I could do to restore my immune function to normal. My intuition and medical experience told me that I could find a better way, and once I did, I wanted to shout it to the world. One by one, my patients came to see me with another doctor's diagnosis of a lifetime of prescription medication and pain. They were told they would get used to living that way and that this would be their new normal. But I knew different. I became committed to guiding each one of them who came to see me because they didn't want that way of life—and I didn't want that for them, either. I decided to write this book because I don't want that life for *you*!

It has become my passion to share what I've learned so that you and so many others are not held back by autoimmune disease but, rather, use it as a way to improve your lives. Taking care of yourself and recovering your immune system will be a lifelong journey. It is one that I personally take steps along each day and one that *does* get easier as you travel it. There are ups and downs, but you are never alone, which is also why I wrote this book. My goal has been to offer you hope, along with many answers. I want to empower you to take charge of your own health and get the care you need. I want you to be the captain of your own ship because I *know* that if we take the necessary steps, we can improve not only our own lives but those of our friends, family, and the world at large.

You can't wait to make the life changes that I have outlined in this book. You can't wait for the government or the medical system to adopt different policies or to clean up the environment. No one else can help you but *you*. You need to take control of your health and make changes *now*. That said, I know this book contains a lot of information and the plan asks a lot of you. But don't get overwhelmed. Take your time and work your way through it at your own pace. This isn't a sprint; it's a marathon.

There is a quote that says, "The journey of a thousand miles begins with a single step." I am glad that you have chosen to take those first steps with me, and I am sure that if you keep following this plan, you will have a healing journey that leads you down the road to better health. You can do it. I know you can!

—Susan Blum, M.D.
November 2012

Acknowledgments

Writing this book was a true labor of love. But it was made so much easier because I had an amazing writing partner, Michele Bender. We worked in rhythm, sending chapters back and forth, and I think this experience was as painless as it could possibly have been because of her. I am also forever grateful to my agent, Janis Donnaud, whose advice and guidance at the beginning of this process was so necessary and helpful. I also want to thank our publisher, Susan Moldow, who, along with our editor, Whitney Frick, immediately understood the importance of what I was trying to say. Thank you, Whitney, for your humor, passion, and excellent suggestions, which helped us shape and create a book that we hope will help millions.

Thank you to all my patients for opening my eyes to the need to tell this story. My vision for bringing functional medicine to those suffering with chronic disease began as a simple medical practice where I worked with and helped hundreds, now thousands, of people. It became clear to me that I was on to something, because my patients with "incurable" conditions got better.

Of course, I couldn't have learned to practice medicine this way without my colleagues and teachers at the Institute for Functional Medicine. Jeffrey Bland, Ph.D., Mark Hyman, M.D., David Jones, M.D., Joel Evans, M.D., David Perlmutter, M.D., Patrick Hanaway, M.D., and Dan Lukaczer, M.D., opened the doors for me and many others. I also need to give a shout-out to my friend and colleague Adria Rothschild, who has traveled this path with me and reviewed and gave me feedback for "Using Food as Medicine."

A special thanks to Mark Hyman for including me as one of the "Fantastic Four Disease Detectives" on the *Dr. Oz* show. My gratitude to the many producers I have worked with and to Mehmet Oz, M.D., for the opportunity to be on the show.

In addition to my focus in functional medicine, I have been living and working closely with the Center for Mind-Body Medicine for many years. I will always be indebted to James Gordon, M.D., the founder and director, who has been my greatest teacher and friend. The faculty members at CMBM are my best friends. They have supported my personal growth and helped me become who I am today, so thank you to Kathy Farah, Lynda Richtsmeier-Cyr, Jerrol Kimmel, Amy Shinal, Kelsey Menehan, Toni Bankston, Claire Wheeler, Monique Class, Debra Kaplan, Lora Matz, Bob Buckley, and the rest of the team for helping me bloom. Also, a special thanks to Jim and Amy, who gave me feedback on "Understanding the Stress Connection," and to Jo Cooper, for supporting me and my efforts to incorporate CMBM's concept of food as medicine at Blum Center for Health and in this book. I know there are countless others in this field to thank, but there isn't enough room. You came before me, and I am so grateful to be one of you now.

Two years ago, I took a big leap to fulfill a dream and open Blum Center for Health, where under one roof I have integrated our functional medicine clinic with a lifestyle education center, including a teaching kitchen and meditation room. To my dedicated and supportive team at Blum Center for Health, I am grateful for and amazed at what we have accomplished together in this time. It has been truly magical, and this book is an extension of all that we are and have learned. Thank you to my committed assistant, Sabrina De Gregorio, who has been by my side since the beginning, sharing the ups and downs and never wavering in her dedication; Elizabeth Greig, M.S.N., F.N.P., my fellow clinician and sounding board for all things medical; Marti Wolfson, our culinary director, who created all the wonderful recipes in this book; and Dana Epstein, our director of media and branding, who's guided me since the beginning of this project. To more of my team, which includes Bernadette Valcich, Mary Beth Weisner, Elspeth Beier, and Gary Goldman, you are always willing to jump in when needed and support me in every way possible, and I appreciate this more than words can say.

They say it takes a village; for me that is certainly true. Blum Center for Health and this book have been dreams of mine for as long as I can remember, and neither would have been possible without the support of my family. I am grateful first and foremost to my husband, Bruce, who cheered me on every step of the way. He not only helped me with financing and the business plan but put up with many weekends where I was huddled in my office immersed in writing. He became my greatest fan, preaching to everyone about the virtues of a whole-foods diet and never wavering in his support. I also want to say thank-you to my sons, Jeremy,

Corey, and especially Avery, who was still living at home while I wrote this book and never complained when I was distracted by the enormousness of this project. I know you weren't always happy with the food in the house, but you will thank me someday!

I will be eternally indebted to my mother-in-law, Carol Blum, who designed and built Blum Center for Health and gave me invaluable business advice; to my sister, Cindy Conroy, who has been my CFO and chief go-to business partner; to David Bender, my brother-in-law, who has designed all things Blum; to my nephew Adam, a key member of our team who is in charge of the website; and finally to Keith Warner, who helped me at the very beginning. To my parents, Barbara and Donald Spanton, my siblings, Diane and Andrew, and my in-laws, Anita and Yale Roe and Mort Blum, M.D., there is no luckier girl than me to have a family like you to support me in every way. The list goes on and on. But one thing I know for certain is that there have been many people behind me, which means they are all behind you now, too.

Appendix I:
Helpful Books, CDs, At-Home Programs, and Destination Programs

NUTRITION AND COOKBOOKS

- *BlumKitchen Nutrition Guide and Cookbook,* www.immuneprogram.com
- *Clean Start* and *Clean Food* by Terry Walters
- *Healing with Whole Foods* by Paul Pitchford
- *How to Cook Everything Vegetarian* by Mark Bittman
- *Vegetarian Cooking for Everyone* by Deborah Madison
- *Nourishing Traditions* by Sally Fallon
- *The Blood Sugar Solution* by Mark Hyman
- *The Body Ecology Diet* by Donna Gates
- *The China Study* by T. Colin Campbell
- *Primal Body, Primal Mind* by Nora T. Gedgaudas
- *The Slow Down Diet* by Marc David
- *The Whole-Food Guide to Strong Bones* by Annemarie Colbin, Ph.D.
- *Wheat Belly* by William Davis, M.D.

TOOLS FOR LEARNING TO RELAX

Kits that include books and CDs

- Learn to Relax Kit by Blum Center for Health, www.immuneprogram.com
- Best of Stress Management Kit by the Center for Mind-Body Medicine, www.cmbm.org
- *Meditation for Beginners* by Jack Kornfield, includes book and CD

Recommended Books

- *10 Simple Solutions to Stress* by Claire Michaels Wheeler, M.D., Ph.D.
- *Unstuck: Your Guide to the Seven-Stage Journey Out of Depression* by James S. Gordon, M.D.
- *50 Ways to Soothe Yourself Without Food* by Susan Albers, Psy.D.
- *Flip the Switch: 40 Anytime, Anywhere Meditations in 5 Minutes or Less* by Eric Harrison
- *Guided Imagery for Self-Healing* by Martin L. Rossman, M.D.
- *I Can Do It* by Louise L. Hay
- *Why People Don't Heal and How They Can* by Carolyn Myss, Ph.D.

Recommended CDs

- *Empowerment for Mind and Body* by Claire Wheeler, M.D.
- *Relax and Renew Guided Stress Management* by Amy Shinal
- *Learn to Relax* CD by Blum Center for Health
- From www.healthjourneys.com, choose from hundreds of titles. You can listen to a sample of the voice and music before you purchase
- www.soundstrue.com
- www.thehealingmind.org
- *Breathing* by Andrew Weil, M.D.
- *Guided Mindfulness Meditation* by Jon Kabat-Zinn, Ph.D.
- *Creative Visualization Meditations* by Shakti Gawain

DESTINATION PROGRAMS

I often suggest that my patients spend a weekend at these wonderful places that offer delicious, health-supportive food and terrific programs to choose from. You can find accommodations and price ranges from rustic to luxurious. It is so helpful to find a teacher who can get you started or deepen your practice. In addition to mind-body-spirit programs, the following also offer nutrition, food, and healing options.

- Kripalu Center for Yoga & Health in Lenox, Massachusetts
- Omega Institute in Rhinebeck, New York
- Canyon Ranch in Lenox, Massachusetts, or Tucson, Arizona

- Spirit Rock Meditation Center in Woodacre, California
- Menla Mountain Retreat in Phoenicia, New York, www.menla mountain.org
- The Chopra Center in Carlsbad, California, www.chopra.com/ meditationweekend

Appendix II:
Supplement and Herb Guide

What follows is a list of the specific supplements and herbs that I use with my patients at Blum Center for Health to work through the four-step Immune System Recovery Plan as you are doing in this book. There are many wonderful companies and products out there; however, these are the ones that I am familiar with and therefore feel comfortable recommending. There are four different product lists. Each one corresponds to one of the four workbooks.

CHAPTER 2: USING FOOD AS MEDICINE
Antioxidants and Immune Support

Product	Manufacturer
Ultra Potent C	Metagenics
Stellar C	Designs for Health
E Complex	Metagenics
Zinc Picolinate	Thorne
Selenium Picolinate	Thorne
Vitamin D3 2000	Xymogen
Vitamin D3 1000	Metagenics
Vitamin D3 5000	Metagenics
Bio-D-Emulsion Forte	Biotics
Oxygenics	Metagenics
Silymarin (Milk Thistle)	Designs for Health, Metagenics
EGCG	Designs for Health
Celapro	Metagenics

(continued on next page)

Product	Manufacturer
GlutaClear	Metagenics
N-acetyl cysteine (NAC)	Designs for Health
Detox Antioxidants	Designs for Health
Lipoic Acid Supreme	Designs for Health
ALAmax (Extended Release Lipoic Acid)	Xymogen
Fish Oil High Concentrate Liquid	Pharmax
Fish Oil EPA/DHA 720	Metagenics
GLA Forte	Metagenics
ProEFA Liquid	Nordic Naturals
Immune and Antioxidant Packets	Blum Center for Health
Protein Drinks	
Immune Support Powder	Blum Center for Health
BioPure Whey	Metagenics

CHAPTER 5: UNDERSTANDING THE STRESS CONNECTION

These are the products I recommend and use to support the adrenal glands and a healthy stress response. I am also including my favorite supplements for sleep.

Product	Manufacturer
Adreset	Metagenics
Adrenal Support	Blum Center for Health
Cortico B5B6	Metagenics
AdreCor	Neuroscience
Cortisol Manager	Integrative Therapeutics
DHEA	Vital Nutrients
Serenagen	Metagenics
MyoCalm P.M.	Metagenics
Somnolin	Metagenics

CHAPTER 9: HEALING YOUR GUT WORKBOOK

Supplements to Support Digestion

Product	Manufacturer
Complete Digestion Support	Blum Center for Health
Enzyme Support	Blum Center for Health
GastrAcid	Xymogen
Vital-Zymes Complete	Klaire Labs
Iberogast	Medical Futures, Inc

Supplements to Treat Dysbiosis

Product	Manufacturer
GI Cleansing Herbs	Blum Center for Health
A.D.P. Oregano	Biotics
Formula SF722	Thorne
GI Microb-X	Designs for Health
Tricycline	Allergy Research Group
CandiBactin BR and AR	Metagenics

Probiotics and Prebiotics

Product	Manufacturer
Flora Support	Blum Center for Health
Ther-Biotic complete	Klaire Labs
Ultra Flora IB	Metagenics
Ultra Flora Plus DF Capsules	Metagenics
Sacharomyces Boulardii	Klaire Labs
BiotaGen	Klaire Labs
Endefen	Metagenics
Protein Drinks	
GI Support Protein Powder	Blum Center for Health
Immune Support Protein Powder	Blum Center for Health

Supplements to Repair the Stomach and Intestinal Lining

Product	Manufacturer
DGL Chewable Licorice	Natural Factors
GI Lining Support Capsules	Blum Center for Health
GI Revive Capsules	Vital Nutrients
GI Protect Powder	Xymogen
Glutagenics Powder	Metagenics
Glutamine Powder and Capsules	Xymogen, Designs for Health, Thorne
IgG 2000 Powder and Capsules	Xymogen
Protein Drinks	
GI Repair Protein Powder	Blum Center for Health
UltraInflamX Protein Powder	Metagenics

CHAPTER 12: SUPPORTING YOUR LIVER WORKBOOK

Supplements to Improve Detoxification

Product	Manufacturer
AdvaClear	Metagenics
Silymarin	Metagenics, Designs for Health
Amino D-Tox	Klaire Labs
DIM-Avail	Designs for Health
BroccoProtect	Designs for Health
Methyl-Guard Plus	Thorne
Methyl Protect	Xymogen
Intrinsi B12 Folate	Metagenics
Modified Citrus Pectin Powder	Thorne
Liver Protect	Xymogen
MetalloClear	Metagenics
Chelex	Xymogen
GlutaClear	Metagenics
LV-GB Complex	Designs for Health
N-Acetyl Cysteine	Designs for Health
Detox Booster	Blum Center for Health

Daily Detox Support	Blum Center for Health
Detox Fiber Blend	Blum Center for Health
Protein Drinks	
UltraClear Plus	Metagenics
I5	Xymogen
PaleoCleanse	Designs for Health
MeDiclear	Thorne
Liver Support Powder	Blum Center for Health

Appendix III: Tips for Healthy Eating and Grocery Shopping List

There is a lot of confusion these days about what to eat. Once you've completed all four steps recommended in *The Immune System Recovery Plan*, we advise adhering to a few basic tips and techniques when you're planning your weekly meals and shopping for food.

SUGGESTIONS

- Try to avoid processed food, including gluten-free products.
- Make a pot of soup, a large salad, and extra chicken. It is smart to have prepared food on hand so that you do not reach for food that is not allowed.
- Use leftovers.
- Eat often. We do not recommend a calorie-restricted diet—although many people using the plan recommended in this book have lost weight.
- It is important to keep your blood sugar stable. Carry food such as a small bag of nuts and seeds with you when you leave the house.
- If there are foods that you know you do not tolerate well and they are on the "Food to Include" list, please avoid them also.
- Eat colorful vegetables (5–7 servings per day) and fruits (2–3 servings per day). Be conscious of this and try to eat a detoxifying vegetable and a carotenoid vegetable daily.
- Choose organically grown fruits and vegetables, because they are not sprayed with pesticides.
- Hormone- and antibiotic-free poultry and grass-fed lamb are best as well.
- If you are a vegetarian, be sure to get enough protein from legumes and grains such as rice, quinoa, amaranth, teff, millet, and 100 percent buckwheat.
- Drink lots of plain, filtered water. This will help your body flush out toxins.

SHOPPING LIST

When you're making your grocery list, we encourage you to pick from the items listed here. Items in **bold** are great detoxifiers—indulge daily.

Fruits

Flavonoid family: detoxifiers, anti-inflammatory, and anti-cancer	**Blueberries** **Blackberries** Cherries Cranberries (not dried) Currants Figs (fresh) Gooseberries Grapes, red skin Plums **Pomegranates** Prunes **Raspberries** **Strawberries**
Carotenoid family: immune-enhancing	Apricots (fresh) Cantaloupe Mangoes Nectarines Papayas Peaches Persimmons Watermelon
Citrus family: antioxidants	**Grapefruits** Kumquats Lemons Limes Tangerines
Other fruits	Apples Bananas Kiwis Pears Pineapples

Vegetables

(If you have arthritis, avoid nightshades, in *italics*.)

Cruciferous/Brassica family: detoxifiers	**Arugula** **Bok choy** **Broccoflower** **Broccoli** **Broccoli rabe** **Broccoli sprouts** **Brussels sprouts** **Cabbage** **Cauliflower** **Collard greens** **Kale** **Kohlrabi** **Mustard greens** **Napa cabbage** **Radishes** **Swiss chard** **Turnips** **Watercress**
Carotenoid family: immune-enhancing	Avocados Beets Carrots Pumpkins Radicchio *Red peppers* Romaine lettuce Spinach Sweet potatoes and yams *Tomatoes, fresh* *Tomato sauce* Winter squashes (butternut, acorn, delicata, spaghetti) Yams

Allium family: detoxifiers	**Chives** **Garlic** **Leeks** **Onions** **Shallots** **Scallions**

Other Vegetables

(If you have arthritis, avoid nightshades, in *italics*.)

Artichokes
Asparagus
Burdock
Celery
Cucumbers
Eggplants
Fennel
Green beans
Jicama

Mushrooms
Okra
Parsnips
Peas
Potatoes
Sea vegetables—seaweed, kelp
Summer squashes
Zucchini

Starch/Bread/Cereal

(non-gluten)

Amaranth
100 percent buckwheat
Millet
Oat bran

Oats—gluten-free
Quinoa
Rice—brown, white, wild
Teff

Legumes

Aduki beans
Black beans
Chick peas
Kidney beans
Lentils

Lima beans
Mung beans
Pinto beans
Split peas

Nuts and Seeds

(and their butters)

Almonds
Cashews
Pumpkin seeds

Sesame (tahini)
Sunflower seeds
Walnuts

Meats and Fish

(Choose low-mercury fish and organic, grass-fed,
hormone-free, and antibiotic-free meat)

Black sea bass
Chicken
Lamb
Light tuna
Sardines
Scallops
Sole

Tilapia (USA)
Trout
Turkey
Whitefish
Wild game
Wild salmon

Dairy Products and Milk Substitutes

Almond milk
Coconut milk
Hazelnut milk

Hemp milk
Oat milk
Rice milk

Fats

(cold-pressed)

Almond

Canola

Coconut

Flaxseed

Olive

Pumpkin

Safflower

Sesame

Sunflower

Walnut

Beverages

Filtered water

Herbal tea

Spring water

Vegetable juice

Herbs, Spices, and Condiments

Basil

Black pepper

Cilantro

Cinnamon

Cumin

Dandelion

Dill

Dry mustard

Garlic

Ginger

Mustard (made with apple cider vinegar)

Nutmeg

Nutritional yeast

Oregano

Parsley

Pure vanilla extract

Rosemary

Salt-free herbal blends

Tarragon

Thyme

Turmeric

Sweeteners

(small amounts)

Honey	Rice syrup
Maple syrup	Stevia
Molasses	

Appendix IV:
Healthy Anti-Inflammatory Snacks for Detoxification Support

- Hummus with celery and carrot sticks (hummus can be made with many types of beans, such as white beans or lima beans)
- Nuts, nut butters
- Olives
- Edamame
- Coconut kefir, plain, with berries
- Lettuce/kale/nori wrap with turkey
- Whole fruit—apple, pear, berries
- Raw or lightly steamed veggies
- Blum Kitchen Almond Flour Muffins with blueberries or apples
- Sunflower seeds, pumpkin seeds, and ground flaxseeds
- Gluten-free oatmeal with a scoop of protein powder
- Gluten-free crackers, rice cakes, or rice crackers with hummus, tahini, avocado, or nut butter
- Coconut milk smoothie
- Mixed nuts with dried fruit and shredded coconut
- Tahini dip with lightly steamed veggies
- Bean dips, especially homemade
- Fruit with nuts or nut butters
- Granola, gluten-free, with coconut yogurt, coconut milk, or almond milk
- Whole foods bar, like a Lärabar, with nuts and fruit

Notes

Chapter 1: Autoimmune Disease Basics

1. Fourth National Report on Human Exposure to Environmental Chemicals. Centers for Disease Control. www.cdc.gov/exposurereport/pdf/FourthReport_Executive Summary.pdf.

Chapter 2: Using Food as Medicine

1. Anna Sapone et al. Spectrum of gluten-related disorders: consensus on new nomenclature and classification. *BMC Medicine* 2012;10:13.
2. William Davis, M.D. *Wheat Belly: Lose the Wheat, Lose the Weight, and Find Your Path Back to Health.* Rodale Books, 2011.
3. L. Paimela et al. Gliadin immune reactivity in patients with rheumatoid arthritis. *Clin Exp Rheumatol* 1995 Sep–Oct;13(5):603–607.
4. Amy C. Brown. Gluten sensitivity: problems of an emerging condition separate from celiac disease. *Expert Rev Gastroenterol Hepatol* 2012;6(1):43–55.
5. Yolanda Gonzalez et al. High glucose concentrations induce TNF-alpha production through the down-regulation of CD33 in primary human monocytes. *BMC Immunology* 2012;13:19, DOI: 10.1186/1471-2172-13-19.
6. Olaf Adam et al. Anti-inflammatory effects of a low arachidonic acid diet and fish oil in patients with rheumatoid arthritis. *Rheumatol Int* 2003;23:27–36, DOI 10.1007/s00296-002-0234-7.
7. Deborah Rothman, Pamela DeLuca, and Robert B. Zurier. Botanical lipids: effects on inflammation, immune responses and rheumatoid arthritis. *Semi Arthritis Rheu* 1995 Oct;25(2):87–96.
8. Emeir M Duffy et al. The clinical effect of dietary supplementation with omega-3 fish oils and/or copper in systemic lupus erythematosus. *J Rheumatol* 2004;31:1551–1556.
9. D. J. Birmingham et al. Evidence that abnormally large seasonal declines in vitamin D status may trigger SLE flare in non–African Americans. *Lupus* 2012;21(8):855–864.
10. Joost Smoldersa et al. Vitamin D as an immune modulator in multiple sclerosis, a review. *J Neuroimmunol* 2008;194:7–17.
11. A. Vasquez, G. Manso, and J. Cannell. The clinical importance of vitamin D (cholecalciferol): a paradigm shift with implications for all healthcare providers. *Altern Ther Health Med* 2004;10:28–36.
12. Anna Velia Stazi and Biagino Trinti. Selenium status and over-expression of interleukin-15 in celiac disease and autoimmune thyroid diseases. *Ann Ist Super Sanita* 2010;46(4):389–399, DOI: 10.4415/Ann_10_04_06.

13. Diana Stoye et al. Zinc aspartate suppresses T cell activation in vitro and relapsing experimental autoimmune encephalomyelitis in SJL/J mice. *Biometals*, DOI 10.1007/s10534-012-9532-z.
14. Dayong Wu et al. Green tea EGCG, T cells, and T cell-mediated autoimmune diseases. *Mol Aspects Med* 2012;33:107–118.
15. Carmen P. Wonga et al. Induction of regulatory T cells by green tea polyphenol EGCG. *Immunol Lett* 2011;139:7–13.

Chapter 5: Understanding the Stress Connection

1. Susan J. Torres and Caryl A Nowson. Relationship between stress, eating behavior, and obesity. *Nutrition* 2007;23:887–894.
2. Linda Witek-Janusek et al. Psychological stress, reduced NK cell activity, and cytokine dysregulation in women experiencing diagnostic breast biopsy. *Psychonacroendocrinology* 2007;32:22–35.
3. Mirjana Dimitrijevic et al. End-point effector stress mediators in neuroimmune interactions: their role in immune system homeostasis and autoimmune pathology. *Immunol Res*, DOI 10.1007/s12026-012-8275-9.
4. M. Skamagas and E. B. Geer. Autoimmune hyperthyroidism due to secondary adrenal insufficiency: resolution with glucocorticoids. *Endocr Pract* 2011 Jan–Feb;17(1):85–90.
5. Michelle A. Petri et al. Effects of prasterone on corticosteroid requirements of women with systemic lupus erythematosus. *Arthritis Rheum* 2002 Jul;46(7):1820–1829.
6. A. Booji et al. Androgens as adjuvant treatment in postmenopausal female patients with rheumatoid arthritis. *Ann Rheum Dis* 1996;55:811–886.
7. M. Lyte, L. Vulchanova, and D. R. Brown. Stress at the intestinal surface: catecholamines and mucosa-bacteria interactions. *Cell Tissue Res* 2011 Jan;343(1):23–32.
8. Femke Lutgendorff, Louis M. A. Akkermans, and Johan D. Söderholm. The role of microbiota and probiotics in stress-induced gastrointestinal damage. *Curr Mol Med* 2008;8:282–298.
9. Y. Tache and S. Brunnhuber. From Hans Selye's discovery of biological stress to the identification of corticotropin-releasing factor signaling pathways: implication in stress-related functional bowel diseases. *Ann N Y Acad Sci* 2008 Dec;1148:29–41.

Chapter 6: Understanding the Stress Connection Workbook

1. C. Potagas et al. Influence of anxiety and reported stressful life events on relapses in multiple sclerosis: a prospective study. *Multiple Sclerosis* 2008;14:1262–1268.

Chapter 8: Healing Your Gut

1. Lauren Steele. Lloyd Mayer, and M. Cecilia Berin. Mucosal immunology of tolerance and allergy in the gastrointestinal tract. *Immunol Res*, DOI 10.1007/s12026-012-8308-4.
2. Denise Kelly, Shaun Conway, and Rustam Aminov. Commensal gut bacteria: mechanisms of immune modulation. *Trends Immunol* 2005 Jun;26(6).
3. Laurence Macia et al. Microbial influences on epithelial integrity and immune function as a basis for inflammatory diseases. *Immunol Rev* 2012 Jan;245(1):164–76, DOI: 10.1111/j.1600-065X.2011.01080.x.

4. Hsin-Jung Wu and Eric Wu. The role of gut microbiota in immune homeostasis and autoimmunity. *Gut Microbes* 2012 Jan–Feb;3(1):1–11.
5. S. Grenham et al. Brain-gut-microbe communication in health and disease. *Front Physiol* 2011;2:94.
6. Graham A. W. Rook. Hygiene hypothesis and autoimmune diseases. *Clin Rev Allerg Immu* 2012 Feb;42(1):5–15, DOI: 10.1007/s12016-011-8285-8.
7. J. Thorens et al. Bacterial overgrowth during treatment with omeprazole compared with cimetidine: a prospective randomised double blind study. *Gut* 1996 Jul;39(1):54–59.
8. Christophe E. M. De Block, Ivo H. De Leeuw, and Luc F. Van Gaal. Autoimmune gastritis in type 1 diabetes: a clinically oriented review. *J Clin Endocrinol Metab* 2008;93:363–371.
9. M. Lyte, L. Vulchanova, and D. R. Brown. Stress at the intestinal surface: catecholamines and mucosa-bacteria interactions. *Cell Tissue Res* 2011 Jan;343(1):23–32.
10. Femke Lutgendorff, Louis M. A. Akkermans, and Johan D. Söderholm. The role of microbiota and probiotics in stress-induced gastro-intestinal damage. *Curr Mol Med* 2008;8:282–298.
11. Francisco Guarner, et al. World Gastroenterology Organisation global guidelines probiotics and prebiotics October 2011. *J Clin Gastroenterol* 2012 Jul;46(6).
12. Saranna Fanning et al. Bifidobacterial surface-exopolysaccharide facilitates commensal-host interaction through immune modulation and pathogen protection. *PNAS* 2012 Feb 7;109(6), DOI: 10.1073/pnas.1115621109.
13. A. Fasano. Leaky gut and autoimmune diseases. *Clin Rev Allergy Immunol* 2012 Feb;42(1):71–78.
14. Linda Chia-Hui Yu et al. Host-microbial interactions and regulation of intestinal epithelial barrier function: from physiology to pathology. *World J Gastrointest Pathophysiol* 2012 Feb 15;3(1):27–43.
15. Katherine R. Groschwitz and Simon P. Hogan. Intestinal barrier function: molecular regulation and disease pathogenesis. *J Allergy Clin Immunol* 2009;124:3–20.

Chapter 11: Supporting Your Liver

1. Centers for Disease Control. Fourth National Report on Human Exposure to Environmental Chemicals. www.cdc.gov/exposurereport/pdf/FourthReport_Executive Summary.pdf.
2. Environmental Working Group. Human Toxome Project, Mapping the Pollution in People. www.ewg.org/sites/humantoxome.
3. United States Environmental Protection Agency, Toxics Release Inventory Program. www.epa.gov/TRI.
4. Lyn Patrick. Mercury toxicity and antioxidants: part I: role of glutathione and alpha-lipoic acid in the treatment of mercury toxicity. *Altern Med Rev* 2002;7(6):456–471.
5. Campaign for Safe Cosmetics. Lead in lipstick. http://safecosmetics.org/article .php?id=223.
6. Environmental Working Group. Skin Deep Cosmetics Database. www.ewg.org/skindeep.
7. Environmental Working Group. Bisphenol A. www.ewg.org/chemindex/chemicals/bisphenolA.
8. Environmental Working Group. Pharmaceuticals pollute tapwater. www.ewg.org/node/26128.

9. Ahmad Movahedian Attar et al. Serum mercury level and multiple sclerosis. *Trace Elem Res* 2012;146:150–153.

10. A. Fulgenzi et al. A case of multiple sclerosis improvement following removal of heavy metal intoxication: lessons learnt from Matteo's case. *Biometals* 2012 Jun;25(3):569–576.

11. Gilbert J. Fournié et al. Induction of autoimmunity through bystander effects: lessons from immunological disorders induced by heavy metals. *J Autoimm* 2001;16:319–326.

12. Benjamin Rowley and Marc Monestier. Review: mechanisms of heavy metal-induced autoimmunity. *Mol Immunol* 2005;42:833–838.

13. Glinda S. Cooper et al. Occupational risk factors for the development of systemic lupus erythematosus. *J Rheumatol* 2004;31:1928–1933.

14. J. F. Nyland et al. Biomarkers of methylmercury exposure immunotoxicity among fish consumers in Amazonian Brazil. *Environ Health Perspect* 2011 Dec;119(12):1733–1738.

15. F. C. Arnett et al. Urinary mercury levels in patients with autoantibodies to U3-RNP (fibrillin). *J Rheumatol* 2000 Feb;27(2):405–410.

16. Carolyn M. Gallagher and Jaymie R. Meliker. Mercury and thyroid autoantibodies in U.S. women, NHANES 2007–2008. *Environ Int* 2012;40:39–43.

17. L. Tomljenovic and C. A. Shaw. Mechanisms of aluminum adjuvant toxicity and autoimmunity in pediatric populations. *Lupus* 2012;21:223–230.

18. Cecilia Chighizola and Pier Luigi Meroni. The role of environmental estrogens and autoimmunity. *Autoimmun Rev* 2012;11:A493–A501.

19. Aisha Lateef and Michelle Petri. Hormone replacement and contraceptive therapy in autoimmune diseases. *J Autoimmun* 2012 May;38(2–3):J170–J176.

20. Christine G. Parks. Insecticide use and risk of rheumatoid arthritis and systemic lupus erythematosus in the Women's Health Initiative Observational Study. *Arthritis Care Res* 2011 Feb;63(2):184–194, DOI 10.1002/acr.20335.

21. T. E. McAlindon et al. Indole-3-carbinol in women with SLE: effect on estrogen metabolism and disease activity. *Lupus* 2001;10:779–783.

22. Yi Wang et al. An investigation of modifying effects of metallothionein single-nucleotide polymorphisms on the association between mercury exposure and biomarker levels. *Environ Health Perspect* 2012 April;120(4):530–534.

23. T. Uchikawa et al. Chlorella suppresses methylmercury transfer to the fetus in pregnant mice. *J Toxicol Sci* 2011 Oct;36(5):675–680.

24. G. Park et al. *Coriandrum sativum L.* protects human keratinocytes from oxidative stress by regulating oxidative defense systems. *Skin Pharmacol Physiol* 2012;25:93–99.

25. [No authors listed]. DMSA. *Altern Med Rev* 2000 Jun;5(3):264–267.

26. F. Bamonti et al. Metal chelation therapy in rheumatoid arthritis: a case report. Successful management of rheumatoid arthritis by metal chelation therapy. *Biometals* 2011 Dec;24(6):1093–1098.

Chapter 14: Infections and Specific Autoimmune Conditions

1. M. Larsen et al. Exhausted cytotoxic control of Epstein-Barr virus in human lupus. *Plos Pathog* 2011 Oct;7(10):e1002328.

2. F. A. Luque and S. L. Jaffe. Cerebrospinal fluid analysis in multiple sclerosis. *Int Rev Neurobiol* 2007;79:341–56.

3. Siddharama Pawate and Subramaniam Sriram. The role of infections in the pathogenesis and course of multiple sclerosis. *Ann Indian Acad Neurol* 2010 Apr–Jun;
13(2):80–86.

4. H. Lassmann et al. Epstein-Barr virus in the multiple sclerosis brain: a controversial
issue—report on a focused workshop held in the Centre for Brain Research of the
Medical University of Vienna, Austria. *Brain* 2011 Sep;134(Pt 9):2772–2786.

5. Joost Smoldersa et al. Vitamin D as an immune modulator in multiple sclerosis, a
review. *J Neuroimmunol* 2008;194:7–17.

6. Brian D. Poole et al. Epstein-Barr virus and molecular mimicry in systemic lupus
erythematosus. *Autoimmunity* 2006 Feb;39(1):63–70.

7. Michael P. Pender, Review article: CD8+ T-cell deficiency, Epstein-Barr virus infection, vitamin D deficiency, and steps to autoimmunity: a unifying hypothesis. *Autoimmune Dis* 2012, DOI: 10.1155/2012/189096.

8. Taha Rashid and Alan Ebringer. Autoimmunity in rheumatic diseases is induced
by microbial infections via crossreactivity or molecular mimicry. *Autoimmune Dis*
2012, DOI:10.1155/2012/539282.

9. Nathalie Balandraud, Jean Roudier, and Chantal Roudier. Epstein-Barr virus and
rheumatoid arthritis. *Autoimmunity Rev* 2004;3:362–367.

10. Barbara L. Goldstein et al. Epstein-Barr virus serologic abnormalities and risk of
rheumatoid arthritis among women. *Autoimmunity*, 2012 Mar;45(2):161–168.

11. Clio P. Mavragani et al. Endocrine alterations in primary Sjögren's syndrome: An
overview. *J Auto-immunity* 2012, DOI: 10.1016/j.jaut.2012.05.011.

12. Eric Toussirot and Jean Roudier. Epstein-Barr virus in autoimmune diseases. *Best
Pract Res Cl Rh* Vol. 22, 2008;22(5):883–896, DOI: 10.1016/j.berh.2008.09.007.

13. Rachel Desailloud and Didier Hober. Viruses and thyroiditis: an update. *Virology J*
2009;6:5.

Additional References

CHAPTER 1:
AUTOIMMUNE DISEASE BASICS

Afzali, B., G. Lombardi, R. I. Lechler, and G. M. Lord. The role of T helper 17 (Th17) and regulatory T cells (Treg) in human organ transplantation and autoimmune disease. *Clin Exp Immunol* 2007 Apr;148(1):32-46.

Afzali, B., P. Mitchell, R. I. Lechler, S. John, and G. Lombardi. Translational mini-review series on Th17 cells: induction of interleukin-17 production by regulatory T cells. *Clin Exp Immunol* 2010 Feb;159(2):120-30.

Chia-Hui Yu, Linda, Jin-Town Wang, Shu-Chen Wei, and Yen-Hsuan Ni. Host-microbial interactions and regulation of intestinal epithelial barrier function: from physiology to pathology. *World J Gastrointest Pathophysiol* 2012 Feb 15;3(1):27-43, ISSN 2150-5330.

Cooper, Glinda S., and Christine G. Parks. Occupational exposures and risk of systemic lupus erythematosus: a review of the evidence and exposure assessment methods in population and clinic based studies. *Lupus* 2006;15:728–736.

Cooper, Glinda S., Christine G. Parks, Edward L. Treadwell, E. William St. Clair, Gary S. Gilkeson, and Mary Anne Dooley. Occupational risk factors for the development of systemic lupus erythematosus. *J Rheumatol* 2004;31:1928–1933.

Dimitrijevic, Mirjana, Stanislava Stanojevic, Natasa Kustrimovic, Gordana Leposavic. End-point effector stress mediators in neuroimmune interactions: their role in immune system homeostasis and autoimmune pathology. *Immunol Res* 2012 Apr;52(1–2):64–80, DOI: 10.1007/s12026-012-8275-9.

Fasano, Alessio. Leaky gut and autoimmune diseases. *Clinic Rev Allerg Immunol* 2012;42:71–78, DOI: 10.1007/s12016-011-8291-x.

Pender, Michael P. CD8+ T-cell deficiency, Epstein-Barr virus infection, vitamin D deficiency, and steps to autoimmunity: a unifying hypothesis *Autoimmune Diseases* 2012;2012:16 pages, DOI:10.1155/2012/189096.

Ramos-Casals, M., P. Brito-Zerón, and J. Font. The overlap of Sjögren's syndrome with other systemic autoimmune diseases. *Semin Arthritis Rheum* 2007 Feb;36(4):246–255.

Rashid, Taha, and Alan Ebringer. Review article autoimmunity in rheumatic diseases is induced by microbial infections via crossreactivity or molecular mimicry. *Autoimmune Diseases* 2012; Article ID 539282: 9 pages, DOI:10.1155/2012/539282.

Rowley, Benjamin, and Marc Monestier. Mechanisms of heavy metal-induced autoimmunity. *Molecular Immunology* 42 (2005):833–838.

Sapone, Anna, Julio C. Bai, Carolina Ciacci, Jernej Dolinsek, Peter H. R. Green, Marios Hadjivassiliou, Katri Kaukinen, Kamran Rostami, David S. Sanders, Michael

Schumann, Reiner Ullrich, Danilo Villalta, Umberto Volta, Carlo Catassi, and Alessio Fasano. Spectrum of gluten-related disorders: consensus on new nomenclature and classification. *BMC Medicine* 2012;10:13, http://www.biomedcentral.com/1741-7015/10/13.

Saranac, L., S. Zivanovic, B. Bjelakovic, H. Stamenkovic, M. Novak, and B. Kamenov. Why is the thyroid so prone to autoimmune disease? *Horm Res Paediatr* 2011;75:157–165, DOI: 10.1159/000324442.

Selmi, Carlo, Anna Maria Papini, Piera Pugliesi, Maria Claudia Alcaro, and M. Eric Gershwin. Environmental pathways to autoimmune diseases: the cases of primary biliary cirrhosis and multiple sclerosis. *Arch Med Sci* 2011;7(3): 368–380, DOI: 10.5114/aoms.2011.23398.

Tlaskalova-Hogenova, Helena, Ludmila Tuckova, Renata Stepankova, Tomas Hudcovic, Lenka Palova-Jelinkova, Hana Kozakova, Pavel Rossman, Daniel Sanchez, Jana Cinova, Tomas Hrnoir, Miloslav Kverka, Lenka Frolova, Holm Uhlig, Fiona Powrie, and Paul Bland. Involvement of innate immunity in the development of inflammatory and autoimmune diseases. *Ann NY Acad Sci* 2005;1051:787–798, DOI: 10.1196/annals.1361.122.

Toussirot, Eric, and Jean Roudier. Epstein–Barr virus in autoimmune diseases. *Best Practice Res Clin Rheum* 2008;22(5):883–896, DOI:10.1016/j.berh.2008.09.007.

Weyand, Cornelia, Hiroshi Fujii, Lan Shao, and Jörg J. Goronzy. Rejuvenating the immune system in rheumatoid arthritis. *Nat. Rev. Rheumatol* 2009;5:583–588, DOI:10.1038/nrrheum.2009.180.

CHAPTER 2

USING FOOD AS MEDICINE

Eisenmann A, C. Murr, D. Fuchs, M. Ledochowski. Gliadin IgG antibodies and circulating immune complexes. *Scand J Gastroenterol* 2009;44(2):168-171.

Kang, Jing X. The coming of age of nutrigenetics and nutrigenomics. *J Nutrigenet Nutrigenomics* 2012;5:I–II.

Krzyżowsk, M., A. Wincenciak, A.Winnicka, K. Baranowski, J. Jaszczak, M. Zimny, M. Niemiałtowski. The effect of multigenerational diet containing genetically modified triticale on immune system in mice. *Pol J of Vet Sci* 2010;13(3):423–430.

Ruuskanen, Anitta, Katri Kaukinen, Pekka Collin, Heini Huhtala, Raisa Valve, Markku Maki, and Liisa Luostarinen. Positive serum antigliadin antibodies without celiac disease in the elderly population: does it matter? *Scand J of Gastr.* 2010 Oct;45(10):1197–1202.

Smolders, J., J. Damoiseaux, P. Menheere, R. Hupperts. Vitamin D as an immune modulator in multiple sclerosis, a review. *J Neuroimmunol* 2008;194(1–2):7–17.

Ventura, Alessandro, Giuseppe Magazzu, and Luigi Greco. Duration of exposure to gluten and risk for autoimmune disorders in patients with celiac disease. *Gastroenterology* 1999;117:297–303.

Volta, Umberto, Alessandro Granito, Claudia Parisi, Angela Fabbri, Erica Fiorini, Maria Piscaglia, Francesco Tovoli, Valentina Grasso, Paolo Muratori, Georgios Pappas, and Roberto De Giorgio. Deamidated gliadin peptide antibodies as a routine test for celiac disease. *J Clin Gastroenterol* 2010 Mar;44(3):186–190.

Zurier, R. B. Fatty acids, inflammation and immune responses. *Prostaglandins Leukotrienes and Essential Fatty Acids* 1993;48:57–62.

CHAPTER 5
UNDERSTANDING THE STRESS CONNECTION

Ader, R., and N. Cohen. Behaviorally conditioned immunosuppression. *Psychosom Med* 1975;37(4):333–340.

Ader, R., N. Cohen, and D. Felten. Psychoneuroimmunology: interactions between the nervous system and the immune system. *Lancet* 1995; 345(8942):99–103.

Bennett, M. P., J. M. Zeller, L. Rosenberg, and J. McCann. The effect of mirthful laughter on stress and natural killer cell activity. *Altern Ther Health Med* 2003;9(2): 38–45.

Blalock, J. E. The syntax of immune-neuroendocrine communication. *Immunol Today* 1994;15(11):504–511.

Cutolo, Maurizio, and Rainer H. Straub. Insights into endocrine-immunological disturbances in autoimmunity and their impact on treatment. *Arthritis Research & Therapy* 2009;11:218.

Elenkov, Ilia J., and George P. Chrousos. Stress hormones, Th1/Th2 patterns, pro/antiinflammatory cytokines and susceptibility to disease. *Trends in Endocrinology & Metabolism* 1999 Nov;10(9):359–368, ISSN 1043-2760, DOI: 10.1016/S1043-2760(99)00188-5.

Elenkov, Ilia J., Ronald L. Wilder, Georger P. Chrousos, and E. Sylvester Vizi. The sympathetic nerve—an integrative interface between two supersystems: the brain and the immune system. *Pharmacol Rev* 2000;52(4):595–638, DOI: 41/865371.

Epel, E., E. Blackburn, J. Lin, F. Dhabhar, N. Adler, J. Morrow, and R. Cawthon. Accelerated telomere shortening in response to life stress. *PNAS* 2004;101(49):17312–17315.

Fabre, B., H. Grosman, O. Mazza, C. Nolazco, N. Fernandez Machulsky, V. Mesch, L. Schreier, Y. Gidron, and G. Berg. Relationship of cortisol and life events to the metabolic syndrome in men. *Stress* 2012 Mar 14 (epub ahead of print).

Field, Tiffany. Yoga clinical research review. *Comp Ther Clin Prac* (2011);17:1–8.

Fry, R. W., J. R. Grove, A. R. Morton, P. M. Zeroni, S. Gaudieri, and D. Keast. Psychological and immunological correlates of acute over-training. *Brit J of Sports Med* 1994 Dec;28(4):241–246.

Glaser, R. Stress-associated immune dysregulation and its importance for human health: a personal history of psychoneuroimmunology. *Brain, Behav, and Imm* 2005; 19:3–11.

Godbout, J., and R. Glaser. Stress-induced immune dysregulation: implications for wound healing, infectious disease and cancer. *J Neuroimmune Pharmacol* 2006 Dec;1(4):421–427.

Grenham, S., G. Clarke, J. F. Cryan, T. G. Dinan. Brain-gut-microbe communication in health and disease. *Front Physiol* 2011;2:94.

Irwin, M., M. Daniels, S. C. Risch, E. Bloom, H. Weiner. Plasma cortisol and natural killer cell activity during bereavement. *Biol Psychiatry* 1988;24(2):173–178.

Kiecolt-Glaser, J. K., L. McGuire, T. F. Robles, R. Glaser. Negative emotions and stressful experiences stimulate production of proinflammatory cytokines. *Psychosom Med* 2002 Jan–Feb;64(1):15–28.

Maier, S. F., L. R. Watkins, M. Fleshner. Psychoneuroimmunology: the interface between behavior, brain, and immunity. *Am Psychol* 1994;49(12):1004–1017.

Potagas, C., C. Mitsonis, L. Watier, G. Dellatolas, A. Retziou, P. Mitropoulos, C. Sfagos, and D. Vassilopoulos. Influence of anxiety and reported stressful life events on relapses in multiple sclerosis: a prospective study. *Mult Scler* 2008 Nov;14(9):1262–1268 (epub August 28, 2008).

Sternberg, E. M. Neurendocrine regulation of autoimmune/inflammatory disease. *J Endocrinol* 2001;169:429–435.

Witek-Janusek, Linda, Sheryl Gabram, and Herbert L. Mathews. Psychologic stress, reduced NK cell activity, and cytokine dysregulation in women experiencing diagnostic breast biopsy. *Psychoneuroendocrinology* 2007 Jan;32(1):22–35, ISSN 0306-4530, DOI: 10.1016/j.psyneuen.2006.09.011.

Wright, B. J. Effort-reward imbalance is associated with salivary immunoglobulin a and cortisol secretion in disability workers. *J Occup Environ Med* 2011 Mar;53(3):308–312.

CHAPTER 8:
HEALING YOUR GUT

Apperloo-Renkema, H. Z., H. Bootsma, B. I. Mulder, C. G. Kallenberg, and D. Van Der Waajj. Host-microflora interaction in systemic lupus erythematosus (SLE): colonization resistance of the indigenous bacteria of the intestinal tract. *Epidemiol Infect* 1994;112:367–373.

Apperloo-Renkema, H. Z., H. Bootsma, B. I. Mulder, C. G. Kallenberg, and D. Van Der Waajj. Host-microflora interaction in systemic lupus erythematosus (SLE): circulating antibodies to the indigenous bacteria of the intestinal tract. *Epidemiol Infect* 1995;114:133–141.

Berer, Kerstin, and Gurumoorthy Krishnamoorthy. Commensal gut flora and brain autoimmunity: a love or hate affair? *Acta Neuropathol* 2012;123:639–651, DOI: 10.1007/s00401-012-0949-9.

Berer, Kersten, Marsilius Mues, Michail Koutrolos, Zakeya Al Rasbi1, Marina Boziki, Caroline Johner, Hartmut Wekerle, and Gurumoorthy Krishnamoorthy. Commensal microbiota and myelin autoantigen cooperate to trigger autoimmune demyelination. *Nature* 2011 Oct 26;479(7374):538–541, DOI: 10.1038/nature10554.

Christophe E. M., Ivo H. De Block, and Luc F. Van Gaal. Autoimmune gastritis in type 1 diabetes: a clinically oriented review. *J Clin Endocrinol Metab* 2008 Feb 1;93(2):363–371.

Fanning, Saranna, Lindsay J. Hall, Michelle Cronin, Aldert Zomer, John MacSharry, David Goulding, Mary O'Connell Motherway, Fergus Shanahan, Kenneth Nally, Gordon Dougan, and Douwe van Sinderen. Bifidobacterial surface-exopolysaccharide facilitates commensal-host interaction through immune modulation and pathogen protection. *PNAS* 2012 Feb 7;109(6), www.pnas.org/cgi/doi/10.1073/pnas.1115621109.

Fasano A. Systemic autoimmune disorders in celiac disease. *Curr Opin Gastroenterol* 2006 Nov;22(6):674–679.

Kono, Hiroshi, Hideki Fujii, Masami Asakawa, Akira Maki, Hidetake Amemiya, Yu Hirai, Masanori Matsuda, and Masayuki Yamamoto. Medium-chain triglycerides enhance secretory IgA expression in rat intestine after administration of endotoxin. *Am J Physiol Gastrointest Liver Physiol* 2004;286:G1081–G1089, DOI:10.1152/ajpgi.00457.2003.

Lahner, Edith, Marco Centanni, Giacoma Agnello, Lucilla Gargano, Lucy Vannella, Carlo Iannoni, Gianfranco Delle Fave, Bruno Annibale. Occurrence and risk factors for autoimmune disease in patients with atrophic body gastritis. *Amer J Med* 2008 Feb;121(2):136–141, ISSN 0002-9343, DOI: 10.1016/j.amjmed.2007.09.025.

Miceli, Emanuela, Marco Vincenzo Lenti, Donatella Padula, Ombretta Luinetti, Claudia Vattiato, Claudio Maria Monti, Michele Di Stefano, and Gino Roberto Corazza. Common features of patients with autoimmune atrophic gastritis. *Clin Gastroenterol and Hepatol* 2012 Mar;ISSN 1542-3565, DOI: 10.1016/j.cgh.2012.02.018.

Mora, J. R., and U. H. von Andrian. Role of retinoic acid in the imprinting of gut-homing IgA-secreting cells. *Semin Immunol* 2009 Feb;21(1):28–35.

Peltonen, R., M. Nenonen, T. Helve, O. Hanninen, P. Toivanen, and E. Eerola. Faecal microbial flora and disease activity in rheumatoid arthritis during a vegan diet. *Br J Rheumatol* 1997;36:64–68.

Rapin, J. R., and N. Wiernsperger. Possible links between intestinal permeability and food processing: a potential therapeutic niche for glutamine. *Clinics* 2010;65(6):635–643.

Steele, Lauren, Lloyd Mayer, and M. Cecilia Berin. Mucosal immunology of tolerance and allergy in the gastrointestinal tract. *Immunol Res,* DOI 10.1007/s12026-012-8308-4.

Weiner, Howard L., Andre Pires da Cunha, Francisco Quintana, and Henry Wu. Oral tolerance. *Imm Rev* 2011;241:241–259.

CHAPTER 11
SUPPORTING YOUR LIVER

Ahmed, Sattar Ansar. The immune system as a potential target for environmental estrogens (endocrine disrupters): a new emerging field. *Toxicology* 2000;150:191–206.

Bang, So-Young, Kyoung-Ho Lee, Soo-Kyung Cho, Hye-Soon Lee, Kyung Wha Lee, and Sang-Cheol Bae. Smoking increases rheumatoid arthritis susceptibility in individuals carrying the HLA–DRB1 shared epitope, regardless of rheumatoid factor or anti–cyclic citrullinated peptide antibody status. *Arth & Rheum* 2010 Feb;62(2):369–377, DOI: 10.1002/art.27272.

Caldas, Cezar Augusto Muniz, and Jozélio Freire de Carvalho. The role of environmental factors in the pathogenesis of non-organ-specific autoimmune diseases. *Best Prac Clin Rheum* 2012;26:5–11.

Cooper, Glinda S., Joan Wither, Sasha Bernatsky, Jaime O. Claudio, Ann Clarke, John D. Rioux, and Paul R. Fortin. Occupational and environmental exposures and risk of systemic lupus erythematosus: silica, sunlight, solvents. *Rheumatology* 2010;49:2172–2180.

Cooper, Glinda S., Susan L. Makris, Paul J. Nietert, and Jennifer Jinot. Evidence of autoimmune-related effects of trichloroethylene exposure from studies in mice and humans. *Environ Health Persp* 2009 May;117(5).

Cousins, R. J. Absorption, transport, and hepatic metabolism of copper and zinc: special reference to metallothionein and ceruloplasmin. *Physiol Rev* 1985 Apr;65(2):238–309.

Duntas, Leonidas H. Environmental factors and autoimmune thyroiditis. *Endocrinol Metab* 2008 Aug;4(8).

Elinder, Carl-Gustaf. Epidemiology and toxicity of cadmium. April 2012. http://www .uptodate.com/contents/epidemiology-and-toxicity-of-cadmium?source=search _result&search=cadmium+toxicity&selectedTitle=1%7E150.

Flora, S. J. S., Megha Mittal, and Ashish Mehta. Heavy metal induced oxidative stress & its possible reversal by chelation therapy. *Indian J Med Res* 2008 Oct;128:501–523.

Gundacker, Claudia, Martin Gencik, and Markus Hengstschla. The relevance of the individual genetic background for the toxicokinetics of two significant neurodevelopmental toxicants: mercury and lead. *Mutation Research* 2010;705:130–140.

Hybenova, M., P. Hrda, J. Procházková, V. Stejskal, I. Sterzl. The role of environmental factors in autoimmune thyroiditis. *Neuro Endocrinol Lett* 2010;31(3):283–289.

Langer, P., M. Tajtakova, G. Fodor, A. Kocan, P. Bohov, J. Michalek, and A. Kreze. Increased thyroid volume and prevalence of thyroid disorders in an area heavily polluted by polychlorinated biphenyls. *Euro J Endocrinol* 1998;139:402–409.

Minich, Deanna M., and Jeffrey S. Bland. A review of the clinical efficacy and safety of cruciferous vegetable phytochemicals. *Nutrition Reviews* 2007 Jun;65(6[I]):259–267.

Parks, C. G., and G. .S Cooper. Occupational exposures and risk of systemic lupus erythematosus: a review of the evidence and exposure assessment methods in population- and clinic-based studies. *Lupus* 2006;15:728–736.

Söderlin, M. K., I. F. Petersson, S. Bergman, and B. Svensson. Smoking at onset of rheumatoid arthritis (RA) and its effect on disease activity and functional status: experiences from BARFOT, a long-term observational study on early RA. *Scand J Rheumatol* 2011;40:249–255.

Sonnenschein, Carlos, and Ana M. Soto. An updated review of environmental estrogen and androgen mimics and antagonists. *J. Steroid Biochem Molec Biol* 1998;65 (1–6):143–150.

CHAPTER 14:
INFECTIONS AND SPECIFIC AUTOIMMUNE CONDITIONS

For this chapter, please note that many references for specific diseases were used in earlier chapters in the book and are not repeated here.

Multiple Sclerosis

Benito-León, J., D. Pisa, R. Alonso, P. Calleja, M. Díaz-Sánchez, and L. Carrasco. Association between multiple sclerosis and Candida species: evidence from a case-control study. *Eur J Clin Microbiol Infect Dis* 2010;29:1139–1145, DOI: 10.1007/s10096-010-0979-y.

Berer, Kerstin, and Gurumoorthy Krishnamoorthy. Commensal gut flora and brain autoimmunity: a love or hate affair? *Acta Neuropathol* 2012;123:639–651, DOI: 10.1007/s00401-012-0949-9.

Berer, Kerstin, Marsilius Mues, Michail Koutrolos, Zakeya Al Rasbi, Marina Boziki, Caroline Johner, Hartmut Wekerle, and Gurumoorthy Krishnamoorthy. Commensal microbiota and myelin autoantigen cooperate to trigger autoimmune demyelination. *Nature* 2011 Oct 26;479(7374):538–541, DOI: 10.1038/nature10554.

Chen, Xiaohong, Xiaomeng Ma, Ying Jiang, Rongbiao Pi, Yingying Liu, and Lili Ma. The prospects of minocycline in multiple sclerosis. *J Neuroimmunol* 2011;235:1–8.

Contini, Carlo, Silva Seraceni, Rosario Cultrera, Massimiliano Castellazzi, Enrico Granieri, and Enrico Fainardi. Chlamydophila pneumonia infection and its role in neurological disorders. *Interdiscip Perspect Infect Dis* 2010;2010.

Deretzi, G., J. Kountouras, S. S. A. Polyzos, C. Zavos, E. Giartza-Taxidou, E. Gavalas, I. Tsiptsios, and G Deretzi. Gastrointestinal immune system and brain dialogue implicated in neuroinflammatory and neurodegenerative diseases. *Curr Mol Med* 2011 Nov;11(8):696–707.

Fainardi, Enrico, Massimiliano Castellazzi, Carmine Tamborino, Silva Seraceni, Maria

Rosaria Tola, Enrico Granieri, and Carlo Contini. Chlamydia pneumoniae–specific intrathecal oligoclonal antibody response is predominantly detected in a subset of multiple sclerosis patients with progressive forms. *J NeuroVirol* 2009;15:425–433.

Fazakerley, John K., and Robert Walker. Virus demyelination. *J NeuroVirol* 2003;9:148–164.

Filippi, Massimo, and Maria Assunta Rocca. MRI evidence for multiple sclerosis as a diffuse disease of the central nervous system. *J Neurol* 2005;252 (Suppl 5):V/16–V/24, DOI: 10.1007/s00415-005-5004-5.

Giuliania, Fabrizio, Sue Anne Fu, Luanne M. Metz, and V. R. Wee Yong. Effective combination of minocycline and interferon-h in a model of multiple sclerosis. *J Neuroimmunol* 2005;165:83–91.

Kaushansky, Nathali, Miriam Eisenstein, Rina Zilkha-Falb, and Avraham Ben-Nun. The myelin-associated oligodendrocytic basic protein (MOBP) as a relevant primary target autoantigen in multiple sclerosis. *Autoimmunity Reviews* 2010;9:233–236.

Kuusisto, H., H. Hyöty, S. Kares, E. Kinnunen, and I. Elovaara. Human herpes virus 6 and multiple sclerosis: a Finnish twin study. *Mult Scler* 2008;14:54.

Lünemann, Jan D., Thomas Kamradt, Roland Martin, and Christian Münz. Epstein-Barr virus: environmental trigger of multiple sclerosis? *J Virol* 2007 Jul;81(13):6777–6784, DOI: 10.1128/JVI.00153-07.

Morelli, Alessandro, Silvia Ravera, Daniela Calzia, and Isabella Panfoli. Impairment of heme synthesis in myelin as potential trigger of multiple sclerosis. *Medical Hypotheses* 2012;78:707–710.

Riccio, P. The molecular basis of nutritional intervention in multiple sclerosis: a narrative review. *Compl Ther Med* 2011;19:228–237.

Selmi, Carlo, Anna Maria Papini, Piera Pugliese, Maria Claudia Alcaro, and M. Eric Gershwin. Environmental pathways to autoimmune diseases: the cases of primary biliary cirrhosis and multiple sclerosis. *Arch Med Sci* 2011;7(3): 368–380, DOI: 10.5114/aoms.2011.23398.

Van Meeteren, M. E., C. E. Teunissen, C. D. Dijkstra, and E. A. F. van Tol. Antioxidants and polyunsaturated fatty acids in multiple sclerosis. *Euro J Clin Nutr* 2005; 59:1347–1361.

Yao, S. Y., C. W. Stratton, W. M. Mitchell, and S. Sriram. CSF oligoclonal bands in MS include antibodies against *Chlamydophila* antigens. *Neurology* 2001 May 8;56(9): 1168-1176.

Systemic Lupus Erythematosus (SLE or Lupus)

Crispín, Jose C., Maria Ines Vargas-Rojas, Adriana Monsiváis-Urenda, and Jorge Alcocer-Varela. Phenotype and function of dendritic cells of patients with systemic lupus erythematosus. *Clin Immunol* 2012;143:45–50.

Fagan, Thomas F., and Denise L. Faustman. Sex differences in autoimmunity. *Adv Cell Biol* 2004;34:295–306, DOI:10.1016/S1569-2558(03)34020-2.

Harley, John B., and Judith A. James. Epstein-Barr virus infection induces lupus autoimmunity. *Bulletin of the NYU Hospital for Joint Diseases* 2006;64(1–2).

Lyons, Robert. Effective use of autoantibody tests in the diagnosis of systemic autoimmune disease. *Ann NY Acad Sci* 2005;1050:217–228, DOI: 10.1196/annals.1313.023.

McMurray, Robert W. Estrogen, prolactin, and autoimmunity: actions and interactions. *International Immunopharmacol* 2001Jun;1(6):995–1008.

Niller, H. H., H. Wolf, and J. Minarovits. Regulation and dysregulation of Epstein-Barr virus latency: implications for the development of autoimmune diseases. *Autoimmunity* 2008 May;41(4):298–328.

Celiac Disease

Fasano, A. Systemic autoimmune disorders in celiac disease. *Curr Opin Gastroenterol* 2006 Nov;22(6):674–679.

Mirza, N., E. Bonilla, and P. E. Phillips. Celiac disease in a patient with *systemic lupus erythematosus:* a case report and review of literature. *Clin Rheumatol* 2007;26:827–828, DOI: 10.1007/s10067-006-0344-9.

Sollid, Ludvig M., and Bana Jabri. Is celiac disease an autoimmune disorder? *Curr Opin Immunol* 2005;17:595–600.

Ventura, Alessandro, Giuseppe Maguzzo, and Luigi Greco. Duration of exposure to gluten and risk for autoimmune disorders in patients with celiac disease. *Gastroenterology* 1999;117:297–303.

Rheumatoid Arthritis

Bamonti, F., A. Fulgenzi, C. Novembrino, and M. E. Ferrero. Metal chelation therapy in rheumathoid arthritis: a case report: successful management of rheumathoid arthritis by metal chelation therapy. *Biometals* 2011 Dec;24(6):1093-1098.

Ebringer, Alan, Taha Rashid, and Clyde Wilson. Rheumatoid arthritis: proteus, anti-CCP antibodies and Karl Popper. *Autoimmunity Reviews* 2010;9:216–223.

Fasano, A. Leaky gut and autoimmune diseases. *Clin Rev Allergy Immunol* 2012 Feb;42(1):71–78.

Hasni, S., A. Ippolito, G. G. Illei. Helicobacter pylori and autoimmune diseases. *Oral Diseases* 2011;17:621–627.

Peltonen, R., M. Nenonen, T. Helve, O. Hanninen, P. Toivanen, and E. Eerola. Faecal microbial flora and disease activity in rheumatoid arthritis during a vegan diet. *Br J Rheumatol* 1997;36:64–68.

Scher, Jose U., Carlos Ubeda, Michele Equinda, Raya Khanin, Yvonne Buischi, Agnes Viale, Lauren Lipuma, Mukundan Attur, Michael H. Pillinger, Gerald Weissmann, Dan R. Littman, Eric G. Pamer, Walter A. Bretz, and Steven B. Abramson. Periodontal disease and the oral microbiota in new-onset rheumatoid arthritis. *Arthritis & Rheumatism,* DOI: 10.1002/art.3453.

Wu, Hsin-Jung, and Eric Wu. The role of gut microbiota in immune homeostasis and autoimmunity. *Gut Microbes* 2012 Jan–Feb;3(1), 1–11.

Sjögren's Syndrome

Laine, Mikael, Pauliina Porola, Lene Udby, Lars Kjeldsen, Jack B. Cowland, Niels Borregaard, Jarkko Hietanen, Mona Ståhle, Antti Pihakari, and Yrjo T. Konttinen. Low salivary dehydroepiandrosterone and androgen-regulated cysteine-rich secretory protein 3 levels in Sjögren's syndrome. *Arthritis Rheum* 2007 Aug;56(8):2575–2584.

Ramos-Casals, Manuel, Pilar Brito-Zerón, and Josep Font. The overlap of Sjögren's syndrome with other systemic autoimmune diseases. *Semin Arthritis Rheum* 36:246–255.

Tzioufas, Athanasios G., Efstathia K. Kapsogeorgou, Haralampos M. Moutsopoulos. Pathogenesis of Sjögren's syndrome: what we know and what we should learn. *J Autoimmun* 2012 Aug;39(1–2):1–116, DOI: 10.1016/j.jaut.2012.01.002.

Autoimmune Thyroid Diseases: Graves' Disease and Hashimoto's Thyroiditis

Ahmed, Rania, Safa Al-Shaikh, and Mohammed Akhtar. Hashimoto's Thyroiditis: a century later. *Adv Anat Pathol* 2012;19:181–186.

Boelaert, Kristien, Paul R. Newby, Matthew J. Simmonds, Roger L. Holder, Jacqueline D. Carr-Smith, Joanne M. Heward, Nilusha Manji, Amit Allahabadia, Mary Armitage, Krishna V. Chatterjee, John H. Lazarus, Simon H. Pearce, Bijay Vaidya, Stephen C. Gough, and Jayne A. Franklyn. Prevalence and relative risk of other autoimmune diseases in subjects with autoimmune thyroid disease. *Amer J Med* 2010;123:183.e1–183.e9.

Canning, M.O., C. Ruwhof, and H. A. Drexhage. Aberrancies in antigen-presenting cells and T cells in autoimmune thyroid disease: a role in faulty tolerance induction. *Autoimmunity* 2003 Sept–Nov;36 (6–7):429–442.

Duntas, Leonidas. Environmental factors and autoimmune thyroiditis. *Endocrinol & Metab* 2008 Aug;4(8):454–460.

Gallagher, Carolyn M., and Jaymie R. Meliker. Mercury and thyroid autoantibodies in U.S. women, NHANES 2007–2008. *Environment International* 2012;40:39–43.

Hybenova, M., P. Hrda, J. Prochazkova, V. Stejskal, and I. Sterzl. The role of environmental factors in autoimmune thyroiditis. *Neuro Endocrinol Lett* 2010;31(3):283-289.

Langer, P., M. Tajtakova, G. Fodor, A. Kocan, P. Bohov, J. Michalek, and A. Kreze. Increased thyroid volume and prevalence of thyroid disorders in an area heavily polluted by polychlorinated biphenyls. *Euro J Endocrinol* 1998;139:402–409.

Morshed, Syed A., Rauf Latif, and Terry F. Davies. Delineating the autoimmune mechanisms in Graves' disease. *Immunol Res* 2012, DOI: 10.1007/s12026-012-8312-8.

Prochazkova, J., I. Sterzl, H. Kucerova, J. Bartova, and V. D. Stejskal. The beneficial effect of amalgam replacement on health in patients with autoimmunity. *Neuro Endocrinol Lett* 2004 Jun;25(3):211–218.

Saranac, L., S. Zivanovic, B. Bjelakovic, H. Stamenkovic, M. Novak, and B. Kamenov. Why is the thyroid so prone to autoimmune disease? *Horm Res Paediatr* 2011;75:157–165, DOI: 10.1159/000324442.

Skamagas, M., and E. B. Geer. Autoimmune hyperthyroidism due to secondary adrenal insufficiency: resolution with glucocorticoids. *Endocr Pract* 2011 Jan–Feb;17(1): 85–90.

Stazi, Anna Velia, and Biagino Trinti. Selenium status and over-expression of interleukin-15 in celiac disease and autoimmune thyroid diseases. *Ann Ist Super Sanita* 2010;46(4):389–399, DOI: 10.4415/Ann_10_04_06.

Sterzl, I., J. Prochazkova, P. Hrda, P. Matucha, J. Bartova, V. D. Stejskal. Removal of dental amalgam decreases anti-TPO and anti-Tg autoantibodies in patients with autoimmune thyroiditis. *Neuro Endocrinol Lett* 2006 Dec;27 (Suppl 1):25–30.

Tomer, Yaron. Genetic susceptibility to autoimmune thyroid disease: past, present, and future. *Thyroid* 2010 Jul;20(7):715–725, DOI: 10.1089/thy.2010.1644.

Tomer, Yaron, and Amanda Huber. The etiology of autoimmune thyroid disease: a story of genes and environment. *J Autoimmun* 2009;32:231–239.

Recipe Index

Index

Q&A with Dr. Susan Blum

BY KRISTY OJALA

In *The Immune System Recovery Plan*, Dr. Susan Blum, one of the most sought-after experts in the field of functional medicine, shares the four-step program she used to treat her own serious autoimmune condition and help countless patients reverse their symptoms, heal their immune systems, and prevent future illness. I found her quizzes and tips very helpful and I wanted to find out more about how we can live better—and be nicer to our poor, poor guts.

First of all, thank you for your book. If I hadn't picked it up at work, I wouldn't have been able to start taking charge of some major health issues I was not aware of. Your quizzes are very helpful. Why are so many of us in the dark about our diet and the importance of a "healthy gut"?

Dr. Susan Blum: Because we are in the midst of an obesity epidemic, and also a self-image crisis, everyone is very focused on being thin and counting calories. This is just the wrong way to look at food. One of my favorite sayings is that "all calories are not created equal." A 100-calorie apple and a 100-calorie snack bag of pretzels cause a completely different series of reactions in the body. The apple results in less inflammation and the pretzels are the opposite. We need to shift our thinking away from calories to the idea that food has function, and we need to choose our food based on the information it brings into the body. This is a new field called functional nutrition and when practiced by a doctor is called nutritional medicine. Eating this way has the power to prevent and treat disease, and this is the approach I use in my medical practice. Many registered dieticians are still behind the times, and so many people don't understand this yet. But the word is definitely getting out.

The importance of a healthy gut has become news in the last decade. While those of us in functional medicine have known this for longer, recent studies have shown the medical community conclusive evidence that the health of the gut has the power to drive inflammation throughout the body—certainly for autoimmune diseases, but also for other inflammatory conditions like osteoarthritis and fibromyalgia. These conditions are on the rise, in epidemic numbers. One of the reasons is that we have been very cavalier about doing things that harm our intestinal flora: taking lots of antibiotics and antacids, for example. Not to mention all the medication like Advil and other NSAIDS, alcohol, and stress. As a nation, our guts are a mess, and we are just now seeing conclusive evidence of the fallout.

But at the end of the day, one of the main reasons that people are in the dark about the role of food and gut health is that most physicians aren't trained to understand this connection, or taught skills to teach nutrition or treat the gut in this way. Medical schools still don't teach nutrition, and conventionally trained rheumatologists don't know anything about the gut connection to arthritis, for example. If people don't hear it from their doctor, where will they learn about this and believe it is true? While the Internet is very helpful, when your doctor doesn't believe or know about this, a lot of people don't get on board either.

Autoimmune disease is on the rise. What is the biggest challenge to overcome when you're diagnosed with an autoimmune disease?
The biggest challenge to overcome when you are first diagnosed is the attitude of the conventional medical community. You are usually told there is nothing you can do, that there is no hope of a cure, and the best you are offered is medication to try to control the symptoms. People become passive and give up and feel hopeless and depressed. This is not the road to healing! People need hope, they need to know that there *is* something they can do to find the cause of their illness, and cure the cause, and then they will feel better and improve without medication. They need to feel empowered.

Is the popularity of a gluten-free diet helpful or harmful?
I would say the popularity of a gluten-free diet is both helpful and harmful. It is helpful because in most areas (except in rural areas, perhaps) there are so many gluten-free products available in the supermarket or health food stores that you can adopt a gluten-free diet relatively easily. And there isn't much stigma associated with eating this way.

I suppose one way it can be harmful is that some people dismiss it as a fad just to sell expensive food. But I think there are so many people who obviously feel better on a gluten-free diet that this is irrelevant.

There is so much evidence in the research that gluten causes inflammation and autoimmunity in the body, that it is hard to dismiss this as a fad. So, I would support the positive side and say it's good that it's popular.

Many of us have had amalgam fillings all of our lives. Dr. Oz recently did a show on the dangers of mercury in our mouths, and my own (integrative) M.D. strongly recommended I remove all of my amalgam fillings ASAP. My dentist scoffed during my first appointment, but I am proceeding all the same. Why is there so much controversy over the safety of mercury fillings?

I think that most people agree that mercury from fillings can leach into the body and cause problems. There is also mercury "vapor" that can be released and inhaled. The controversy seems to be that after having the same fillings in your mouth for many years, most dentists believe there isn't much mercury vapor being released anymore and that removing the fillings is therefore unnecessary. The problem is, this attitude isn't really based in fact because it is hard to know which fillings are a health hazard and which ones aren't. There have been studies that have looked at silver fillings and autoimmune thyroid disease, with a drop in mercury levels and an improvement in antibodies when the fillings were removed.

I am a believer that they should be removed, especially in people with thyroid disease, because the mouth sits right next to the neck, where the thyroid is located.

What is self-care, and why is it essential to our overall health?

Self-care means that you are fully engaged in activities that are good for you, and making time for yourself to do these activities. Examples of self-care are eating healthy, meditating or practicing other relaxation techniques, and exercise. These kinds of activities are essential to your overall health because stress, eating poorly, and too little exercise contribute to 80 percent of all our chronic disease in this country. In order to treat and reverse illness, lifestyle change is crucial, and this isn't something that a doctor can just give you a pill for.

And this is the other part of the definition of self-care: You are a partner with your health care provider. You need to do your part. It turns out that people who are fully engaged in helping themselves in this way heal faster and do better than people who take a passive role and expect to be "fixed" by someone else.

How much are all the plastic products we're using every day affecting our health? I realize that in the course of a day—despite my best efforts—I drink from plastic, eat from plastic, throw away receipts made of plastic, use a phone made from plastic, work on a plastic computer with a plastic mouse and write with a plastic pen, and carry a ton of plastic in my purse. Then I get home and try to remove plastic from my household and my pets' food. It's exhausting.

I like to use the concept of total toxic load to think about environmental exposures. These things are cumulative. Your liver is in charge of removing toxins from your body, and it needs lots of nutrients, like greens, antioxidants, protein, and cruciferous veggies, to do its job effectively. Plastics have toxins that leak out into the food, and for some people it might not be as big of a deal if they don't have a lot of other environmental exposures like pesticides, heavy metals, or air pollution, to name a few. The liver has to deal with all of it. If you have a high exposure to many things, adding plastics to the list can just be too much. Some symptoms of having an overload of toxins are fatigue, brain fog, weight gain, feeling puffy and swollen.

The best strategy is to go to a website like ewg.org and try to reduce the toxins in your world. Couple that with eating lots of veggies to support your liver detox processes, and you can increase your protection from all those things you can't see.

Can you please explain what the rotational diet is, and why it is being recommended more frequently by medical professionals such as yourself?

Rotation diets are used to treat food sensitivities. Here is the definition of a food sensitivity: You feel worse when you eat it and better when you don't. There is more and more understanding now that eating the same foods day after day can increase the possibility that your body will become sensitized to that food. By doing a rotation diet, you can reduce the immune reaction to a particular food by not eating it every day.

I found it interesting that you said "going more than four hours without eating activates your stress system." When is it best to eat our main

meals, and how often should we be eating? Do you recommend small meals over three main meals?

Cortisol, the stress hormone, helps regulate your blood sugar. So when you haven't eaten for more than four hours, your blood sugar can drop, triggering a release of cortisol to bring it back up. If you are trying to restore balance to your stress system, for example when treating adrenal fatigue, you don't want to add this stressor. Therefore, I recommend eating breakfast, lunch, snack, dinner, with some form of protein (veggie included) at each meal. I think every four hours is a good rhythm, so if you eat an early breakfast you might also need a snack midmorning.